Diagnostic DSM-5-TR Workbook

1400 True/False, 1120 Multiple Choice Questions, 140 Case Studies, and 840 Matching Exercises to Improve Your Clinical Practice and Test Your Knowledge

Edward Reed

Table of Contents

Disclaimer

This workbook has been developed to provide a practical and interactive resource for studying the DSM-5-TR. However, it does not replace or replicate the original diagnostic manual. It is important to note that this book is not approved, endorsed, or sponsored by the American Psychiatric Association (APA), the organization responsible for the publication of the DSM-5-TR.

What this book is not:

- It is not a substitute for the DSM-5-TR. For a comprehensive and in-depth understanding of diagnostic criteria and clinical descriptions, you should refer to the original manual.
- It does not provide definitive guidance for clinical diagnoses or treatments. The exercises and content in this book are intended solely for educational and training purposes.
- It does not guarantee any certification or clinical competence; its use is entirely at the reader's discretion.

A message to the reader:

This book is designed to support your learning process, making it more interactive and practical. However, the DSM-5-TR remains the only official source for diagnostic criteria and detailed information on mental disorders. I invite you to use this workbook as a bridge between theory and practice, helping you gain greater confidence and clarity in your studies.

Disclaimer of liability:

The author and publisher assume no responsibility for any misinterpretation or misuse of the content of this book. It is intended solely for educational purposes and should not be used as a clinical guide or as the basis for diagnostic or therapeutic decisions.

Preface

The primary aim of this manual is to provide a practical and interactive resource for anyone seeking to gain a deeper understanding of the mental disorders described in the DSM-5-TR. Specifically, it is designed to foster the development of diagnostic, clinical, and critical thinking skills, allowing readers to become familiar with diagnostic criteria through targeted exercises, multiple-choice questions, true/false items, matching activities, and illustrative case studies.

The manual's modular and systematic structure is intended to guide readers step by step as they explore and interpret different disorders, highlighting key features and common challenges along the way. Both students and professionals will find it a valuable tool for in-depth learning, knowledge consolidation, and the development of essential clinical competencies.

In addition, the manual seeks to make DSM-5-TR content more accessible and understandable, given that it is often perceived as complex and information-heavy. By emphasizing active learning, this text offers readers the opportunity to immediately put theoretical knowledge into practice. Each disorder is presented with concrete examples and realistic clinical scenarios, helping to bridge diagnostic concepts and real-world situations.

Lastly, the manual is designed to fit seamlessly into various educational and professional development programs: it can serve as a helpful supplement to theoretical texts, support material for university courses or specialized workshops, and a useful resource for clinicians wishing to keep their skills current. The goal is to contribute to the education of confident and competent professionals and students who are adept at diagnosing and treating mental disorders, promoting evidence-based practices grounded in a solid foundation.

Who Is This Manual For?

This manual is intended for anyone looking to enhance their diagnostic skills regarding mental disorders as outlined in the DSM-5-TR, through a hands-on, interactive approach. In particular, it serves as a valuable resource for:

- **University students and undergraduates** in Psychology, Psychiatry, Nursing, or related fields who need focused exercises to strengthen their grasp of diagnostic criteria and become more familiar with diverse clinical presentations.
- **Residents and trainees** in health professions (Clinical Psychology, Psychiatry, Counseling, Social Work, etc.) aiming to reinforce their theoretical knowledge with practical exercises and specially crafted case studies.
- **Mental health professionals** (psychologists, psychiatrists, physicians, nurses, social workers, and other healthcare providers) who can use the question sets, exercises, and case studies to keep their skills up to date and integrate broader clinical perspectives into their daily practice.
- **Teachers and educators**, who can draw from a wide range of exercises and case examples to enrich their lessons, workshops, and seminars, encouraging active student participation.

- **Readers with a keen interest in the field**, such as educators, consultants, or those working in the non-profit sector, who want to gain a clearer understanding of DSM-5-TR diagnostic criteria and the clinical dynamics of mental disorders.

By emphasizing practical application and problem-solving, the manual equips readers with the tools needed to immediately apply their newly acquired knowledge, fostering a deeper understanding and promoting a critical mindset geared toward accurate diagnostic evaluation.

Who I Am and Why I Wrote This Book

My name is Edward Reed, and my journey into the study of mental health began years ago. I found myself diving into complex and highly technical texts like the DSM-5, a vital resource for anyone seeking to deeply understand mental disorders and how to address them. Navigating its content was not easy—it was often challenging to retain the information, especially without a structured approach to make the connections between theory and practice clearer. Over time, I began developing a method to better organize and internalize the material. At first, it was simply a collection of tools that helped me remember and apply concepts more effectively. Multiple-choice questions, true/false exercises, matching activities, and case studies became my way of turning a dense text into something understandable, useful, and, most importantly, applicable in clinical practice.

When I shared this approach with colleagues, students, and friends who were on a similar path, I realized I wasn't alone in needing practical support. Time and time again, I heard how valuable these tools were. That's when I understood that what I had created for myself could become a resource for many others. This book was born from that realization. It is not intended to replace the DSM-5-TR but to serve as a companion. It has been designed to help you navigate its pages, make the concepts clearer and more accessible, and provide you with a structured guide to follow step by step. The exercises in this workbook are not just a way to test your knowledge—they are tools to help you deepen your understanding and apply theory in real-world contexts.

The goal of this book is not to oversimplify but to make the learning process less overwhelming and more productive. I want it to be a resource that supports you, helps you turn complexity into clarity, and transforms theory into action. What you hold in your hands is the result of years of work and the refinement of a method that I hope will be useful to anyone seeking to better understand the world of mental health. Whether you are a student, a professional in training, or simply someone passionate about these topics, this book is designed to help you make progress, step by step, without ever feeling lost. As you work through the exercises and turn these pages, remember that every small step forward is a success. My hope is that this workbook will not only help you learn but also equip you with the tools to approach complexity with confidence, clarity, and precision.

Before you begin this journey, I want to say something: I know that tackling a complex topic like mental health can feel overwhelming at times. Whether you're here for study, work, or personal interest, know that every step you take on this path matters. This workbook isn't a race to the finish line or a test to pass. It's a companion designed to help you find clarity, discover connections, and turn complex concepts into practical tools. Some exercises might feel easy, while others may challenge you—and that's exactly how it should be. Take your time, reflect, and don't hesitate to revisit sections as needed. There's no right or wrong way to approach this; there's only your way. Mental health is a subject that deserves our full attention and dedication, but also kindness toward ourselves as we explore it. This book is the result of years of work and refinement, and I hope it becomes a valuable tool for you—not just to learn, but to grow.

I wish you a meaningful journey, and I thank you for choosing to take it with me.

With gratitude,

Edward Reed

DSM 5 Fundamentals

Introduction and Historical Context

The history of the Diagnostic and Statistical Manual of Mental Disorders (DSM) dates back to the first half of the twentieth century, driven by an increasingly pressing need for a systematic, shared means of defining and classifying mental disorders. In the United States, the push for diagnostic standardization initially stemmed from administrative and statistical goals: documenting the number of psychiatric inpatients and gathering data on a national scale. Following some early attempts at classification, the American Psychiatric Association (APA) published the first edition of the DSM, known as DSM-I, in 1952.

Influenced heavily by psychoanalytic models, DSM-I offered broad descriptions of mental disorders, often consistent with the prevailing psychodynamic theories of the time. Minor revisions appeared in DSM-II (1968), but the approach remained largely descriptive and still carried certain conceptual ambiguities. A major turning point arrived with the DSM-III (1980), when the push for clearer, operational criteria led to a system based on observable descriptions, aiming to reduce subjective interpretations. DSM-III also introduced the controversial yet influential multi-axial system, which organized diagnostic information across several axes (clinical, personality, medical, psychosocial, etc.).

DSM-IV (1994) and its revision, DSM-IV-TR (2000), continued to refine diagnostic criteria and integrate emerging clinical and neuroscientific findings. Nonetheless, debates persisted on various fronts: for instance, the rigidity of certain diagnostic categories, the risk of overdiagnosis, and the need for more robust consideration of cultural factors.

In 2013, DSM-5 marked another evolutionary milestone: although it kept a categorical approach, the manual offered increased openness to dimensional models (such as measuring symptom severity) and reorganized certain disorders to align more closely with neuroscientific insights. Notable changes included the addition of new diagnoses, the repositioning of existing ones, and an emphasis on cross-cutting measures that span multiple diagnostic categories.

The text revision, DSM-5-TR, introduced further updates and clarifications to the criteria and terminology without radically altering DSM-5's core structure. Its aim is to reflect the latest research advances while addressing some contentious points raised in clinical practice. In particular, there has been greater attention to diagnostic language, increased cultural sensitivity, and stronger epidemiological data.

Over the course of more than half a century, the DSM has undergone significant transformations, shaped by both evolving psychopathological theories and the practical needs of clinicians, researchers, and policymakers. The manual's history can be seen as an ongoing quest to balance simplicity with complexity, combining the need for workable diagnostic categories with the recognition that psychological distress is often varied and nuanced. Today, DSM-5-TR stands as the most recent step in this continuum—a shared, continually evolving tool designed to guide diagnosis and encourage clear communication among mental health professionals.

Structure and Organization of the DSM-5-TR

The Diagnostic and Statistical Manual of Mental Disorders, Fifth Edition, Text Revision (DSM-5-TR) largely retains the framework introduced in DSM-5, with certain updates and clarifications. Disorders are arranged in a way that reflects increasing clinical complexity and, at the same time, groups together conditions with similar neurobiological and symptomatic profiles. Compared to previous editions, this organization aims to offer a more integrated approach consistent with current scientific evidence.

One of the most notable features is how Neurodevelopmental Disorders are positioned at the beginning of the manual. This reflects the importance of early identification and intervention for conditions that typically emerge in childhood, such as Specific Learning Disorders, Attention-Deficit/Hyperactivity Disorder (ADHD), and Autism Spectrum Disorder. By placing these diagnoses at the forefront, the DSM-5-TR emphasizes how genetic, biological, and environmental factors can influence developmental trajectories and, often, the onset of other mental health conditions later in life.

Following the section on Neurodevelopmental Disorders, the manual presents Schizophrenia Spectrum and Other Psychotic Disorders, which includes Schizophrenia, Schizoaffective Disorder, Brief Psychotic Disorders, and psychotic conditions induced by substances or medical conditions. It then moves on to major diagnostic categories such as Bipolar Disorders, Depressive Disorders, Anxiety Disorders, Obsessive-Compulsive and Related Disorders, Trauma- and Stressor-Related Disorders, and so forth. This layout creates a logical progression based on clinical manifestations, grouping diagnostic categories that frequently overlap or share certain symptoms (for instance, anxiety and obsessive-compulsive patterns).

A distinctive aspect introduced with DSM-5—and maintained in the DSM-5-TR—is the dedicated section for Substance-Related and Addictive Disorders, comprising both substance use disorders (alcohol, opioids, stimulants, etc.) and behavioral addictions, such as pathological gambling. This reflects growing awareness of the profound societal and health implications of addiction, as well as the need to group all forms of dependence under a single nosological umbrella.

Towards the end of the manual, you will find Personality Disorders, arranged into three clusters (A, B, and C) based on shared clinical traits, and the Paraphilic Disorders, which involve specific patterns of sexual interest or arousal that are considered unusual or problematic. Additional chapters address Medication-Induced Movement Disorders and Other Conditions That May Be a Focus of Clinical Attention, encompassing relational, occupational, or academic issues that often co-occur with, or complicate, a primary disorder.

Finally, the DSM-5-TR places emphasis on sections pertaining to assessment and differential diagnosis, referencing Cross-Cutting Symptom Measures and other scales designed to capture the severity and pervasive nature of certain symptoms (such as anxiety, depression, or suicidal ideation) that can appear across multiple disorders. Overall, the manual's structure is intended as a comprehensive diagnostic map that still allows for dimensional interpretations and the use of screening tools or more in-depth evaluations. The ultimate goal is to guide clinicians in identifying the disorder(s) that best match a patient's presentation, while also integrating cultural context, comorbidities, and neurobiological factors into the diagnostic process.

Categorical vs. Dimensional Logic

Like its predecessors, the DSM-5-TR relies primarily on a categorical approach, describing each disorder through well-defined diagnostic criteria that specify the nature of symptoms, their duration, the age of onset (when relevant), and the level of functional impairment. This approach provides clinicians with a clear reference framework to determine if and when certain signs and symptoms meet the threshold for a formal diagnosis. For instance, with a condition such as Major Depressive Disorder, the DSM-5-TR clearly states how many symptoms (and of which type) must be present over a specific time frame, as well as how these symptoms impact an individual's daily functioning.

This so-called "categorical" method emerged largely from the need for a standardized classification system in clinical, academic, and research settings. Dividing disorders into distinct categories promotes communication among professionals, facilitates epidemiological and clinical studies, and supports the development of treatment guidelines. However, concerns about the rigidity of this approach have long been recognized: psychiatric symptoms often defy strict boundaries, presenting with varying degrees of severity and combinations of signs that extend beyond classic categorizations.

For this reason, DSM-5 (and, by extension, the DSM-5-TR) incorporates certain dimensional components, introducing tools and concepts designed to capture the transdiagnostic variability of symptoms. One notable example is the use of cross-cutting measures, which assess the presence and severity of symptoms such as depression, anxiety, or suicidal ideation, regardless of a patient's primary diagnostic category. Although these measures are not formal diagnostic criteria, they offer clinicians valuable insights into a patient's overall condition and help identify symptom dimensions that might span multiple disorders.

In addition, the DSM-5-TR sometimes requires assessing symptom severity through dedicated scales, allowing for more nuanced diagnostic judgments based on the degree of impairment. This is particularly important in areas such as Autism Spectrum Disorders or Depressive Disorders, where recognizing varying intensities of symptoms is crucial for tailoring the most appropriate clinical intervention.

In summary, while the categorical logic remains the foundation of diagnostic practice, integrating dimensional elements offers a clearer picture of the complexity and variability of clinical presentations. This combination aims to maintain an operational and reliable classification system while acknowledging that mental disorders are often multifaceted and nuanced.

General Principles of Diagnosis and Assessment

In the DSM-5-TR, establishing a diagnosis involves a structured process aimed at collecting and integrating clinical, historical, and contextual information. These general diagnostic and assessment principles rest on several key pillars:

1. Adherence to Diagnostic Criteria

First and foremost, it's essential to compare the patient's clinical presentation with the specific criteria outlined in the manual. This involves more than simply checking off symptoms: clinicians must evaluate their duration, intensity, age of onset, and impact on functioning. For example, to confirm an anxiety disorder, generic worries alone aren't enough—certain features must be identified (such as excessive anxiety in multiple settings over a minimum specified period) alongside significant impairment in everyday life.

2. Ruling Out Other Causes or Conditions

A cornerstone of the DSM assessment process involves excluding alternative explanations for the symptoms, whether they stem from medical, neurological, or substance-related factors. Many psychiatric presentations can be mimicked by physical conditions (e.g., hypothyroidism can sometimes resemble depression) or by medication side effects. It's also crucial to consider cultural and linguistic factors that may influence how psychological distress is expressed, avoiding overdiagnosis due to normal cultural variations or specific belief systems within a given context.

3. Evaluating Overall Functioning

In addition to identifying symptoms, clinicians must examine how severely the patient's personal, social, occupational, or academic functioning is compromised. For many disorders, the level of functional impairment is a central criterion. Understanding how symptoms affect the patient's life—limiting their ability to maintain relationships, perform job duties, or handle daily responsibilities—often plays a decisive role in diagnosis. Various tools, such as rating scales and structured interviews, can help quantify severity and track the disorder's evolution over time.

4. A Multidimensional Assessment Approach

Although the DSM-5-TR adopts a categorical structure, a truly comprehensive evaluation requires multiple sources of information and a range of instruments. The clinical interview remains the core of assessment, but it can be supplemented by psychological tests, screening scales, and discussions with family members or other informants. Increasingly, dimensional assessments (like cross-cutting measures) are recommended to capture both the presence and severity of transdiagnostic symptoms.

5. Individualization and Case Formulation

Finally, diagnosis must account for each patient's unique life context and personal history. Factors such as cultural background, family environment, recent stressors, past trauma, or physical health conditions all influence how disorders manifest. The ultimate goal goes beyond assigning a diagnostic label; it involves understanding how these issues emerge and persist, in order to create a targeted and specific intervention plan.

Cross-Cutting Symptom Measures and Other Resources

One of the noteworthy features introduced in DSM-5, and carried over into DSM-5-TR, is the focus on Cross-Cutting Symptom Measures. These are broad assessment tools designed to identify and monitor symptoms that often appear across multiple disorders. Typically divided into two levels (Level 1 and Level 2), these questionnaires provide an overview of recurring symptoms (e.g., depressed mood, anxiety, irritability, sleep issues) and, if necessary, offer a more detailed follow-up evaluation of specific areas.

The underlying concept is that clinically relevant symptoms can cut across diagnostic boundaries. For instance, a patient with Major Depressive Disorder may also exhibit significant anxiety, while someone with Generalized Anxiety Disorder could show signs of "masked" depression. Incorporating this transdiagnostic view allows the clinician to gain a more comprehensive picture of the patient's condition, guiding both evaluation and treatment more effectively.

Cross-Cutting Symptom Measures usually take the form of short self-report questionnaires (or, in some cases, clinician-administered tools) in which the patient rates the presence and severity of certain symptoms over the past week or two weeks. If high scores emerge in key areas (e.g., elevated anxiety, suicidal ideation, memory or concentration problems), the clinician can opt to use second-level (Level 2) scales for a more detailed assessment of those specific domains.

In addition to Cross-Cutting Symptom Measures, DSM-5-TR encourages the use of other diagnostic and clinical support tools, such as:

- Structured and semi-structured interviews (e.g., the SCID-5, Structured Clinical Interview for DSM-5), which guide clinicians through a systematic exploration of each diagnostic category.

- Specific psychological tests targeting certain domains, such as the PHQ-9 for depression severity or the GAD-7 for anxiety.
- Self-assessment instruments for particular concerns, such as sleep quality, substance use, or post-traumatic symptoms.
- Observation logs and clinical diaries, helpful for tracking daily or weekly changes in symptoms and behavioral patterns.

This overall approach, as outlined in the DSM-5-TR, extends beyond simply assigning a single diagnostic label. Instead, it aims to capture a multifaceted understanding of the patient by leveraging as many tools as possible to pinpoint strengths, areas of concern, and potential comorbidities. Using Cross-Cutting Symptom Measures and complementary resources is thus crucial to ensuring accurate assessment, a well-grounded case formulation, and a treatment plan that meets the patient's actual needs.

From Theory to Practice

The exercises in this manual—spanning multiple-choice and true/false questions, matching tasks, and clinical case studies—are designed to sharpen the clinical insight of students, trainees, and professionals in psychology and psychiatry. Rather than providing further theoretical explanations (already well covered by existing literature), the aim here is to offer a practical tool that reinforces the ability to recognize diagnostic criteria, capture important nuances, and understand how symptoms can present in overlapping or varied ways.

To get the most out of this approach, it is helpful to combine reading the DSM-5-TR criteria with systematically working through the exercises, so you can solidify key concepts and clinical dynamics. If you encounter a doubt or make a mistake while answering a question, it's worth investigating the root cause of that discrepancy: often, it stems from an overlooked detail or a missed interpretation that could lead to new insights. Discussing your results with colleagues or classmates can further encourage a constructive exchange of ideas, revealing perspectives that might not emerge during solitary study.

When reviewing answers, paying close attention to why a certain option is correct or incorrect helps strengthen your recall of diagnostic criteria and supports the association of clinical situations with specific symptom patterns. This ongoing practice also makes it easier to identify crucial elements such as symptom duration, level of functional impairment, or relevant cultural factors. Over time, this method of study boosts confidence in real clinical contexts, where the complexity of individuals and the variability of settings demand flexible, clear-headed reasoning.

Ultimately, the value of a practice-based approach lies in its capacity to turn theory into a thoughtful, hands-on diagnostic process. Regularly grappling with diverse clinical profiles, reflecting on errors, and breaking down challenges into their core components fosters a strong foundation of skills. In this way, using the DSM-5-TR becomes not just a technical step in "naming" a disorder, but a dynamic process of observation, analysis, and understanding—one that leads to more targeted and effective interventions.

How to Use This Book

This manual follows a standardized, practice-focused format designed to help students and clinical practitioners refine their diagnostic skills through a variety of exercises. Unlike other books that provide extensive theoretical overviews for each disorder, this one is almost exclusively practical: each chapter is devoted to a single disorder and presents a recurring structure of multiple-choice questions, true/false questions, matching exercises, and a clinical case study with corresponding questions, culminating in answer keys with explanations. Below are some guidelines to help you get the most out of the book.

Chapter Structure:

Each disorder is introduced simply with its title (for example, "Tic Disorders," "Schizotypal Personality Disorder," "Major Depressive Disorder," etc.). Immediately after the title, you will find five sections, always in the following order:

1. Multiple-Choice Questions
2. True/False
3. Matching Exercise
4. Case Study
5. Answers

Each section is designed to test and strengthen different aspects of diagnostic comprehension, ranging from basic knowledge of DSM-5-TR criteria to practical application in realistic clinical scenarios.

Multiple-Choice Questions

The first section provides a list of multiple-choice questions, each with four options (A, B, C, D). These questions are intended to evaluate your command of diagnostic criteria, as well as your understanding of relevant specifiers, etiological factors, differential diagnoses, or main treatment options. Sometimes the answer choices might be quite similar, helping you hone your ability to discern subtle clinical nuances or distinguishing criteria.

Tips for Success

- Read each question carefully and consider whether it relates to a specific DSM criterion or a commonly recognized clinical feature of the disorder.
- Avoid jumping to the answer that merely "sounds" right: check the other options to ensure there isn't a more precise or DSM-accurate choice.
- If you have doubts, make a note of them and compare your thoughts with the answer key at the end of the chapter.

True/False

The second section presents a list of statements to be marked as true (✓) or false (✗). These statements range from basic criteria to less obvious clinical features, offering a quick and focused review of key information about each disorder.

Making the Most of True/False Questions:

- If a statement seems partially correct but contains an inaccuracy, it's likely "false." Always double-check the details (e.g., age of onset, minimum symptom duration, diagnostic variants).
- Use these statements as "review triggers": a single true/false item can summarize a crucial piece of information distinguishing one disorder from another (for instance, "For Disorder X, the age of onset is always before age 10").

Matching Exercise

In the third section, you will match different elements—such as definitions, symptoms, behaviors, or diagnostic criteria—with a list of concepts. For example, you may see a set of clinical terms that must be matched to their corresponding descriptions, or particular symptoms to the correct diagnostic label.

Why Matching Matters:

- It develops quick recognition skills: in clinical practice, being able to link a symptom to a criterion or disorder swiftly is essential.
- Pay close attention to descriptions that appear very similar: this will help you identify the key detail that makes the difference in a correct diagnosis.

Case Study

The fourth and final section of each chapter features a clinical case: a short description of a patient (including age, gender, main symptoms, sociocultural context, and other relevant diagnostic information), followed by 2–3 multiple-choice questions. Here you can apply everything you've learned about the disorder's criteria, typical presentations, and clinical reasoning. The goal is to simulate a diagnostic assessment and explore the various nuances of the disorder.

Recommended Approach:

- Read the case carefully, noting all symptoms and any contextual details (duration, age of onset, family background, possible stressors, etc.).
- Try to identify key points that link to the DSM-5-TR diagnostic criteria: recognize which symptoms are "core" and which might be nonspecific.
- Answer the questions as though you were evaluating the individual in an actual clinical setting, considering comorbidities, the exclusion of other possible conditions, the meaning of symptoms, and so forth.

Answer Keys and Explanations

At the end of each chapter, you'll find a summary of the correct answers to all questions (Multiple Choice, True/False, Matching), along with commentary on the case study responses. It's crucial not to look at the answers right away: try to complete the exercises on your own and jot down any uncertainties or guesses. This helps you maximize the self-assessment process, gaining a clear grasp not only of which answers are correct, but also why they are correct.

If certain points remain unclear after reading the explanations, you may want to consult the DSM-5-TR or other reference texts for additional theoretical detail. This manual is intended as a hands-on complement to theoretical study, focusing on the "how" of recognizing, differentiating, and evaluating disorders rather than the "why" or "how they develop."

Study Methods and Suggestions

1. **Focus on one disorder at a time**: devote enough time to complete all sections of a chapter (Multiple Choice, True/False, Matching, Case Study, and answers) before moving on.
2. **Take notes**: if you find certain aspects confusing while answering the questions, write them down and revisit them when checking the answer key. Then consult theoretical texts or discuss them with classmates, instructors, or colleagues if necessary.
3. **Pair results with theoretical study**: although this is a practical manual, a thorough understanding often requires periodic review of the DSM-5-TR criteria. If you're a student, you might alternate reading a theory-based text with working through these exercises.
4. **Use the manual in groups**: in academic or training contexts, discussing responses and diagnostic reasoning with others can make learning more dynamic and engaging.
5. **Leverage case studies for diagnostic synthesis**: if you already work in a clinical setting, try adapting the book's case studies into a diagnostic format similar to what you would use professionally (e.g., including notes about psychological testing or medical examinations).

Neurodevelopmental Disorders

Neurodevelopmental Disorders involve a group of conditions that begin early in life, affecting various aspects of an individual's personal and social functioning. Although each disorder has its own distinct features, they share a disruption of key processes needed for cognitive, language, motor, emotional, or relational development. In the DSM-5-TR, this category typically refers to disorders that emerge at a young age and significantly influence a child's progress in learning, behavior, and social interactions.

One noteworthy point is the variability in how symptoms present. Even within the same diagnosis, they can appear with differing levels of severity and in different forms. For instance, in Autism Spectrum Disorder, some children have pronounced difficulties with verbal communication, while others can speak but encounter social challenges or focus intensely on a narrow range of interests. Communication Disorders can involve issues with articulation, fluency, or the practical use of language. In Attention-Deficit/Hyperactivity Disorder (ADHD), the triad of inattention, hyperactivity, and impulsivity can manifest to varying degrees and affect daily functioning in different ways.

Another common aspect is the need for ongoing observation over time. A child's developmental stages are shaped by environmental, genetic, and cultural factors, so recognizing a Neurodevelopmental Disorder often requires information from multiple sources—parents, teachers, specialists, as well as neuropsychological or cognitive assessments. Monitoring how symptoms evolve can lead to adjustments in intervention strategies and educational choices, especially when additional diagnoses are involved. For example, a Specific Learning Disorder may occur alongside anxiety, or Autism Spectrum Disorder may be paired with language difficulties.

Early identification and management of these disorders can influence a child's quality of life and participation in key environments, including school and family. Timely rehabilitative or psychoeducational interventions can alter the course of the condition and encourage better adjustment. Neurodevelopmental Disorders are placed at the beginning of the DSM-5-TR to emphasize how important it is to address potential warning signs at an early stage.

From a diagnostic standpoint, it's essential to consider overlap with other conditions such as anxiety or mood issues, particularly during adolescence. A thorough differential diagnosis, including the possibility of medical or sensory causes (for example, hearing problems mistaken for inattention), is a critical step. This approach helps clarify how and to what extent neurological factors affect the child's learning, communication, and social development, which in turn supports more precise interventions and better overall outcomes.

Intellectual Disability

Multiple-Choice Questions

1. Which of the following is a necessary criterion for diagnosing Intellectual Disability according to the DSM-5?
   - An IQ below 100 and difficulties in adaptive functioning
   - Deficits in intellectual functioning and adaptive behavior, with onset during the developmental period
   - Only an IQ below 70, disregarding adaptive functioning
   - Intellectual functioning below average but with adequate social skills
2. According to the DSM-5, the severity (mild, moderate, severe, profound) of Intellectual Disability is primarily determined by:
   - IQ score alone
   - Impairments in adaptive functioning across conceptual, social, and practical domains
   - The presence of co-occurring medical conditions
   - The same age thresholds used for motor development milestones
3. Which of the following does not fall under the main domains assessed when determining the severity of Intellectual Disability?
   - Conceptual domain
   - Social domain
   - Practical domain
   - Biological domain
4. Which statement about Intellectual Disability is correct?
   - It can only be diagnosed after age 18
   - It is characterized by deficits in intellectual and adaptive functioning, with onset during the developmental period
   - It only includes cognitive deficits due to traumatic brain injury in adulthood
   - It excludes any possibility of comorbidity with other neurodevelopmental disorders
5. In a child with mild Intellectual Disability, which of the following is most likely observed?
   - An inability to learn basic academic skills
   - A constant need for supervision regarding personal hygiene
   - An ability to develop social and work-related skills with minimal support
   - No difficulties in adaptive functioning
6. A crucial aspect in evaluating Intellectual Disability is:
   - Measuring only the IQ using standardized tests
   - Assessing adaptive abilities in practical, social, and conceptual domains
   - Omitting the patient's clinical history
   - Relying on a single, non-standardized test
7. Which of the following best describes comorbidity in Intellectual Disability?
   - It cannot coexist with Autism Spectrum Disorder
   - It can coexist with other neurodevelopmental or psychiatric disorders
   - It always includes a motor disorder
   - It rules out any other medical or psychiatric diagnosis

True/False Questions

		T	F
1	Intellectual Disability can be diagnosed solely on the basis of IQ scores.		
2	Social adaptation and autonomy are key factors in the diagnosis.		
3	The onset of Intellectual Disability must occur after age 18.		
4	In the DSM-5, severity is mostly determined by adaptive skills.		
5	A child with mild Intellectual Disability can achieve a decent level of independence with proper support.		
6	A medical condition (e.g., Down syndrome) is the only cause of Intellectual Disability.		
7	Environmental factors (such as early stimulation) can influence the development of adaptive skills.		
8	Difficulties with abstract reasoning and problem-solving are examples of intellectual deficits.		
9	Intellectual Disability excludes the possibility of attending school successfully, even with support.		
10	Diagnosis requires standardized testing and clinical observation.		

Matching Exercise

1. Conceptual domain [ ]
2. Social domain [ ]
3. Practical domain [ ]
4. Mild Intellectual Disability [ ]
5. Severe Intellectual Disability [ ]
6. Comorbidity [ ]

Descriptions:

- A. Significant deficits in daily problem-solving skills, requiring constant support in nearly all activities.
- B. Can learn basic academic skills, with possible moderate independence if minimal support is provided.
- C. Involves abilities such as reasoning, memory, language, and academic knowledge.
- D. Relates to effectiveness in interacting with others, understanding social cues, and interpersonal communication.
- E. Co-occurrence of other psychiatric or neurodevelopmental disorders in addition to Intellectual Disability.
- F. Includes personal care, household management, and using tools and technology in daily life.

Case Study

Martina is an 8-year-old girl in the third grade. Her parents and teachers report that she struggles to acquire basic reading and writing skills and requires repeated instructions to carry out daily tasks. Although she is shy, she tries to interact with peers but often has trouble understanding group game rules and more nuanced aspects of communication (such as irony). Her parents say that from early childhood, she reached developmental milestones (walking, talking) later than expected, despite no significant physical issues. Standardized tests indicate below-average intellectual functioning for her age, and her adaptive skills—especially at school—are markedly compromised.

1. Which element is central to diagnosing Intellectual Disability according to the DSM-5?
    - A. Significant deficits in social interactions only
    - B. Below-average intellectual functioning with no impairment in adaptive behavior
    - C. Deficits in intellectual functioning and adaptive behavior, with onset in the developmental period
    - D. Difficulty exclusively in basic reading and writing skills
2. Which condition should be ruled out first in Martina's case?
    - A. Academic difficulties due to inadequate instruction
    - B. Sensory disorders (e.g., hearing impairment)
    - C. Generalized Anxiety Disorder
    - D. ADHD
3. What is the most appropriate treatment plan for Martina?
    - A. Immediate antipsychotic medication
    - B. Placement in a personalized educational program, family support, and speech therapy
    - C. No support measures, as the condition is transient
    - D. Psychoeducational intervention in an inpatient setting only

Answers

Multiple Choice Questions

1. B
2. B
3. D
4. B
5. C
6. B
7. B

True/False Questions

1. False
2. True
3. False
4. True
5. True
6. False
7. True
8. True
9. False
10. True

Matching Exercise

1. C
2. D
3. F
4. B
5. A
6. E

Case Study Answers and Explanations

1. C – Explanation: According to the DSM-5, the essential diagnostic features of Intellectual Disability include both deficits in intellectual functioning (e.g., reasoning, problem-solving) and deficits in adaptive behavior (e.g., practical daily life skills), with onset in the developmental period.
2. B – Explanation: It is crucial to rule out organic or sensory causes (e.g., hearing impairment) that might affect learning and adaptive functioning before confirming Intellectual Disability.
3. B – Explanation: A multimodal approach is indicated for mild Intellectual Disability, including tailored educational support, family involvement, and, if needed, specialized interventions (e.g., speech therapy) to address communication challenges.

Communication Disorders

Multiple-Choice Questions

1. Which of the following is a key feature for diagnosing a Language Disorder according to the DSM-5?
    - A. Persistent difficulties in the social use of language
    - B. Persistent difficulties acquiring and using language in all forms (spoken, written, sign language)
    - C. Intellectual deficits that fully explain the language difficulties
    - D. Relational conflicts unrelated to language issues
2. Which of the following is a typical sign of Childhood-Onset Fluency Disorder (Stuttering)?
    - A. Excessive speed of speech without comprehension problems
    - B. Fear of public speaking without any blocks or repetitions
    - C. Repetitions or prolongations of sounds and syllables, possibly accompanied by involuntary pauses
    - D. Complete absence of verbal communication
3. According to the DSM-5, Social (Pragmatic) Communication Disorder is primarily characterized by:
    - A. Pronunciation errors not resolved by age 4
    - B. Difficulties with the social use of language and understanding conversational rules
    - C. Stuttering combined with tics or muscle spasms
    - D. Adequate language skills but accompanied by a mood disorder
4. Which of the following is not typically included in a Speech Sound Disorder (Phonological Disorder)?
    - A. Persistent errors in producing sounds (e.g., omissions, substitutions)
    - B. Specific difficulties forming syntactically correct sentences
    - C. Pronunciation errors not due to motor or sensory factors (e.g., deafness)
    - D. Difficulty articulating one or more phonemes in a manner appropriate for the child's age
5. When do the symptoms of a Language Disorder become most evident?
    - A. While learning a foreign language
    - B. In both expressing and comprehending everyday language, especially in more complex situations
    - C. Only when reading aloud
    - D. Exclusively in written interactions
6. Which of the following is a possible comorbidity associated with Communication Disorders?
    - A. Autism Spectrum Disorder
    - B. Agoraphobia with no history of communication issues
    - C. Substance dependence as the only symptom
    - D. Brief Psychotic Disorder
7. Which aspect is most important to assess when differentiating a Communication Disorder from a delay caused by environmental deprivation?
    - A. Whether language difficulties appear only in a school setting
    - B. The child's motivation to learn
    - C. The level of stimulation and learning opportunities provided by the environment
    - D. The parents' age at the child's birth

True/False Questions

		T	F
1	In Language Disorder, deficits appear in both language expression and comprehension.		
2	Stuttering is exclusively characterized by social anxiety, with no blocks or repetitions.		
3	A child with a Phonological Disorder might consistently substitute "r" with "l."		
4	Social (Pragmatic) Communication Disorder can involve difficulty respecting conversational turn-taking.		
5	Communication Disorders always disappear by adolescence, without exception.		
6	The etiology of a Communication Disorder can include genetic and neurobiological factors.		
7	An audiological evaluation is often recommended to rule out hearing problems that could underlie language difficulties.		
8	Repetition of syllables (e.g., "pa-pa-ball") is a typical example of stuttering.		
9	If a child's language difficulties are explained by a low IQ, a Language Disorder is not diagnosed.		
10	Effective social interaction also depends on understanding the conversational context.		

Matching Exercise

1. Language Disorder [ ]
2. Speech Sound Disorder (Phonological Disorder) [ ]
3. Childhood-Onset Fluency Disorder (Stuttering) [ ]
4. Social (Pragmatic) Communication Disorder [ ]
5. Repetition or prolongation of sounds [ ]
6. Environmental deprivation [ ]

Descriptions:

- A. A disorder involving persistent difficulty in pronouncing phonemes, with errors such as substitution or omission.
- B. A situation where the child does not receive adequate linguistic or educational stimulation.
- C. Persistent difficulty acquiring and using language in all its forms (both expression and comprehension).
- D. Stuttering, characterized by repetitions and prolongations of sounds, as well as potential blocking.
- E. Difficulty adhering to the pragmatic rules of conversation, such as turn-taking or contextual cues.
- F. A typical symptom of stuttering (e.g., "Ma-ma-mommy").

Case Study

Oliver, a 6-year-old boy in first grade, often confuses certain sounds during conversation (e.g., saying "pato" instead of "gatto" in his native language) and sometimes omits entire syllables. He seems to understand what's said to him, yet some classmates struggle to follow his speech. According to his parents, Oliver talks a lot at home, but his words frequently sound distorted or unclear. No sensory or neurological issues have been identified, and his home environment appears to be sufficiently stimulating.

1. What is the most likely diagnosis for Oliver?
   - A. Language Disorder
   - B. Childhood-Onset Fluency Disorder (Stuttering)
   - C. Speech Sound Disorder (Phonological Disorder)
   - D. Selective Mutism
2. What should be ruled out before confirming the diagnosis?
   - A. Significant intellectual disability
   - B. Lack of proper environmental stimulation
   - C. Attention-Deficit/Hyperactivity Disorder (ADHD)
   - D. Anatomical malformations (e.g., issues with the speech apparatus)
3. Which initial intervention is most appropriate?
   - A. A program to enhance vocabulary and syntax without focusing on pronunciation
   - B. Speech therapy targeting the most difficult or confusing sounds
   - C. Mild anxiolytics to reduce stuttering
   - D. Family therapy in a group setting with no speech intervention

Answers

Multiple-Choice Questions
1. B
2. C
3. B
4. B
5. B
6. A
7. C

True/False Questions
1. True
2. False
3. True
4. True
5. False
6. True
7. True
8. True
9. True
10. True

Matching Exercise
1. C
2. A
3. D
4. E
5. F
6. B

Case Study Answers and Explanations
1. C - Explanation: Oliver has difficulties pronouncing certain sounds (substitutions and omissions) but does not exhibit major problems with comprehension. This pattern is characteristic of a Speech Sound Disorder.
2. B - Explanation: It is essential to rule out that Oliver's language difficulties are not due to environmental deprivation or insufficient linguistic stimulation.
3. B - Explanation: Therapy focused on articulation, phoneme production, and overall pronunciation is the most appropriate initial approach, given that there are no other identified comorbidities.

Autism Spectrum Disorder

Multiple-Choice Questions

1. According to the DSM-5, which of the following best characterizes Autism Spectrum Disorder (ASD)?
    - A. Language deficits only, with no social impairment
    - B. Persistent deficits in communication and social interaction, along with restricted interests and repetitive behaviors
    - C. Primarily oppositional and defiant behaviors
    - D. Complete absence of any interaction with peers
2. Which of the following is a typical feature of the restricted and repetitive behaviors seen in ASD?
    - A. Automatically imitating other people's gestures
    - B. Engaging in a wide variety of age-appropriate pretend play
    - C. Intense interest in specific topics, repetitive use of objects or phrases
    - D. Easily transitioning between activities
3. In Autism Spectrum Disorder, symptoms must be present:
    - A. Only during adolescence
    - B. Before age 3
    - C. From early childhood, though they may not become clearly evident until social demands exceed the individual's abilities
    - D. Only after completing elementary school
4. Which of the following factors should be ruled out before making an ASD diagnosis?
    - A. Genetic conditions (e.g., Fragile X Syndrome)
    - B. Isolated anxiety disorders that do not affect social interaction
    - C. A neurological or sensory condition that could explain social and communication deficits
    - D. Sleep-wake disorders present since birth
5. Which of the following approaches is commonly used to treat ASD?
    - A. Behavioral techniques (Applied Behavior Analysis, ABA) and psychoeducational interventions
    - B. Pharmacotherapy alone
    - C. Complete withdrawal from school and social settings to reduce stress
    - D. No intervention is useful, as the condition is irreversible
6. Under the DSM-5 classification, the severity of Autism Spectrum Disorder is determined by:
    - A. The child's IQ score alone
    - B. The level of support needed for social-communication skills and the degree of restricted/repetitive behaviors
    - C. The presence or absence of mutism
    - D. Whether there are coexisting vision or hearing problems
7. Which statement best describes how ASD symptoms evolve?
    - A. They resolve spontaneously by preadolescence
    - B. They can vary over time, with possible improvements through targeted interventions
    - C. They inevitably become more severe and debilitating with age
    - D. They are always associated with severe cognitive impairment

True/False Questions

		T	F
1	Children with ASD always have an intellectual disability.		
2	An intense, absorbing interest in certain topics is common in ASD.		
3	Social skill impairments can range from mild to very severe.		
4	The absence of repetitive behaviors rules out an ASD diagnosis.		
5	Reduced eye contact is a possible but not universal sign.		
6	Early intervention can help improve social and communication abilities.		
7	A temporary loss (regression) of certain language and social skills can occur in some ASD cases.		
8	Interventions based on Applied Behavior Analysis (ABA) are never recommended.		
9	Hypersensitivity to sounds or lights can be part of ASD's sensory symptoms.		
10	Autism Spectrum Disorder only affects males.		

Matching Exercise

1. Deficits in social communication [ ]
2. Repetitive, stereotyped behaviors [ ]
3. Behavioral intervention [ ]
4. Language regression [ ]
5. Required level of support [ ]
6. Sensory hypersensitivity [ ]

Descriptions:

- A. A technique that uses reinforcement and modeling (e.g., ABA) to improve social-communication skills.
- B. The varying degree of assistance (from mild to extensive) depending on symptom severity and functional limitations.
- C. The loss of previously acquired abilities, such as words a child used to speak.
- D. Lack of emotional reciprocity, difficulty maintaining or understanding conversational context.
- E. Repetitive movements, behavioral rigidity, insistence on sameness.
- F. Overreactions or avoidance related to auditory, tactile, or visual stimuli.

Case Study

Ethan, a 7-year-old boy in second grade, struggles to interact with classmates: he does not respond to greetings, avoids eye contact, and shows a nearly exclusive interest in dinosaurs, on which he has extensive knowledge. When he speaks, he often repeats phrases from cartoons, without using them appropriately. His gross motor skills are adequate, but during recess he prefers spinning in circles or lining up objects. His parents report that Ethan started saying a few words around age 2, then stopped for a while, resuming speech only later. No significant sensory or cognitive impairments have been noted, but he requires constant help adapting to new situations.

1. Which DSM-5 feature is most central to Ethan's presentation, suggesting Autism Spectrum Disorder?
    - A. A preference for non-social play but no repetitive behaviors
    - B. Persistent deficits in social communication/interaction and restricted, repetitive patterns of behavior
    - C. Brief psychotic symptoms triggered by stress
    - D. Early advanced language skills and no need for behavioral support
2. Which factor must be ruled out before confirming an ASD diagnosis?
    - A. Lack of adequate linguistic stimulation within the family
    - B. Intellectual disability that alone could account for social and communication deficits
    - C. Situational anxiety
    - D. Major depressive disorder in early childhood
3. Which initial intervention strategy is generally recommended for Ethan?
    - A. Complete withdrawal from school to avoid stressful stimuli
    - B. A pharmacological regimen aimed at reducing his interest in dinosaurs
    - C. A multimodal intervention that includes behavioral therapies, educational support, and family involvement
    - D. No intervention—simply wait for social skills to improve on their own

Answers

Multiple-Choice Questions
1. B
2. C
3. C
4. C
5. A
6. B
7. B

True/False Questions
1. False
2. True
3. True
4. False
5. True
6. True
7. True
8. False
9. True
10. False

Matching Exercise
1. D
2. E
3. A
4. C
5. B
6. F

Case Study Answers and Explanations
1. B – Explanation: ASD involves social communication deficits and restricted, repetitive behaviors per DSM-5 criteria.
2. B – Explanation: Exclude intellectual disability sufficient to explain social/communication deficits alone.
3. C – Explanation: A multimodal approach (behavioral therapies, educational support, family training) is recommended early for ASD.

Attention-Deficit/Hyperactivity Disorder

Multiple-Choice Questions

1. Which of the following best describes ADHD according to the DSM-5?
    - A. Primarily intellectual deficits
    - B. A persistent pattern of inattention and/or hyperactivity-impulsivity that impairs functioning or development
    - C. Acute episodes of hallucinations and delusions
    - D. Excessive sensitivity to auditory stimuli
2. According to the DSM-5, ADHD symptoms must:
    - A. Appear in only one setting (e.g., only at school or only at home)
    - B. Be present before age 12
    - C. Occur exclusively during adolescence
    - D. Begin after age 16 if behavioral issues persist
3. Which of the following symptoms is typical of the inattention seen in some ADHD subtypes?
    - A. An inability to remain seated in class and a tendency to run or climb excessively
    - B. Talking continuously without listening to others
    - C. Difficulty sustaining attention on tasks or play activities, frequent careless mistakes
    - D. Struggling with frustration and social anxiety
4. Hyperactivity in a child with ADHD often manifests as:
    - A. Apathy and extreme passivity
    - B. Excessive movement or restlessness, difficulty remaining seated or calm
    - C. Constant fear of making mistakes and avoidant behavior
    - D. Depressed mood and social withdrawal
5. Which of the following is crucial for differentiating ADHD from other disorders?
    - A. The presence of psychotic phenomena
    - B. The frequency and intensity of inattention and/or hyperactivity symptoms across multiple settings (school, home, etc.)
    - C. A single IQ test
    - D. Dietary factors or food allergies
6. Which statement is correct regarding ADHD comorbidity?
    - A. ADHD can never co-occur with other neurodevelopmental disorders
    - B. Comorbidity with Oppositional Defiant Disorder or Conduct Disorder is common
    - C. ADHD cannot occur alongside anxiety or depressive disorders
    - D. ADHD always implies co-occurring Autism Spectrum Disorder
7. For an ADHD diagnosis, it is necessary to:
    - A. Show a developmental delay of at least 2 years in motor milestones
    - B. Confirm that symptoms are not better explained by another disorder (e.g., mood disorder, anxiety disorder)
    - C. Rely solely on the opinion of the child's teacher
    - D. Exclude any form of support or intervention before making the diagnosis

True/False Questions

		T	F
1	ADHD is always associated with below-average intellectual functioning.		
2	ADHD symptoms may change over time; for example, hyperactivity can decrease while impulsivity or inattention becomes more prominent.		
3	It is possible to diagnose ADHD in adulthood if there is evidence of symptoms before age 12.		
4	Only children can have ADHD; it never occurs in adolescents or adults.		
5	A common comorbidity of ADHD is with Specific Learning Disorders.		
6	Impulsivity may present as difficulty taking turns in conversation or play activities.		
7	ADHD can appear in three subtypes: predominantly inattentive, predominantly hyperactive-impulsive, or combined.		
8	Excessive use of digital devices is the only proven cause of ADHD.		
9	Before diagnosing ADHD, it is important to rule out severe environmental deprivation as the cause of symptoms.		
10	A multimodal treatment approach (pharmacological and behavioral) is often recommended for ADHD.		

Matching Exercise

1. Inattention [ ]
2. Hyperactivity [ ]
3. Impulsivity [ ]
4. Combined subtype [ ]
5. Comorbidity [ ]
6. Multimodal intervention [ ]

Descriptions:

- A. Characterized by excessive movement, difficulty staying still or calm.
- B. Both inattention and hyperactivity-impulsivity at clinically significant levels.
- C. Trouble sustaining attention, distractibility, frequently losing items.
- D. The co-occurrence of other disorders (e.g., Oppositional Defiant Disorder, Specific Learning Disorder).
- E. A treatment plan that includes behavioral strategies and, when necessary, medication.
- F. Acting without thinking of the consequences, interrupting others, difficulty waiting one's turn.

Case Study

Aiden, an 8-year-old boy in third grade, has long struggled to finish his assignments: he frequently loses school materials, seems easily distracted, and jumps from one activity to another without completing any of them. In class, Aiden constantly gets up from his seat, talks to classmates while the teacher is explaining a lesson, and interrupts conversations. He has no cognitive deficits or sensory issues. However, he appears restless even in situations that require calm, such as during meals or while waiting his turn to play. His parents report that these behaviors have been present since early childhood and occur both at home and at school.

1. Which factor best distinguishes ADHD from typical childhood restlessness?
   - A. Restlessness that appears only in one setting (e.g., at home but not at school)
   - B. Occasional fidgeting or mild inattention limited to boring tasks
   - C. Persistent inattention and/or hyperactivity across multiple settings, clearly impairing functioning
   - D. High energy levels on playground activities, but normal attention when seated
2. Which factor must be ruled out before confirming the diagnosis?
   - A. Neurological or sensory problems that could explain his inattention
   - B. Difficulties in reading and writing as his only symptom
   - C. Above-average IQ
   - D. Adequate behavior at home
3. Which intervention is most appropriate to start with?
   - A. Medication-only therapy with antipsychotics
   - B. A multimodal approach involving behavioral interventions, possible medication, and family support
   - C. Withdrawing him from school for 6 months, waiting for symptoms to resolve spontaneously
   - D. No intervention; hyperactive behaviors will disappear as he grows up

Answers

Multiple-Choice Questions

1. B
2. B
3. C
4. B
5. B
6. B
7. B

True/False Questions

1. False
2. True
3. True
4. False
5. True
6. True
7. True
8. False
9. True
10. True

Matching Exercise

1. C
2. A
3. F
4. B
5. D
6. E

Case Study Answers and Explanations

1. **C** – Explanation: ADHD involves persistent inattention/hyperactivity across different settings (e.g., home and school), significantly impacting daily functioning—more than normal childhood restlessness.
2. **A** – Explanation: Before diagnosing ADHD, alternative causes (e.g., hearing issues, neurological conditions) must be ruled out.
3. **B** – Explanation: A multimodal approach typically combines behavioral strategies, family support, and—if necessary—pharmacological treatment (e.g., stimulants).

Specific Learning Disorder (SLD)

Multiple-Choice Questions

1. According to the DSM-5, which of the following best characterizes a Specific Learning Disorder?
    - A. Persistent and significant difficulties in one specific domain (reading, writing, or math) not explained by intellectual disability or sensory deficits
    - B. Exclusively delayed language in preschool
    - C. Frequent unexplained absences from school
    - D. Disruptive classroom behaviors
2. Which of the following is not recognized as a subtype of SLD under the DSM-5?
    - A. Reading Disorder (Dyslexia)
    - B. Math Disorder (Dyscalculia)
    - C. Written Expression Disorder (which may include spelling and handwriting difficulties)
    - D. Generalized Social Adaptation Disorder
3. Which sign is most typical of a child with a Reading Disorder (Dyslexia)?
    - A. Difficulty only with mental calculation
    - B. Slowness and/or errors when reading text and words, including decoding mistakes
    - C. Oppositional behaviors aimed at teachers
    - D. No reading problems but difficulty understanding text
4. Which of the following must be ruled out before diagnosing a Specific Learning Disorder?
    - A. Access to schooling appropriate for the child's age
    - B. Sensory impairments (e.g., deafness) or a low IQ that alone could account for the deficit
    - C. A family environment of average socioeconomic level
    - D. A comorbid anxiety disorder
5. Which statement best describes the prognosis of Specific Learning Disorders?
    - A. There is no spontaneous improvement; symptoms remain unchanged throughout life
    - B. With early and appropriate intervention, many individuals can significantly compensate for their difficulties
    - C. Medication is the only way to improve these disorders
    - D. Specific Learning Disorder always disappears automatically at the start of adolescence
6. Which of the following manifestations might indicate a Written Expression Disorder?
    - A. Persistent difficulty pronouncing certain phonemes
    - B. Frequent spelling mistakes, poorly structured sentences, difficulty organizing written text
    - C. Slowness in written calculation but good reading skills
    - D. Difficulty maintaining attention for long periods
7. Which of the following strategies is helpful in addressing Specific Learning Disorders?
    - A. Avoiding any academic support to prevent "labeling" the child
    - B. Tailored psychoeducational interventions, including compensatory tools and supportive measures
    - C. Relying solely on pharmacological treatment
    - D. Withdrawing from school to reduce anxiety

True/False Questions

		T	F
1	A Specific Learning Disorder is always accompanied by below-average IQ.		
2	Dyslexia is a reading difficulty that may involve accuracy, speed, and/or comprehension.		
3	Dyscalculia refers to difficulties in learning and using arithmetic or numerical concepts.		
4	Dysorthographia involves primarily difficulty understanding written text, without spelling errors.		
5	Proper educational intervention can significantly improve a child's performance in SLD.		
6	Specific Learning Disorders can never coexist with ADHD or other neurodevelopmental disorders.		
7	Reading or spelling errors must be evaluated against the child's chronological age and level of instruction.		
8	Early identification of an SLD can facilitate more timely and effective intervention.		
9	The use of compensatory tools (such as text-to-speech or a calculator) is never recommended.		
10	Environmental and instructional factors should also be considered when diagnosing a Specific Learning Disorder.		

Matching Exercise

1. Dyslexia [ ]
2. Dysgraphia [ ]
3. Dyscalculia [ ]
4. Compensatory tools [ ]
5. Support measures ("dispensatory" adjustments) [ ]
6. Comorbidity [ ]

Descriptions:

- A. A writing disorder at the executive and motor level, resulting in illegible handwriting.
- B. The possibility of reducing certain academic demands (e.g., excessive written assignments) to help the student cope.
- C. Difficulty mastering and fluidly using math and numerical reasoning skills.
- D. A reading disorder that may involve speed, accuracy, and/or comprehension.
- E. The use of concept maps, text-to-speech software, audiobooks, or calculators to support specific needs.
- F. The presence of additional disorders (e.g., ADHD) alongside SLD.

Case Study

Megan, a 9-year-old in the fourth grade, struggles to read texts fluently; she makes decoding errors (for instance, confusing similar letters like "b" and "d") and reads very slowly. However, she seems to understand the content when it's read aloud to her. She also makes frequent spelling errors and has trouble organizing sentences. Neither parents nor teachers have noticed any evident cognitive or sensory impairments, and Megan is actually very curious and interested in many topics. Nonetheless, there is a high level of frustration during homework and when reading textbooks.

1. Which detail best distinguishes Megan's reading and spelling difficulties from a general intellectual deficit?
    - A. She is anxious about speaking in public but shows no decoding problems
    - B. She struggles with reading and writing despite normal intelligence and no sensory issues
    - C. She has occasional motor tics that interfere with her handwriting
    - D. She compensates well if texts are read to her, though her IQ is below average
2. Which factor should be ruled out before confirming this diagnosis?
    - A. Low IQ that alone explains the reading and writing problems
    - B. Difficulty speaking in public due to shyness
    - C. Occasional motor tics
    - D. Occasional family conflicts
3. What is the first recommended intervention for Megan?
    - A. A stimulant-based medication regimen
    - B. Intensive individual psychotherapy focused on performance anxiety
    - C. Targeted educational strategies, compensatory tools, and speech/psychoeducational support
    - D. Temporary withdrawal from school to reduce frustration

Answers

Multiple-Choice Questions
1. A
2. D
3. B
4. B
5. B
6. B
7. B

True/False Questions
1. False
2. True
3. True
4. False
5. True
6. False
7. True
8. True
9. False
10. True

Matching Exercise
1. D
2. A
3. C
4. E
5. B
6. F

Case Study Answers and Explanations
1. B – Explanation: For an SLD, reading/writing issues persist despite normal intelligence and absence of sensory deficits.
2. A – Explanation: Before diagnosing SLD, it's important to rule out that the difficulties are fully explained by low IQ or sensory deficits.
3. C – Explanation: The most appropriate approach includes specialized educational interventions, compensatory tools (e.g., concept maps, text-to-speech), and speech/psychoeducational support.

Motor Disorders

Multiple-Choice Questions

1. Which of the following best describes Developmental Coordination Disorder (DCD) according to the DSM-5?
    - A. Motor difficulties primarily due to neurological conditions (e.g., cerebral palsy)
    - B. Persistent difficulties in acquiring and executing motor skills not attributable to medical or intellectual conditions
    - C. No coordination problems, with age-appropriate motor skills
    - D. Both motor and vocal tics occurring simultaneously
2. In Stereotypic Movement Disorder, stereotypies are:
    - A. Repetitive, seemingly purposeless motor behaviors that may result in self-injury
    - B. Brief episodes of motor amnesia with loss of muscle tone
    - C. Intentional movements aimed at reaching an object
    - D. Always associated with a Psychotic Disorder
3. Which of the following statements is true regarding motor stereotypies?
    - A. They occur only in adulthood and rarely in childhood
    - B. They may present as muscle-tone fluctuations without repetitive movements
    - C. If they cause physical harm, they are specified as "with self-injurious behavior"
    - D. They are always accompanied by cognitive delay
4. Developmental Coordination Disorder is often associated with:
    - A. Moderate to severe intellectual disability as the primary cause
    - B. Age-appropriate motor performance but co-occurring attention problems
    - C. Difficulties with daily activities requiring coordination (e.g., writing, using utensils, tying shoelaces)
    - D. Psychotic episodes in adolescence
5. To distinguish Developmental Coordination Disorder from a simple developmental delay, it is important to:
    - A. Assess whether the motor difficulties are consistent with the child's age and level of education
    - B. Use only verbal intelligence tests
    - C. Assume that all clumsy children have Developmental Coordination Disorder
    - D. Rely solely on parental observations
6. Which factor must be ruled out before diagnosing Stereotypic Movement Disorder?
    - A. That the repetitive movements are not due to the physiological effects of a substance or another medical condition
    - B. That the child shows excellent coordination in complex activities
    - C. That the motor behavior occurs only at school
    - D. That the child's social skills are impaired
7. Which of the following interventions is considered helpful for Motor Disorders?
    - A. Avoiding any specific intervention, as the problem resolves on its own
    - B. Occupational therapy and/or physical therapy targeting deficient motor skills
    - C. Antipsychotic medication in all cases of stereotypies
    - D. Completely isolating the child to reduce external stimuli

True/False Questions

		T	F
1	Developmental Coordination Disorder is often diagnosed only in the presence of intellectual disability.		
2	Motor stereotypies can include self-injurious behaviors, such as repeatedly hitting one's head.		
3	Stereotypic Movement Disorder requires that these movements not be attributable to other medical conditions or substances.		
4	Children with Developmental Coordination Disorder typically struggle with activities such as running, jumping, or handling objects.		
5	Motor stereotypies never cause distress or impair daily functioning.		
6	A child with Developmental Coordination Disorder may have difficulty participating in age-appropriate sports.		
7	Motor stereotypies are always linked to autism spectrum disorders.		
8	A child with Developmental Coordination Disorder may appear clumsier and more awkward than peers.		
9	Early intervention offers no benefit in improving motor skills.		
10	Some children with Stereotypic Movement Disorder experience a reduction in these movements as they get older.		

Matching Exercise

1. Developmental Coordination Disorder [ ]
2. Stereotypic Movement Disorder [ ]
3. Stereotypies with self-injurious behavior [ ]
4. Occupational therapy [ ]
5. Ruling out other medical conditions [ ]
6. Difficulty with fine motor skills [ ]

Descriptions:

- A. Repetitive, seemingly purposeless movements that cause physical harm (e.g., biting or hitting oneself).
- B. A set of interventions aimed at improving coordination and motor skills within daily routines.
- C. Symptoms cannot be explained by cerebral palsy or other conditions that would account for deficits.
- D. A condition in which the child shows clumsiness, slowness, or inaccuracy in daily motor tasks.
- E. Characterized by repetitive movements, which may or may not be self-injurious.
- F. Specific difficulties in tasks such as writing, drawing, using utensils, or tying shoelaces.

Case Study

Kevin, a 7-year-old boy, is brought in for evaluation because his parents and teachers report significant clumsiness and slowness in motor tasks. For example, Kevin takes a long time to dress himself, struggles with cutting paper, and frequently trips when running or playing ball with peers. He has no notable cognitive or sensory deficits and achieved walking and talking milestones at age-appropriate times. At school, he has difficulty with tasks such as cutting shapes or coloring within the lines. His parents report no repetitive or stereotypic movements. His pediatrician has ruled out neurological conditions and other medical issues.

1. Which DSM-5 feature best separates Kevin's presentation from typical childhood clumsiness?
    - A. Repetitive, seemingly purposeless motor movements
    - B. Motor skill deficits that significantly impair daily living, not explained by cognitive or neurological causes
    - C. Loss of previously acquired motor abilities
    - D. Infrequent, minor difficulties in sports only
2. Which factor must be ruled out before confirming the diagnosis?
    - A. An intellectual or sensory deficit that could explain the motor difficulties
    - B. Exceptional ability in drawing or a particular sport
    - C. Recurrent vocal tics
    - D. Family conflicts related to discipline
3. What is the most appropriate initial intervention for Kevin?
    - A. Antipsychotic medication
    - B. Occupational therapy to improve both fine and gross motor skills
    - C. Restricting all physical activities to avoid accidents
    - D. Stricter disciplinary rules without additional support

Answers

Multiple-Choice Questions

1. B
2. A
3. C
4. C
5. A
6. A
7. B

True/False Questions

1. False
2. True
3. True
4. True
5. False
6. True
7. False
8. True
9. False
10. True

Matching Exercise

1. D
2. E
3. A
4. B
5. C
6. F

Case Study Answers and Explanations

1. B – Explanation: Developmental Coordination Disorder involves marked motor skill deficits impairing daily tasks, not accounted for by intellectual or neurological conditions.
2. A – Explanation: Before diagnosing Developmental Coordination Disorder, it is essential to rule out intellectual disability, sensory problems (vision or hearing), or neurological conditions that could account for these deficits.
3. B – Explanation: The most appropriate intervention is occupational therapy (and possibly physical therapy) to strengthen both fine and gross motor abilities.

Tic Disorders

Multiple-Choice Questions

1. Which of the following criteria is required for diagnosing Tourette's Disorder?
    - A. Presence of only motor tics for less than 1 year
    - B. Presence of both motor and vocal tics for at least 1 year, with onset before age 18
    - C. Vocal tics occurring only during stressful situations
    - D. Complete disappearance of tics within 6 months of onset
2. Which of the following statements is not true regarding Persistent (Chronic) Motor or Vocal Tic Disorder?
    - A. It involves either motor tics or vocal tics, but not both
    - B. Symptoms must be present for at least 1 year
    - C. Symptoms can intermittently disappear for several months without losing the diagnosis
    - D. Onset is required exclusively after age 18
3. What differentiates Provisional Tic Disorder from other tic disorders?
    - A. Tics manifest only in social settings
    - B. Tics last less than 1 year and may spontaneously disappear
    - C. Tics must involve both motor and vocal components
    - D. Tics are caused exclusively by medical or neurological factors
4. Which of the following is an example of a complex motor tic?
    - A. Rapid eye blinking
    - B. Repeated shoulder shrugging
    - C. Jumping or repeatedly touching objects
    - D. Throat clearing
5. Which environmental factor often exacerbates tics?
    - A. Consistent daily routines
    - B. Stress or anxiety
    - C. Adequate and regular sleep
    - D. No correlation with external factors
6. Which treatment is considered first-line for managing severe tics?
    - A. Cognitive-Behavioral Therapy (CBT)
    - B. Habit Reversal Therapy (HRT)
    - C. Antipsychotic medication
    - D. Stimulant medication
7. What is the typical age of onset for tic disorders?
    - A. Before age 3
    - B. Between ages 4 and 6
    - C. Between ages 12 and 18
    - D. After age 20

True/False Questions

		T	F
1	In Tourette's Disorder, both motor and vocal tics must be present.		
2	Persistent (Chronic) Motor or Vocal Tic Disorder requires the presence of both motor and vocal tics.		
3	Tics can worsen in response to stress or fatigue.		
4	Provisional Tic Disorder can last for several years without ever meeting criteria for other tic disorders.		
5	The severity of tics typically peaks during adolescence.		
6	Habit Reversal Therapy (HRT) is an evidence-based treatment for tic disorders.		
7	Antipsychotic medications are the first-line treatment for mild tics.		
8	Tic disorders always fully resolve in adulthood.		
9	Tics are often involuntary but can be briefly suppressed.		
10	Vocal tics always involve meaningful words or phrases.		

Matching Exercise

1. Tourette's Disorder [ ]
2. Persistent (Chronic) Motor or Vocal Tic Disorder [ ]
3. Provisional Tic Disorder [ ]
4. Simple motor tics [ ]
5. Complex vocal tics [ ]
6. Habit Reversal Therapy (HRT) [ ]

Descriptions:

- A. Therapy focused on awareness training and competing response strategies to reduce tics.
- B. Motor or vocal tics lasting less than 1 year.
- C. Motor tics such as blinking, shoulder shrugging, or facial grimaces.
- D. Both motor and vocal tics lasting at least 1 year, with onset before age 18.
- E. Motor or vocal tics persisting for more than 1 year, but not both.
- F. Vocal tics involving more elaborate utterances, such as repeating words or phrases.

Case Study

Liam, a 10-year-old boy, has been experiencing repeated eye blinking and throat clearing for about 9 months. These symptoms occur daily and are more intense when he feels anxious or tired. His parents report that the tics have never disappeared for more than one week at a time. Liam has no significant vocal tics and shows no signs of other medical or neurological conditions.

1. Which time-related factor is key in deciding whether Liam's motor tics fit a Provisional Tic Disorder according to the DSM-5?
   - A. Tics must be absent for at least 6 consecutive months
   - B. Tics that persist beyond 1 year
   - C. Tics that last under 1 year, without any break longer than 3 months
   - D. Tics occurring only when the child is anxious or tired
2. Which condition should be ruled out first in Liam's case?
   - A. Anxiety Disorders
   - B. Autism Spectrum Disorder
   - C. Neurological conditions (e.g., epilepsy)
   - D. Obsessive-Compulsive Disorder
3. Which is the most appropriate initial intervention for Liam?
   - A. Habit Reversal Therapy (HRT)
   - B. Antipsychotic medication
   - C. Cognitive-Behavioral Therapy (CBT) for anxiety management
   - D. Observation and reassurance

Answers

Multiple-Choice Questions

1. B
2. C
3. B
4. C
5. B
6. B
7. B

True/False Questions

1. True
2. False
3. True
4. False
5. True
6. True
7. False
8. False
9. True
10. False

Matching Exercise

1. D
2. E
3. B
4. C
5. F
6. A

Case Study Answers and Explanations

1. C – Explanation: Provisional Tic Disorder requires tics lasting under 1 year, typically without any prolonged tic-free period exceeding 3 consecutive months.
2. C – Explanation: It is important to rule out neurological conditions (e.g., epilepsy) that could mimic tic-like movements.
3. D – Explanation: Since Liam's symptoms are mild and relatively brief, an initial approach of observation and reassurance is typically appropriate, especially if symptoms are mild and the child is otherwise functioning well.

Other Neurodevelopmental Disorders

Multiple-Choice Questions

1. Which of the following scenarios would justify using the diagnosis "Other Specified Neurodevelopmental Disorder"?
    - A. When symptoms are fully explained by a sensory deficit
    - B. When there are signs of a neurodevelopmental disorder but not all criteria are met for a specific category, and the clinician wants to specify the reason
    - C. When the child has no symptoms at all
    - D. When an anxiety disorder must necessarily be present
2. In the DSM-5, "Unspecified Neurodevelopmental Disorder" is used when:
    - A. The criteria for a Neurodevelopmental Disorder are clear, but the exact diagnosis is intentionally withheld
    - B. There is insufficient information to provide a more detailed description, but symptoms clearly fall within the neurodevelopmental domain
    - C. Symptoms appear only alongside other medical conditions
    - D. The patient has a psychotic disorder
3. Which of the following examples might call for an "Other Specified" diagnosis within the Neurodevelopmental Disorders?
    - A. A child with motor delays and some language difficulties, yet not fully meeting criteria for either Developmental Coordination Disorder or a Communication Disorder
    - B. An adolescent with marked attention deficits, already diagnosed with ADHD
    - C. A child with severe cognitive delay due to Down Syndrome, already diagnosed with Intellectual Disability
    - D. An individual without any evident academic or social difficulties
4. Which assessment is **most** important to distinguish "Other Specified Neurodevelopmental Disorder" from a more specific diagnosis?
    - A. Basic vision and hearing tests
    - B. Cognitive evaluation, developmental assessment, and examination of communicative, motor, and relational skills
    - C. A single observation at school
    - D. A simple parent-administered questionnaire
5. In which scenario would it be **least** appropriate to use the "Unspecified" category?
    - A. In an emergency room setting where time is limited, but neurodevelopmental problems are suspected
    - B. In a situation where the full criteria for Autism Spectrum Disorder are clearly met
    - C. During an initial screening, before all evaluations have been completed
    - D. If the clinician needs to indicate a neurodevelopmental issue but lacks enough information for a more precise diagnosis
6. Which statement correctly describes the use of "Other Specified" and "Unspecified" diagnoses?
    - A. They are definitive diagnoses that require no further evaluation
    - B. They allow one to avoid any structured diagnostic assessment
    - C. They indicate that the clinical presentation does not fully match any specific disorder but still requires clinical attention
    - D. They always imply a severe and irreversible psychiatric condition

True/False Questions

		T	F
1	"Other Specified" and "Unspecified" are used when criteria are not fully met.		
2	Other Specified Neurodevelopmental Disorder implies no neurodevelopmental issue.		
3	Unspecified is used when a clinician lacks enough information for a specific diagnosis.		
4	These categories still allow interventions or school support recommendations.		
5	Once "Other Specified" is given, there's no need to revisit the case.		
6	These categories help prevent underestimating genuine neurodevelopmental issues.		
7	"Unspecified" means the clinician doesn't wish to disclose the diagnosis.		
8	"Unspecified" is useful for urgent diagnosis when detailed information is lacking.		
9	"Other Specified" includes a description of why full criteria aren't met.		
10	These categories provide flexibility in complex cases.		

Matching Exercise

1. Other Specified [ ]
2. Unspecified [ ]
3. Lack of information [ ]
4. Preliminary screening [ ]
5. Need for further investigation [ ]
6. Suspected comorbidity [ ]

Descriptions:

- A. Used when the clinician has incomplete information but finds signs of a neurodevelopmental disorder.
- B. Indicates that the patient shows symptoms within the Neurodevelopmental Disorders domain but does not fully meet any specific set of criteria, and the clinician specifies why.
- C. A temporary label used while awaiting more extensive evaluation, when signs point to a Neurodevelopmental Disorder but data remain insufficient.
- D. An initial process for identifying potential difficulties; if concerns arise, further testing is carried out.
- E. A situation where more than one disorder is suspected (e.g., mild language difficulties + possible attentional issues) without a clear, definitive picture.
- F. Recognition that targeted diagnostic tests are needed to clarify the clinical picture.

Case Study

Mia, a 6-year-old girl, has been referred by her teacher due to several concerns: she takes longer than average to begin speaking in class and appears inattentive during assignments. She also shows awkward fine motor skills (e.g., cutting with scissors, coloring), but not to a degree that meets criteria for Developmental Coordination Disorder. There are no tics or stereotypic behaviors. The teacher reports that Mia is sociable with classmates but appears to learn more slowly across various areas. According to her parents, there are no noteworthy medical or neurological issues, and cognitively she appears to be developing normally, although no formal testing has been done yet.

1. Why might Mia's mild motor and attention issues be classified as an "Other Specified Neurodevelopmental Disorder"?
    - A. She has a specific, isolated academic deficit
    - B. She meets the full DSM-5 criteria for Autism Spectrum Disorder
    - C. She shows mild but noticeable issues that don't fully match a single neurodevelopmental disorder
    - D. She exhibits tics that started before age 5
2. Which factor should be clarified before confirming the diagnosis?
    - A. The presence of an anxiety disorder that might explain her slow pace
    - B. A possible hearing impairment that could account for her inattentiveness
    - C. Whether Mia already has a family history of Psychotic Disorder
    - D. Her actual IQ, along with standardized assessments of language and motor skills
3. What is the most appropriate initial intervention for Mia?
    - A. No intervention: wait for full neurological maturity
    - B. Anxiolytic medication to improve her attention
    - C. Further diagnostic workup (neuropsychological, speech therapy) and appropriate school support for her current needs
    - D. Immediate withdrawal from school and homeschooling

Answers

Multiple-Choice Questions

1. B
2. B
3. A
4. B
5. B
6. C
7. B

True/False Questions

1. True
2. False
3. True
4. True
5. False
6. True
7. False
8. True
9. False
10. True

Matching Exercise

1. B
2. A
3. C
4. D
5. F
6. E

Case Study Answers and Explanations

1. C – Explanation: Mia shows mild motor and attentional difficulties that do not clearly meet criteria for a single neurodevelopmental disorder, suggesting the "Other Specified" category.
2. D – Explanation: Before assigning an "Other Specified" diagnosis, it is crucial to assess her cognitive functioning and language/motor skills through standardized tests to rule out more specific disorders.
3. C – Explanation: A thorough diagnostic evaluation (e.g., neuropsychological assessment, possible speech therapy referral) plus classroom support tailored to her current challenges is recommended, rather than waiting for spontaneous resolution.

Schizophrenia Spectrum and Other Psychotic Disorders

This category includes disorders marked by psychotic symptoms such as delusions, hallucinations, disorganized thinking, and unusual or bizarre behavior. While there are certain shared features, each disorder has unique aspects related to duration, onset, the prevailing symptoms, and its overall trajectory.

Schizophrenia, for instance, often follows a long-term pattern, with acute episodes during which symptoms become more intense and possible periods of remission or stabilization. Delusions may take various forms—persecutory, referential, grandiose, or somatic—whereas hallucinations typically involve voices that comment on or converse with each other. Disorganized thinking can appear in speech that's hard to follow, abrupt transitions between topics, and at times, behavior lacking coherence. Slowed motor function, reduced emotional expression, and withdrawal from social interactions can also occur, severely affecting overall quality of life and personal relationships.

Within this spectrum, Schizophreniform Disorder presents a clinical picture similar to Schizophrenia, though it tends to last less than six months. Brief Psychotic Disorder usually spans just a few weeks and often emerges in response to highly stressful events, with recovery possible if addressed promptly. Delusional Disorder features false yet relatively organized beliefs (for example, unfounded jealousy or a conviction of being persecuted), which typically do not profoundly undermine everyday functioning, unlike Schizophrenia.

Other conditions include Schizoaffective Disorder, where psychotic symptoms coincide with mood disturbances (depression, mania, or both), as well as Substance/Medication-Induced Psychotic Disorder and psychoses stemming from medical conditions. These require thorough evaluation to rule out substance use or an underlying physical illness. Catatonia, characterized by extreme motor disturbances—from severe immobility to agitation—also appears in this section and may accompany psychotic or mood disorders.

A comprehensive diagnostic process is crucial, not only to exclude neurological, endocrine, or substance-related causes but also to assess cultural and environmental contexts. What may seem "odd" to an external observer could be acceptable within the individual's cultural setting. Clinicians must consider both how long the symptoms have persisted and how they fit into a patient's broader life circumstances.

Therapy often involves antipsychotic medications alongside psychosocial interventions, including cognitive-behavioral approaches, family support, and rehabilitation programs. Early intervention can alter the course of the disorder, reducing the long-term impact on functioning. While some individuals respond well to treatment and achieve or maintain a stable level of functioning, others may need ongoing support. In any case, a detailed understanding of the presenting symptoms helps guide treatment decisions and tailor support measures appropriately.

Schizotypal Personality Disorder

Multiple-Choice Questions

1. Which of the following best describes Schizotypal Personality Disorder according to the DSM-5?
    - A. Intense emotional displays and a constant need for company
    - B. Eccentric behavior, magical or peculiar beliefs, and excessive social anxiety
    - C. Rigid perfectionism and fear of making mistakes
    - D. A tendency toward pathological lying and deceit
2. Which of the following symptoms is most typical of someone with Schizotypal Personality Disorder?
    - A. Recurrent auditory hallucinations of a religious nature
    - B. Marked impulsivity and self-destructive behaviors
    - C. Social difficulties arising from magical thinking and paranoid ideation
    - D. Mood fluctuations, with periods of euphoria followed by depressive episodes
3. How does social anxiety typically manifest in Schizotypal Personality Disorder?
    - A. It occurs only in large public gatherings
    - B. It is linked to visual hallucinations in social contexts
    - C. It is pervasive and mainly driven by paranoid or referential thoughts, rather than simple shyness
    - D. It is exclusively related to fear of work-related judgment
4. Which of the following statements is not correct about Schizotypal Personality Disorder?
    - A. Eccentric beliefs and behaviors are present from early adulthood
    - B. There is a strong tendency toward social isolation and difficulty forming close relationships
    - C. Individuals with Schizotypal Personality Disorder typically have no awareness of their eccentricity
    - D. Magical or superstitious thinking can significantly influence daily life
5. A person with Schizotypal Personality Disorder may exhibit:
    - A. Well-structured persecutory delusions
    - B. Odd sensory perceptions or bodily illusions that do not reach full psychosis
    - C. Multiple auditory hallucinations featuring commenting voices
    - D. Complete apathy and reduced emotional expression without any eccentric beliefs
6. In Schizotypal Personality Disorder, magical thinking refers to:
    - A. Childlike fantasies about imaginary creatures
    - B. Strict logical rules based on science and rationality
    - C. Beliefs or perceptions that link events through superstitious or irrational means, influencing behavior
    - D. Grandiose delusions in which the individual feels omnipotent
7. Which intervention is generally most appropriate for managing Schizotypal Personality Disorder?
    - A. Pharmacotherapy only
    - B. Long-term individual psychotherapy focusing on social skills, addressing paranoid thoughts, and reducing isolation
    - C. Electroconvulsive therapy (ECT) as a first-line treatment
    - D. Confinement in a long-term inpatient setting without external contact

True/False Questions

		T	F
1	A key feature of Schizotypal Personality Disorder is paranoid ideation and bizarre beliefs.		
2	Individuals with Schizotypal Personality Disorder never exhibit psychotic symptoms, not even briefly.		
3	Relationship difficulties often stem from pervasive social anxiety and distorted perceptions of others' intentions.		
4	Schizotypal Personality Disorder can evolve into Schizophrenia in some cases.		
5	The onset of Schizotypal Personality Disorder typically occurs after age 40.		
6	Magical thinking can include superstitions, telepathy, or a "sixth sense," experienced as entirely real by the individual.		
7	Social anxiety in Schizotypal Personality Disorder is often more driven by ideas of reference or paranoia than by straightforward shyness.		
8	There are no effective treatments, as this disorder is invariably resistant to any intervention.		
9	Emotional expression in these individuals can appear inappropriate or constricted.		
10	Long-term psychotherapy focusing on reality testing and interpersonal relationships can be beneficial in some cases.		

Matching Exercise

1. Magical thinking [ ]
2. Social anxiety in Schizotypal Personality Disorder [ ]
3. Ideas of reference [ ]
4. Eccentric behaviors [ ]
5. Awareness of oddity [ ]
6. Supportive psychotherapy [ ]

Descriptions:

- A. A tendency to interpret random external events as specifically referring to oneself, without a solid basis.
- B. Engaging in rituals or wearing unusual attire and mannerisms perceived as odd by observers.
- C. Beliefs or perceptions that link events in superstitious or irrational ways, affecting behavior.
- D. Often accompanied by suspicion or paranoia, rather than mere shyness or overt social judgment.
- E. The individual may be unaware of the eccentric nature of their thoughts or habits, or may view them as normal or even superior.
- F. A long-term approach that can include social skills training and addressing paranoid symptoms.

Case Study

Paige, a 25-year-old who lives alone and works part-time in a metaphysical supply store, often speaks about "subtle" perceptions and believes she can influence events through personal rituals. She interprets certain phrases heard on the radio as hidden messages directed at her and spends considerable time pondering the "true meaning" behind these perceived signals. She has no close friends and reports feeling uneasy in social settings, fearing that others may judge or manipulate her. Affectively, she appears detached, and her emotional reactions sometimes seem out of place given the context. She has not experienced full-blown psychotic episodes, nor do there appear to be signs of other major psychiatric disorders.

1. Which aspect indicates that Paige's eccentric ideas and social unease suggest a personality issue rather than a fully psychotic disorder?
   - A. She frequently experiences full-blown delusions with zero insight
   - B. Her beliefs are odd, yet she remains in touch with reality and has not shown prolonged psychosis
   - C. She displays catatonic behaviors and severe disorganization
   - D. She reports daily auditory hallucinations that guide her actions
2. Which factor is important to rule out before confirming Schizotypal Personality Disorder?
   - A. Severe cognitive decline after age 60
   - B. Major Depressive Disorder with psychotic features
   - C. Ongoing Schizophreniform Disorder with genuine psychotic episodes
   - D. Obsessive-Compulsive Disorder, with clearly ego-dystonic rituals
3. Which intervention would be most appropriate for Paige?
   - A. Immediate electroconvulsive therapy (ECT)
   - B. Ongoing individual therapy focusing on social skills and managing paranoid or referential thinking
   - C. No intervention, since personality disorders are unchangeable
   - D. High-intensity group therapy designed for psychotic patients

Answers

Multiple-Choice Questions

1. B
2. C
3. C
4. C
5. B
6. C
7. B

True/False Questions

1. True
2. False
3. True
4. True
5. False
6. True
7. True
8. False
9. True
10. True

Matching Exercise

1. C
2. D
3. A
4. B
5. E
6. F

Case Study Answers and Explanations

1. C – Although her thinking is peculiar, Paige remains essentially in touch with reality, pointing more toward a personality-based disorder rather than a true psychotic condition.
2. C – It's essential to rule out Schizophreniform Disorder or other conditions involving genuine hallucinations/delusions.
3. B – Long-term supportive psychotherapy, including social skills training and addressing paranoid ideation, is often helpful for this disorder.

Delusional Disorder

Multiple-Choice Questions

1. Which of the following best describes Delusional Disorder according to the DSM-5?
    - A. The presence of bizarre delusions of brief duration, accompanied by prominent hallucinations
    - B. Non-bizarre delusions (plausible real-life situations) persisting for at least 1 month, in the absence of other prominent psychotic symptoms
    - C. Exclusively multiple auditory hallucinations involving voices commenting
    - D. Severe impairment in social and occupational functioning, dominated by psychotic symptoms of a catatonic nature
2. Which of the following **is not** a commonly described subtype of Delusional Disorder?
    - A. Erotomanic
    - B. Paranoid-systemic with multiple hallucinations
    - C. Jealous (delusion of infidelity)
    - D. Somatic
3. In an erotomanic subtype of Delusional Disorder, the person:
    - A. Firmly believes they are being followed by supernatural entities
    - B. Is convinced that someone, often of higher status, is in love with them
    - C. Has delusions of guilt or having committed an unforgivable sin
    - D. Has an irrational fear of contracting illnesses
4. Which of the following elements most clearly distinguishes Delusional Disorder from Schizophrenia?
    - A. Catatonic symptoms are never present in Delusional Disorder
    - B. Delusional Disorder only occurs after age 60
    - C. Absence of prominent psychotic symptoms (such as marked hallucinations or severe disorganization) aside from the delusion itself
    - D. The person can never differentiate their delusion from reality under any circumstances
5. Which aspect of social functioning is often observed in Delusional Disorder?
    - A. Profoundly deteriorated functioning and complete isolation
    - B. Generally adequate social contacts except in areas affected by the delusion
    - C. Total inability to perform any kind of occupational activity
    - D. Frequent substance use as the main issue
6. Which of the following examples could suggest a somatic subtype of Delusional Disorder?
    - A. A belief of having an unbearable body odor not detected by others
    - B. A delusion of being at the center of an international government conspiracy
    - C. A delusion of being dead and decaying (Cotard Syndrome)
    - D. A grandiose delusion of possessing magical powers
7. Which of the following approaches is generally most recommended for treating Delusional Disorder?
    - A. Prescribing high doses of anxiolytics without other interventions
    - B. Supportive psychotherapy, sometimes combined with antipsychotic medication, taking care not to directly undermine the delusion
    - C. Electroconvulsive therapy (ECT) as a first-line treatment
    - D. Long-term inpatient isolation in a psychiatric facility

True/False Questions

		T	F
1	Delusional Disorder is characterized by non-bizarre delusions lasting at least 1 month.		
2	Individuals with Delusional Disorder always present multiple auditory hallucinations.		
3	The somatic subtype involves an unfounded belief regarding one's body or state of health.		
4	Outside the delusional theme, functioning in Delusional Disorder can remain relatively intact.		
5	Delusions in Delusional Disorder are often so bizarre that they are clearly implausible.		
6	The erotomanic subtype is defined by the belief of being loved by someone often of higher or otherwise inaccessible status.		
7	Typical onset of Delusional Disorder is between ages 15 and 20.		
8	People with Delusional Disorder rarely exhibit marked disorganization in their behavior.		
9	The jealousy subtype is characterized by the unfounded conviction that one's partner is unfaithful.		
10	While antipsychotic medication can be helpful, supportive therapy is often needed to improve the therapeutic relationship.		

Matching Exercise

1. Erotomanic subtype [ ]
2. Jealous subtype [ ]
3. Somatic subtype [ ]
4. Non-bizarre delusions [ ]
5. Minimal functional impairment [ ]
6. Supportive psychotherapy [ ]

Descriptions:

- A. The delusion involves having a physical illness or bodily defect (e.g., an unbearable odor, parasites).
- B. The belief of being loved by someone who is often inaccessible, of higher status, or famous.
- C. An unfounded conviction that one's partner is being unfaithful.
- D. Delusions about realistic situations (e.g., being followed, poisoned, or deceived).
- E. The individual maintains adequate social and occupational functioning except in areas touched by the delusion.
- F. An approach that helps build trust, contain anxiety, and address relational issues linked to the delusion.

Case Study

Megan, a 40-year-old who lives alone and works as a government office clerk, has spent about 6 months firmly believing that a former colleague has installed microphones in her apartment to extract work-related secrets. Despite lacking any concrete evidence and receiving reassurances from her employer, she remains certain she's under surveillance. She has changed the locks multiple times and avoids having visitors at home. Outside of this belief, Megan maintains a relatively normal life: she goes to work, manages her finances, and keeps up with a few concerned friends who note no other unusual behavior. No sensory disturbances or additional psychotic symptoms are evident beyond this persecutory delusion.

1. Which feature of Megan's belief best aligns with Delusional Disorder rather than a fully psychotic condition like Schizophrenia?
    - A. She has bizarre delusions involving supernatural entities
    - B. She maintains adequate functioning outside the delusional theme, without major hallucinations or disorganization
    - C. She has repeated auditory hallucinations with multiple voices
    - D. She experiences catatonia and severe social withdrawal
2. Which factor is crucial to rule out before confirming Delusional Disorder?
    - A. Comorbidity with an Anxiety Disorder
    - B. The presence of a real corporate surveillance system
    - C. Signs of severe disorganization or prolonged hallucinations
    - D. A longstanding intellectual impairment
3. What is the most appropriate initial intervention for Megan?
    - A. High doses of anxiolytics to eliminate her anxiety
    - B. Supportive psychotherapy and assessment for potential antipsychotic use, ensuring a trusting therapeutic relationship
    - C. Placing her in a closed psychiatric ward for isolation
    - D. Taking no action and waiting for the delusion to resolve spontaneously

Answers

Multiple-Choice Questions

1. B
2. B
3. B
4. C
5. B
6. A
7. B

True/False Questions

1. True
2. False
3. True
4. True
5. False
6. True
7. False
8. True
9. True
10. True

Matching Exercise

1. B
2. C
3. A
4. D
5. E
6. F

Case Study Answers and Explanations

1. B – Delusional Disorder typically involves a non-bizarre delusion with relatively preserved functioning and no prominent hallucinations or disorganized behavior.
2. C – It's important to rule out Schizophrenia (or other more severe psychotic forms) by confirming the absence of pronounced hallucinations, disorganization, or significant negative symptoms.
3. B – An initial recommended approach is supportive psychotherapy, along with assessing the potential use of antipsychotics. Building therapeutic rapport is essential, avoiding direct confrontation that could be counterproductive.

Brief Psychotic Disorder

Multiple-Choice Questions

1. Which of the following best describes Brief Psychotic Disorder according to the DSM-5?
    - A. Psychotic symptoms (delusions, hallucinations, disorganized thinking) lasting under 1 day
    - B. Intermittent psychotic episodes persisting for over 6 months
    - C. A sudden onset of at least one psychotic symptom, lasting a minimum of 1 day and no more than 1 month, followed by a return to normal functioning
    - D. Gradual cognitive deterioration and a progressive appearance of psychotic deficits
2. Which of the following is a **possible** trigger for Brief Psychotic Disorder?
    - A. Long-term absence of depressive symptoms
    - B. A trauma or major stressful event (e.g., bereavement, natural disasters)
    - C. A common cold causing a mild fever
    - D. Continuous use of low-dose antidepressants
3. In Brief Psychotic Disorder, an individual's functioning:
    - A. Remains severely impaired for at least 6 months following symptom resolution
    - B. Returns to its previous level once symptoms remit, barring other complications
    - C. Never improves, resulting in permanent disability
    - D. Was already severely compromised long before symptom onset
4. Which of the following symptoms may be part of a Brief Psychotic Disorder diagnosis?
    - A. Delusions or hallucinations
    - B. Elimination disorders
    - C. Specific phobias lasting at least 2 years
    - D. Complete lack of insight and contact with reality for more than 6 months
5. Brief Psychotic Disorder with "catatonic features" implies that:
    - A. The person is unaware they are experiencing a psychotic state
    - B. Psychotic symptoms include catatonic manifestations (immobility, mutism, rigidity, or catatonic excitement)
    - C. The person has delirium with constant fluctuations in consciousness
    - D. The individual experiences severe and irreversible cognitive deficits
6. Which of the following would not be a condition to rule out before diagnosing Brief Psychotic Disorder?
    - A. Substance use or withdrawal that could cause psychotic symptoms
    - B. Medical conditions (e.g., epilepsy, brain tumors) that could explain the symptoms
    - C. A Mood Disorder with psychotic features
    - D. Generalized Anxiety Disorder with social phobia
7. Which of the following approaches is most appropriate for the initial management of Brief Psychotic Disorder?
    - A. Electroconvulsive therapy (ECT) as a first-line treatment
    - B. Clinical monitoring, possible short-term use of antipsychotics, and supportive psychotherapy
    - C. Long-term isolation in an inpatient psychiatric setting
    - D. No intervention, since symptoms always disappear on their own

True/False Questions

		T	F
1	In Brief Psychotic Disorder, symptoms last at least 1 month and resolve without leaving any aftereffects.		
2	A single episode of auditory hallucinations, if very short, may be part of a Brief Psychotic Disorder.		
3	Brief Psychotic Disorder can be triggered by highly stressful or traumatic events.		
4	Once symptoms resolve, functioning can return to prior levels if there are no complications.		
5	The presence of prominent negative symptoms (e.g., apathy, alogia) for months is typical of Brief Psychotic Disorder.		
6	Brief Psychotic Disorder is more common in older adults and is linked to primary cognitive decline.		
7	If the psychotic presentation lasts longer than 1 month but less than 6 months, Schizophreniform Disorder should be considered.		
8	Low-dose antipsychotic medication can be helpful for acute symptom management in Brief Psychotic Disorder.		
9	Ruling out schizophrenia involves confirming no prolonged or disorganized symptoms.		
10	In some cases, supportive psychotherapy and reducing environmental stress can lead to rapid symptom remission.		

Matching Exercise

1. Duration of symptoms [ ]
2. Possible trigger [ ]
3. Post-remission functioning [ ]
4. Catatonic features [ ]
5. Need to rule out [ ]
6. Initial treatment [ ]

Descriptions:

- A. Substance use or medical conditions that could explain psychotic symptoms
- B. May return to baseline if no further episodes or complications occur
- C. At least 1 day and under 1 month, with a return to premorbid functioning
- D. Signs such as immobility, mutism, rigid posture, or catatonic agitation
- E. Stressful events, such as bereavement or sudden trauma
- F. Clinical monitoring, short-term antipsychotic medication if needed, and psychological support

Case Study

Ashley, a 22-year-old college student, has displayed unusual behavior over the past 3 days: she reports hearing her professor's voice constantly criticizing her and claims to find hidden messages in a textbook, believing the content has been "encrypted" specifically for her. Symptoms emerged after she learned she would have to retake an important exam. No longstanding mood disturbances or known medical issues have been identified. Though she appears confused, she can still communicate coherently; the symptoms revolve around the idea of being "tested" by others. Only 72 hours have passed since her psychotic symptoms began.

1. Which time-related feature most suggests that Ashley's symptoms could be classified under Brief Psychotic Disorder?
    - A. Psychotic symptoms lasting at least 6 months
    - B. Sudden onset of psychosis lasting less than 1 month
    - C. Delusions lasting for more than 1 year
    - D. Chronic auditory hallucinations from childhood
2. Which factor should be ruled out before confirming the diagnosis?
    - A. Recent use of stimulant substances that might have caused her symptoms
    - B. A long-standing disconnection from reality (exceeding 6 months)
    - C. Lack of any stressful event
    - D. The possibility that she has a higher-than-average IQ
3. Which intervention is initially recommended for Ashley?
    - A. Isolating her in an inpatient psychiatric unit for at least 6 months
    - B. Clinical monitoring, considering short-term antipsychotics if symptoms persist, and offering psychological support
    - C. Electroconvulsive therapy (ECT) as a first-line approach
    - D. No intervention, given the brief duration of her condition

Answers

Multiple-Choice Questions

1. C
2. B
3. B
4. A
5. B
6. D
7. B

True/False Questions

1. False
2. True
3. True
4. True
5. False
6. False
7. True
8. True
9. True
10. True

Matching Exercise

1. C
2. E
3. B
4. D
5. A
6. (F

Case Study Answers and Explanations

1. B – Explanation: Brief Psychotic Disorder involves a sudden onset of psychotic symptoms lasting less than 1 month, often linked to stress.
2. A – Before confirming the diagnosis, it is important to rule out substance-induced or medically induced psychotic states.
3. B – The initial approach includes clinical monitoring; if symptoms persist or worsen, a short course of antipsychotics may be indicated alongside psychological support.

Schizophreniform Disorder

Multiple Choice Questions

1. Which of the following features primarily distinguishes Schizophreniform Disorder from Schizophrenia according to the DSM-5?
   • A. The presence of bizarre delusions
   • B. The overall duration of the disorder
   • C. The absence of negative symptoms
   • D. Higher comorbidity with mood disorders
2. Compared to Brief Psychotic Disorder, Schizophreniform Disorder is mainly differentiated by:
   • A. The mandatory presence of auditory hallucinations
   • B. The fact that symptoms always resolve within 2 weeks
   • C. A duration of symptoms lasting more than 1 month but less than 6 months
   • D. The absence of depressive symptoms
3. During an episode of Schizophreniform Disorder, the patient's social and occupational functioning:
   • A. Is never compromised
   • B. Must be severely compromised for the diagnosis to be made
   • C. Is not a required diagnostic criterion, unlike in Schizophrenia
   • D. Should only be assessed if there are comorbid mood disorders
4. Which positive prognostic factor is commonly associated with Schizophreniform Disorder?
   • A. A gradual, insidious onset of symptoms
   • B. Predominant negative symptoms
   • C. Good social functioning before onset
   • D. Poor family support
5. A patient with Schizophreniform Disorder who presents significant depressive and manic symptoms throughout the active phase of the disorder suggests:
   • A. A possible diagnosis of Schizoaffective Disorder
   • B. That any psychiatric diagnosis should be ruled out
   • C. That mood symptoms do not influence the diagnosis
   • D. A complicated Brief Psychotic Disorder
6. Which duration threshold indicates a possible transition from Schizophreniform Disorder to Schizophrenia?
   • A. 1 month
   • B. 6 months
   • C. 12 months
   • D. There is no specific duration threshold, only severity criteria
7. For Schizophreniform Disorder, psychotic symptoms must be present for:
   • A. At least 1 day but less than 1 month
   • B. At least 2 weeks but less than 1 month
   • C. At least 1 month but less than 6 months
   • D. At least 6 months

True/False Questions

		T	F
1	Schizophreniform Disorder can include catatonic symptoms.		
2	If symptoms persist beyond 6 months, the diagnosis of Schizophreniform Disorder should be reconsidered.		
3	An abrupt and unannounced onset is always excluded in Schizophreniform Disorder.		
4	In Schizophreniform Disorder, social functioning impairment is a decisive diagnostic criterion.		
5	Substance-induced psychotic symptoms automatically rule out Schizophreniform Disorder.		
6	Negative symptoms can be present in Schizophreniform Disorder.		
7	Schizophreniform Disorder is considered part of the Schizophrenia Spectrum.		
8	A history of a previous Brief Psychotic Disorder does not prevent a diagnosis of Schizophreniform Disorder.		
9	Schizophreniform Disorder cannot involve delusional symptoms.		
10	A symptom duration of under 1 month is not sufficient for a Schizophreniform Disorder diagnosis.		

Matching Exercise

1. Duration ranging from 1 to 6 months [ ]
2. Psychotic symptoms present for less than 1 month [ ]
3. May progress to Schizophrenia if symptoms continue beyond 6 months [ ]
4. Presence of negative symptoms [ ]
5. Good premorbid functioning [ ]
6. Absence of mood symptoms during the active episode [ ]

Descriptions:

- A. Characteristic of Brief Psychotic Disorder
- B. Important positive prognostic factor in Schizophreniform Disorder
- C. Characteristic of Schizoaffective Disorder (the absence of mood symptoms is false for this)
- D. Can be observed in both Schizophrenia and Schizophreniform Disorder
- E. The duration range that differentiates Schizophreniform Disorder from Schizophrenia
- F. The reason why, after 6 months, the diagnosis is reconsidered as Schizophrenia

Case Study

A 20-year-old college student began experiencing psychotic symptoms (auditory hallucinations and referential thinking) approximately two months ago. During this time, his grades have slightly dropped, but he has continued attending classes and maintaining some social relationships. He has not shown clear depressive or manic episodes, although he reports a mild loss of interest in previously motivating activities. His family describes him as "always a bit introverted," though they note his behavior has worsened recently. He has a good social support system: his parents and some friends are helping him cope with the situation.

1. Which clinical factor, if well documented, might indicate a favorable prognosis for this patient?
   • A. A history of previous mood disorders
   • B. The presence of catatonia during initial episodes
   • C. Good functioning before the onset of symptoms
   • D. Lack of family support
2. If his symptoms persist continuously for longer than 6 months, which diagnostic adjustment should be considered?
   • A. Switch to Brief Psychotic Disorder
   • B. Schizoaffective Disorder
   • C. Schizophreniform Disorder with mixed features
   • D. Transition to Schizophrenia
3. Which approach would be most helpful in differentiating this clinical picture from a possible Schizoaffective Disorder?
   • A. Assessing for negative symptoms
   • B. Closely monitoring the emergence of mood symptoms during the psychotic phase
   • C. Evaluating whether his social functioning is impaired
   • D. Ordering routine blood tests

Answers

Multiple Choice Questions
1. B
2. C
3. C
4. C
5. A
6. B
7. C

True/False Questions
1. True
2. True
3. False
4. False
5. False
6. True
7. True
8. True
9. False
10. True

Matching Exercise
1. E
2. A
3. F
4. D
5. B
6. C

Case Study Answers and Explanations
1. C – Explanation: Good premorbid functioning (e.g., adequate social adjustment, academic success, and healthy relationships) is often regarded as a positive prognostic factor.
2. D – Explanation: If symptoms continue beyond 6 months, Schizophrenia—rather than Schizophreniform Disorder—should be considered.
3. B – Explanation: Schizoaffective Disorder requires concurrent mood episodes (depressive or manic) during a significant portion of the active psychotic phase. Monitoring for the emergence of mood symptoms helps distinguish the two diagnoses.

Schizophrenia

Multiple Choice Questions

1. Which of the following diagnostic criteria is key to establishing Schizophrenia according to the DSM-5?
    - A. Severe language impairment lasting at least 2 years
    - B. Active psychotic symptoms for at least 1 month and continuous signs of disturbance for at least 6 months
    - C. Exclusive presence of negative symptoms with no delusions or hallucinations
    - D. Delusional manifestations lasting less than 1 month
2. Which of the following is typically considered a negative symptom of Schizophrenia?
    - A. Persecutory delusions
    - B. Disorganized speech
    - C. Flat affect
    - D. Tactile hallucinations
3. In the etiology of Schizophrenia, which of the following factors is thought to play a major role?
    - A. Only environmental factors, such as traumatic events
    - B. A combination of genetic predisposition and environmental factors
    - C. A required history of Brief Psychotic Disorder
    - D. Exclusive comorbidity with personality disorders
4. Which option best describes the concept of a "prodromal phase" in Schizophrenia?
    - A. The period when psychotic symptoms are at their peak
    - B. A phase of gradual functional decline and subclinical symptoms
    - C. A gap in which the patient exhibits no symptoms at all
    - D. The point at which the patient has already reached remission
5. Which of the following is considered a favorable prognostic factor in patients with Schizophrenia?
    - A. Very early onset before age 12
    - B. Regular use of psychoactive substances
    - C. Strong social and family support
    - D. Only negative symptoms present
6. Which of the following statements accurately describes "disorganization" in Schizophrenia?
    - A. Presence of mood symptoms such as mania or depression
    - B. A break in logical thinking with unpredictable behavior
    - C. Complete absence of emotional expression
    - D. The ability to adapt normally to social demands
7. In which situation would Schizophrenia most likely be ruled out?
    - A. When symptoms are directly caused by substance use or another medical condition
    - B. When only referential thinking and extreme shyness are present
    - C. If the patient acknowledges having bizarre thoughts but still considers them plausible
    - D. If the patient shows only a mild decline in social functioning without active psychotic symptoms

True/False Questions

		T	F
1	The "maintenance" phase of Schizophrenia only occurs if positive symptoms persist.		
2	Deterioration in social or occupational functioning is a key aspect of the Schizophrenia diagnosis.		
3	Negative symptoms such as apathy and anhedonia can also appear in other disorders.		
4	First-generation antipsychotics are completely free of extrapyramidal side effects.		
5	A total duration of symptoms of 3 months, including 1 month of active phase, is not enough for a Schizophrenia diagnosis.		
6	The "prodromal phase" can precede the emergence of full-blown psychotic symptoms by months or even years.		
7	A patient must exhibit both delusions and hallucinations for a Schizophrenia diagnosis.		
8	If symptoms persist continuously for over 6 months but with periods of partial improvement, the diagnosis still remains in the Schizophrenia spectrum.		
9	Command auditory hallucinations are among the most frequent symptoms in Schizophrenia.		
10	Active symptoms lasting less than 1 month cannot be classified as Schizophrenia.		

Matching Exercise

1. Prodromal phase [ ]
2. Positive symptoms [ ]
3. Negative symptoms [ ]
4. Chronic course [ ]
5. Persecutory delusions [ ]
6. Comorbidity with substance abuse [ ]

Descriptions:

- A. Involves hallucinations, delusions, and disorganized behavior
- B. Early period of subtle symptoms and behavioral changes
- C. May include flat affect, poverty of speech, and lack of motivation
- D. Can worsen symptom severity and lead to a poorer prognosis
- E. A pervasive sense of being conspired against or threatened
- F. Characterized by repeated episodes and progressive functional decline

Case Study

A 25-year-old man has been showing disorganized behavior and bizarre delusions for about 7 months, with a gradual inability to maintain steady employment. He reports hearing voices accusing him of being untrustworthy and has suddenly withdrawn from his circle of friends. He does not describe any significant mood disturbances. During the first two months, he only experienced mild social withdrawal and unusual thoughts, but in the past five months his psychotic symptoms have intensified.

1. Which time frame criterion does this clinical situation fulfill?
    - A. Insufficient duration for a Schizophrenia diagnosis
    - B. Fits the criteria for Brief Psychotic Disorder
    - C. At least 1 month of active symptoms and a total of at least 6 months of disturbance
    - D. A maximum duration of 3 months before changing the diagnosis
2. Which feature, if present, would make a Schizoaffective diagnosis more likely than straightforward Schizophrenia?
    - A. Bizarre delusions without depressive components
    - B. A significant overlap of manic or depressive episodes with the psychotic phase
    - C. Onset at age 25, typical of Schizophrenia
    - D. A period of spontaneous remission from disorganized symptoms
3. Which psychotherapeutic intervention is commonly recommended alongside medication?
    - A. Psychoanalysis focusing solely on the unconscious
    - B. Social skills training and psychoeducational support for the patient and family
    - C. Regressive hypnosis to eliminate delusions
    - D. Therapy that focuses exclusively on anger management

Answers

Multiple Choice Questions

1. B
2. C
3. B
4. B
5. C
6. B
7. A

True/False Questions

1. False
2. True
3. True
4. False
5. True
6. True
7. False
8. True
9. True
10. True

Matching Exercise

1. B
2. A
3. C
4. F
5. E
6. D

Case Study Answers and Explanations

1. C – Explanation: Schizophrenia requires at least 1 month of active symptoms and a total duration of at least 6 months of disturbance. Here, there have been 7 months of progressive worsening.
2. B – Explanation: Schizoaffective Disorder involves mood episodes (depressive or manic) overlapping significantly with the psychotic phase.
3. B – Explanation: Social skills training and psychoeducation for both the patient and family are widely recognized as supportive interventions alongside pharmacological treatment.

Schizoaffective Disorder

Multiple Choice Questions

1. Which primary feature distinguishes Schizoaffective Disorder from Schizophrenia?
    - A. The presence of delusional symptoms without hallucinations
    - B. Frequent substance use as a triggering factor
    - C. An episode of depression or mania present during the majority of the active phase of the disorder
    - D. An overall duration of less than 6 months
2. Which of the following mood-related symptoms might be present in Schizoaffective Disorder with a bipolar component?
    - A. A slightly low mood
    - B. A full manic episode
    - C. Mild hypochondriasis
    - D. An isolated panic attack
3. What is one of the key time-related criteria for diagnosing Schizoaffective Disorder?
    - A. Psychotic symptoms that completely resolve within 1 month
    - B. Mood symptoms present only during the residual phase
    - C. Psychotic symptoms occurring in the absence of mood disturbances for at least 2 weeks
    - D. No psychotic symptoms at all when mania or depression is present
4. In Schizoaffective Disorder, mood disturbances:
    - A. Are always more severe than psychotic symptoms
    - B. Never occur during the active phase of the disorder
    - C. Occur simultaneously with psychotic symptoms for a significant period
    - D. Are always mild in severity
5. Which of the following statements is accurate regarding the prognosis of Schizoaffective Disorder?
    - A. It is always worse than that of Schizophrenia
    - B. It is generally better than Schizophrenia but worse than pure mood disorders
    - C. It is not influenced by premorbid functioning
    - D. It is always favorable if no manic episodes are present
6. Which factor most clearly differentiates Schizoaffective Disorder from Bipolar Disorder with psychotic features?
    - A. Psychotic symptoms occur only during manic phases
    - B. Psychotic symptoms occur even outside mood episodes
    - C. No negative symptoms are ever present
    - D. Antipsychotic medications are used as part of the treatment
7. Which treatment strategy is most commonly indicated for Schizoaffective Disorder?
    - A. Psychotherapy alone, without medication
    - B. Combined use of antipsychotics and mood stabilizers
    - C. Intervention only in psychiatric emergencies
    - D. Electroconvulsive therapy as a first-line approach

True/False Questions

		T	F
1	In Schizoaffective Disorder, psychotic symptoms can appear even in the absence of mood disturbances.		
2	If mood symptoms are present for only a very brief period, you can still diagnose Schizoaffective Disorder.		
3	The minimum duration required to diagnose Schizoaffective Disorder is 2 years.		
4	A patient with Schizoaffective Disorder can present manic, depressive, or both types of episodes.		
5	Negative symptoms never occur in Schizoaffective Disorder.		
6	The presence of a single manic episode rules out Schizoaffective Disorder.		
7	Schizoaffective Disorder is included in the Schizophrenia Spectrum in the DSM-5.		
8	Good premorbid functioning can positively affect the prognosis of Schizoaffective Disorder.		
9	During remission periods, there may be no psychotic symptoms or mood disturbances.		
10	Treatment can involve both medication and psychotherapeutic interventions.		

Matching Exercise

1. Manic episode [ ]
2. Mood disturbances [ ]
3. Psychotic symptoms in the absence of altered mood [ ]
4. Mood stabilizers [ ]
5. Depressive component [ ]
6. Intermediate prognosis [ ]

Descriptions:

- A. One of the fundamental criteria for differentiating Schizoaffective Disorder from Schizophrenia
- B. A phase marked by elevated mood, increased energy, and sometimes psychotic symptoms
- C. Used in Schizoaffective Disorder to manage mood fluctuations
- D. Allows us to distinguish Schizoaffective Disorder from Brief Psychotic Disorders
- E. Typically includes marked sadness, anhedonia, and feelings of guilt
- F. Better than that of Schizophrenia but not as good as pure mood disorders

Case Study

A 30-year-old man is brought in for psychiatric evaluation because, for about 6 months, he has reported "hearing voices" and has experienced periods of euphoria, increased energy, and reduced need for sleep. In the last few weeks, however, he has shown a marked decrease in mood, yet continues to experience paranoid thoughts and auditory hallucinations. He has never had an extended period without any psychotic symptoms. His family notes that before these episodes, he held a steady job and had an active social life.

1. Which factor most strongly supports a diagnosis of Schizoaffective Disorder rather than Bipolar Disorder with psychotic features?
   - A. Shifts between euphoric phases and low mood
   - B. Hearing voices even when his mood is not markedly altered
   - C. Complete absence of symptoms once the manic episode ends
   - D. A brief overall duration of symptoms
2. Which element might be considered a favorable prognostic factor?
   - A. A later onset after age 45
   - B. Adequate premorbid functioning and a good support network
   - C. Comorbidity with severe anxiety disorders
   - D. The exclusive presence of negative symptoms
3. Which combination of medications is most frequently used for Schizoaffective Disorder?
   - A. Antidepressants combined with hypnotics
   - B. Antipsychotics combined with mood stabilizers
   - C. Only benzodiazepine sedatives
   - D. Long-term anticholinergics

Answers

Multiple Choice Questions

1. C
2. B
3. C
4. C
5. B
6. B
7. B

True/False Questions

1. True
2. False
3. False
4. True
5. False
6. False
7. True
8. True
9. True
10. True

Matching Exercise

1. B
2. D
3. A
4. C
5. E
6. F

Case Study Answers and Explanations

1. B – Explanation: In Schizoaffective Disorder, psychotic symptoms can persist even when mood disturbances are not pronounced, which differentiates it from Bipolar Disorder with psychotic features.
2. B – Explanation: Good functioning prior to the onset of the disorder and strong family support are considered positive prognostic factors.
3. B – Explanation: A combination of antipsychotics and mood stabilizers is commonly used to manage both the psychotic and mood components of Schizoaffective Disorder.

Substance/Medication-Induced Psychotic Disorder

Multiple Choice Questions

1. Which of the following is a key indicator that distinguishes a Substance/Medication-Induced Psychotic Disorder from other psychotic disorders?
   - A. The presence of exclusively visual hallucinations
   - B. The emergence of psychotic symptoms during or immediately after substance or medication use
   - C. The absence of withdrawal symptoms
   - D. A minimum 6-month duration of symptoms
2. Which of the following conditions is most commonly associated with a Substance-Induced Psychotic Disorder?
   - A. Excessive use of analgesics without a prescription
   - B. Receiving vaccines during winter months
   - C. Chronic use of stimulant substances (e.g., cocaine, amphetamines)
   - D. Occasional intake of vitamin supplements
3. According to the DSM-5, before diagnosing a Substance/Medication-Induced Psychotic Disorder, it is necessary to:
   - A. Rule out other possible medical or psychiatric explanations
   - B. Simultaneously diagnose an anxiety disorder
   - C. Demonstrate the absence of mood symptoms
   - D. Obtain an abnormal EEG reading
4. In a Substance/Medication-Induced Psychotic Disorder, psychotic symptoms:
   - A. Must be present for at least 2 years
   - B. Typically resolve within a month after discontinuing the substance or medication, provided there are no complications
   - C. Appear only if there is a concurrent mood disorder
   - D. Are indistinguishable from those of Schizophrenia
5. Which of the following medications or medication classes is most commonly linked to the onset of psychotic symptoms if misused or taken at high doses?
   - A. Antibiotics
   - B. Corticosteroids
   - C. Beta-blockers
   - D. Antacids
6. If psychotic symptoms persist for an extended period after discontinuing the substance, which diagnosis should be considered?
   - A. Bipolar Disorder
   - B. Schizophrenia or another primary psychotic disorder
   - C. Specific Phobia
   - D. Dysthymia
7. Which of the following factors most helps differentiate a Substance/Medication-Induced Psychotic Disorder from Schizophrenia?
   - A. Age of onset
   - B. The presence of bizarre delusions
   - C. The temporal relationship between substance use and symptom onset
   - D. The absence of negative symptoms

True/False Questions

		T	F
1	In Substance/Medication-Induced Psychotic Disorder, psychotic symptoms appear only before substance use.		
2	A diagnosis of Substance/Medication-Induced Psychotic Disorder requires ruling out a general medical condition that could explain the symptoms.		
3	Amphetamine abuse can cause schizophrenia-like psychotic symptoms.		
4	If symptoms appear only after several months of abstinence, it can still be labeled Substance/Medication-Induced Psychotic Disorder.		
5	Long-term use of certain steroids can contribute to delusions or hallucinations.		
6	Alcohol intoxication is rarely associated with psychotic symptoms.		
7	Once the substance is discontinued, psychotic symptoms can never persist for more than 2 weeks.		
8	To diagnose a Substance/Medication-Induced Psychotic Disorder, there must be a clear temporal link between substance use and symptom onset.		
9	A Substance/Medication-Induced Psychotic Disorder can never involve the concurrent use of multiple substances.		
10	Excessive use of nasal decongestants containing sympathomimetic compounds can induce psychotic symptoms.		

Matching Exercise

1. Temporal relationship [ ]
2. Stimulants [ ]
3. Corticosteroids [ ]
4. Spontaneous resolution [ ]
5. Withdrawal effects [ ]
6. Medical evaluation [ ]

Descriptions:

- A. Substances that can induce delusions or hallucinations when abused, such as amphetamines
- B. It is essential to confirm that the condition is not caused by other pathologies or by a primary psychotic disorder
- C. Once intake is stopped, symptoms tend to diminish or disappear within a relatively short period
- D. The connection between substance/medication use and the onset of symptoms
- E. A class of drugs that, in high doses or prolonged use, can contribute to psychosis
- F. A possible period in which psychotic manifestations may emerge after discontinuation of the substance

Case Study

A 28-year-old man arrives at the emergency department displaying marked paranoia and reporting voices insulting him. He admits to having used methamphetamine within the past 24 hours, and his family notes that he has been abusing this substance for a few weeks. He has no previous history of psychotic episodes, and there are no indications of a chronic psychiatric disorder. The man appears agitated and suspicious of the medical staff, but does not report significant depressive or manic symptoms.

1. Which feature most strongly indicates that this is a Methamphetamine-Induced Psychotic Disorder?
    - A. The presence of a slightly depressed mood
    - B. The onset of paranoid symptoms concurrent with substance use
    - C. A history of alcohol abuse dating back to adolescence
    - D. The absence of any negative symptoms
2. If psychotic symptoms persist for more than a month after stopping methamphetamine, which alternative diagnosis becomes more likely?
    - A. Schizoaffective Disorder
    - B. Schizophrenia or another primary psychotic disorder
    - C. Generalized Anxiety Disorder
    - D. Post-Traumatic Stress Disorder
3. Among therapeutic interventions, which measure is often the first priority in Substance/Medication-Induced Psychotic Disorder?
    - A. Continuing the substance at reduced doses
    - B. Initiating a supervised detoxification/tapering program
    - C. Prescribing high-dose hypnotic sedatives without ceasing the substance
    - D. Avoiding any form of pharmacological treatment

Answers

Multiple Choice Questions

1. B
2. C
3. A
4. B
5. B
6. B
7. C

True/False Questions

1. False
2. True
3. True
4. False
5. True
6. False
7. False
8. True
9. False
10. True

Matching Exercise

1. D
2. A
3. E
4. C
5. F
6. B

Case Study Answers and Explanations

1. B – Explanation: The temporal link between methamphetamine use and the onset of psychotic symptoms is a key indicator of a Substance-Induced Psychotic Disorder.
2. B – Explanation: If psychotic symptoms continue well after discontinuation, a primary psychotic disorder becomes a more likely consideration.
3. B – Explanation: In a Substance/Medication-Induced Psychotic Disorder, stopping or gradually reducing the substance and initiating a detox program are often the first crucial steps.

Psychotic Disorder Due to Another Medical Condition

Multiple Choice Questions

1. Which element is essential to diagnose a Psychotic Disorder Due to Another Medical Condition?
    - A. Psychotic symptoms of brief duration (less than 1 month)
    - B. Evidence that a direct pathophysiological mechanism of the medical condition is associated with the onset of psychotic symptoms
    - C. Co-occurrence of a Mood Disorder with psychotic features
    - D. Significantly impaired premorbid functioning
2. Which of the following medical conditions is more likely to provoke psychotic symptoms when associated with certain physiological changes?
    - A. Essential hypertension
    - B. Mild hypothyroidism
    - C. Brain tumors or lesions
    - D. Atopic dermatitis
3. To distinguish a Psychotic Disorder Due to Another Medical Condition from a primary psychotic disorder (e.g., Schizophrenia), it is crucial to:
    - A. Verify that hallucinations are primarily visual
    - B. Check if psychotic symptoms disappear without pharmacological treatment
    - C. Establish a direct causal link between the medical condition and the symptoms
    - D. Administer projective personality tests
4. If psychotic symptoms persist despite effective treatment of the underlying medical condition, which alternative diagnosis becomes plausible?
    - A. Bipolar Disorder with Psychotic Features
    - B. Schizophrenia or another primary psychotic disorder
    - C. Hoarding Disorder with ideas of reference
    - D. Factitious Disorder with psychotic symptoms
5. Which of the following examples might suggest the presence of a Psychotic Disorder Due to Another Medical Condition?
    - A. A patient suspected of stimulant substance abuse
    - B. A patient experiencing intermittent tactile hallucinations during REM sleep
    - C. A patient with a history of temporal lobe epilepsy who suddenly develops delusional episodes
    - D. An adolescent with brief paranoia following stressful events
6. Which of the following statements best describes the temporal relationship between psychotic symptoms and the medical condition?
    - A. Psychotic symptoms begin months after the illness first appears and show no correlation with its course
    - B. Psychotic symptoms emerge at the onset of the medical condition and improve when it is treated
    - C. Psychotic symptoms only occur in response to emotional stress
    - D. The medical condition and the psychotic symptoms are entirely independent
7. A defining feature that distinguishes Psychotic Disorder Due to Another Medical Condition from a Substance-Induced Psychotic Disorder is:
    - A. The absence of demonstrable organic factors
    - B. The lack of any hallucinatory symptoms
    - C. A physiological origin directly tied to a medical problem rather than substance use
    - D. The presence of pronounced negative symptoms

True/False Questions

		T	F
1	In Psychotic Disorder Due to Another Medical Condition, substance use is never involved.		
2	A clear physiological link between the medical pathology and the psychotic symptoms must be demonstrated.		
3	Neurological conditions such as brain tumors or epilepsy can cause psychotic symptoms.		
4	The presence of catatonic symptoms automatically rules out Psychotic Disorder Due to Another Medical Condition.		
5	If psychotic symptoms do not improve after treating the medical condition, a primary psychotic disorder may be suspected.		
6	Finding a hormonal abnormality alone is sufficient to diagnose a Psychotic Disorder Due to Another Medical Condition.		
7	Both delusions and hallucinations may be present.		
8	The onset of psychotic symptoms must coincide with or immediately follow a worsening of the medical condition.		
9	Advanced-stage thyroid disorders can, in some cases, trigger psychotic symptoms.		
10	Psychotic Disorder Due to Another Medical Condition is classified within the schizophrenia spectrum.		

Matching Exercise

1. Direct causal link [ ]
2. Primarily visual hallucinations [ ]
3. Brain tumor [ ]
4. Symptom persistence [ ]
5. Effective treatment of the condition [ ]
6. Absence of psychosocial triggers [ ]

Descriptions:

- A. A classic example of a medical condition that can give rise to a psychotic presentation
- B. In some neurological conditions, one sensory modality may predominate for hallucinations
- C. Psychotic symptoms do not resolve even though the underlying organic illness is adequately controlled
- D. Indicates that the psychotic symptoms stem from the pathophysiological mechanisms of a specific disease
- E. In certain cases, also resolves related psychotic symptoms, if they are dependent on the organic problem
- F. Helps rule out that the psychosis is purely due to psychological stress or trauma

Case Study

A 60-year-old woman with a recent diagnosis of a brain tumor begins experiencing paranoid delusions and auditory hallucinations. These symptoms appear following an increase in tumor size, as evidenced by an MRI. She has never had prior psychotic episodes and exhibits no signs of depression or mania. After surgery significantly reduces the tumor, her symptoms diminish considerably.

1. Which clinical aspect most strongly indicates a Psychotic Disorder Due to Another Medical Condition?
   - A. The patient does not exhibit catatonic symptoms
   - B. The onset of symptoms correlates temporally with the worsening of the tumor
   - C. The patient reports ideas of reference and has never used substances
   - D. Hallucinations are auditory, not visual
2. If, after reducing the tumor mass, the symptoms remained unchanged, which hypothesis would gain more credibility?
   - A. Brief Psychotic Disorder
   - B. Schizoaffective Disorder
   - C. A primary Psychotic Disorder (e.g., Schizophrenia)
   - D. Paranoid Personality Disorder
3. Which intervention is often considered a priority in treating Psychotic Disorder Due to Another Medical Condition?
   - A. Intensive psychotherapy without addressing the medical issue
   - B. Medical or surgical treatment aimed at correcting or reducing the underlying condition
   - C. Only prescribing antipsychotics
   - D. Offering reassurance that the symptoms are "imaginary"

Answers

Multiple Choice Questions
1. B
2. C
3. C
4. B
5. C
6. B
7. C

True/False Questions
1. False
2. True
3. True
4. False
5. True
6. False
7. True
8. True
9. True
10. False

Matching Exercise
1. D
2. B
3. A
4. C
5. E
6. (F

Case Study Answers and Explanations
1. B – Explanation: The temporal relationship between the worsening of a brain tumor and the onset of psychotic symptoms is a hallmark of Psychotic Disorder Due to Another Medical Condition.
2. C – Explanation: If symptoms did not improve after treating the tumor, a primary psychotic disorder would then be considered.
3. B – Explanation: In Psychotic Disorder Due to Another Medical Condition, addressing the organic cause first (e.g., removing or reducing a brain lesion) is crucial, as this may alleviate or resolve the psychotic symptoms.

Catatonia

Multiple Choice Questions

1. Which of the following is a characteristic sign of catatonia?
   - A. Euphoric mood
   - B. A marked reduction in motor activity or passive resistance to movement
   - C. Fluent, confident speech
   - D. Episodes of selective amnesia
2. According to the DSM-5, which of the following catatonia subtypes is recognized?
   - A. Catatonia associated with Depressive Disorders
   - B. Catatonia exclusively in the context of Paranoid Schizophrenia
   - C. Catatonia occurring only during sleep
   - D. Catatonia associated with Panic Disorder
3. What is the primary feature of "catatonic mutism"?
   - A. Rapid, disorganized speech
   - B. Constant repetition of someone else's words (echolalia)
   - C. Complete (or drastically reduced) lack of verbalization despite being physically able to speak
   - D. Substituting words with invented terms
4. In catatonic presentations, the phenomenon of "fixed posture" (catalepsy) can occur. What does this involve?
   - A. Inability to maintain any position, leading to immediate collapse
   - B. A tendency to hold rigid, often uncomfortable postures for long periods, without reacting
   - C. Frenetic, uncoordinated movement of arms and legs
   - D. Partial immobility only during sleep
5. Which of the following is frequently observed in excited catatonia?
   - A. Absence of any agitation
   - B. Repetitive stereotyped movements and intense psychomotor agitation
   - C. Active cooperation with environmental demands
   - D. A consistently euphoric mood
6. Which pharmacological treatment is often considered among the first-line interventions to relieve catatonic symptoms?
   - A. High-dose beta-blockers
   - B. Benzodiazepines (e.g., lorazepam)
   - C. Broad-spectrum antibiotics
   - D. Tricyclic antidepressants
7. If catatonia does not respond to standard pharmacological treatments, which therapeutic approach may be considered?
   - A. Regressive hypnosis
   - B. Electroconvulsive therapy (ECT)
   - C. Herbal remedies and muscle-relaxing massages
   - D. Supportive psychotherapy only

True/False Questions

		T	F
1	Catatonia can occur in both psychotic and mood disorder contexts.		
2	Echolalia is the imitation of someone else's movements, not their words.		
3	Catalepsy involves maintaining fixed postures for an extended period.		
4	In catatonia, mutism is always due to a physical injury of the vocal cords.		
5	Psychomotor agitation may appear in excited catatonia.		
6	Catatonic symptoms can sometimes be mistaken for a neurological or medical disorder.		
7	Benzodiazepines are often considered among the treatment options for catatonia.		
8	Electroconvulsive therapy (ECT) is contraindicated in all cases of catatonia.		
9	Catatonia can present phases of negativism, where the individual passively or actively resists movement.		
10	A catatonic patient always remains aware and responsive to the environment.		

Matching Exercise

1. Mutism [ ]
2. Catalepsy [ ]
3. Echolalia [ ]
4. Negativism [ ]
5. Excited catatonia [ ]
6. Catatonia associated with Mood Disorders [ ]

Descriptions:

- A. Exact repetition of another person's words
- B. Maintaining a rigid posture for a prolonged period
- C. Absence or drastic reduction of speech, not due to a physical deficit in the vocal apparatus
- D. Resistance or non-response to external stimuli or commands
- E. Marked psychomotor agitation, possibly with stereotyped, repetitive movements
- F. Can occur during depressive or manic episodes, as well as in psychotic disorders

Case Study

A 35-year-old man is brought to the emergency department in a state of apparent immobility and with a blank facial expression. He holds the same posture for long periods even when asked to move. He does not speak, but if one of the staff stretches his arms, the patient maintains the new position (imposed posture). At times, he shows brief episodes of agitation in which he engages in repetitive, disorganized movements. There are no indications of substance intoxication or a clear neurological disorder.

1. Which described symptom most strongly suggests a catatonic presentation?
   - A. The presence of complex hallucinations
   - B. The maintenance of imposed postures (waxy flexibility) and persistent immobility
   - C. A tendency to speak excessively and without pause
   - D. The onset of epileptic seizures while being transported in the ambulance
2. If symptoms persist and no other causes are identified, which initial therapeutic approach might be attempted?
   - A. Administering high-dose beta-blockers
   - B. Using benzodiazepines (e.g., lorazepam) to assess the response
   - C. Relying solely on psychodynamic therapy
   - D. Observing passively and waiting for spontaneous remission
3. Which additional sign, if present, would further support a catatonia diagnosis?
   - A. A fixed gaze on a specific point, without shifting focus
   - B. Automatic repetition of words spoken by others (echolalia)
   - C. Ongoing persecutory delusions
   - D. Increased appetite and hyperphagia

Answers

Multiple Choice Questions

1. B
2. A
3. C
4. B
5. B
6. B
7. B

True/False Questions

1. True
2. False
3. True
4. False
5. True
6. True
7. True
8. False
9. True
10. False

Matching Exercise

1. C
2. B
3. A
4. D
5. E
6. F

Case Study Answers and Explanations

1. B – Explanation: Maintaining imposed postures (waxy flexibility) and a complete absence of spontaneous movement are typical signs of catatonia.
2. B – Explanation: Benzodiazepines are often the first-line approach to assess a positive response in catatonic patients.
3. B – Explanation: Echolalia (repeating someone else's words) is another symptom commonly seen in catatonia.

Other Schizophrenia Spectrum and Psychotic Disorders

Multiple Choice Questions

1. Which of the following might fall under the category of "Other Schizophrenia Spectrum and Psychotic Disorders"?
    - A. Delusional Disorder with a specific 5-year duration
    - B. Atypical psychoses that do not fully meet criteria for the main diagnoses
    - C. Schizophrenia manifesting exclusively as negative symptoms
    - D. Obsessive-Compulsive Disorder with poor insight
2. When a psychotic presentation does not fulfill all criteria for Schizophrenia, Schizoaffective Disorder, or other more specific disorders, which diagnosis might be appropriate?
    - A. Psychotic Disorder Due to Another Medical Condition
    - B. Substance/Medication-Induced Psychotic Disorder
    - C. Unspecified Schizophrenia Spectrum and Other Psychotic Disorder
    - D. Bipolar Disorder with Psychotic Features
3. Under what circumstances does the DSM-5 refer to "Other Schizophrenia Spectrum and Psychotic Disorders"?
    - A. When psychotic symptoms are present but there is no functional impairment
    - B. When symptoms do not meet the full temporal or symptomatic criteria for the standard diagnoses
    - C. When the patient is 100% aware that their hallucinations are not real
    - D. When psychotic symptoms begin after age 50
4. Which of the following clinical examples might fall under "Other Schizophrenia Spectrum and Psychotic Disorders"?
    - A. Psychotic symptoms lasting 1 week under severe stress, fully remitting, but lacking a clear context for Brief Psychotic Disorder
    - B. Delusions and hallucinations persisting for 7 months with prominent mood symptoms
    - C. A psychotic disorder strictly related to substance abuse
    - D. A 1-day delusional episode that completely resolved with immediate return to normal functioning
5. In this diagnostic section, the clinician often:
    - A. Has precise, well-defined criteria for each subtype
    - B. Uses the diagnosis for "residual" or "not otherwise specified" presentations
    - C. Cannot use this diagnosis if the patient's symptoms are mild
    - D. Must rule out any form of hallucination
6. The use of the term "Unspecified" or "Not Otherwise Specified (NOS)" for psychotic disorders in DSM-5:
    - A. Has completely disappeared and is never used
    - B. Is reserved only for cases lasting under 2 days
    - C. Indicates atypical presentations that do not meet the criteria for any well-defined disorder
    - D. Automatically replaces the main diagnoses when symptoms are less severe
7. What is typically the goal of diagnosing an "Unspecified Schizophrenia Spectrum and Other Psychotic Disorder"?
    - A. To refer the patient for a neurological evaluation with no psychiatric treatment
    - B. To provide a "bridge" category that allows for re-evaluation when more information becomes available
    - C. To avoid collecting further history or data
    - D. To completely rule out the possibility of Schizophrenia

True/False Questions

		T	F
1	"Other Schizophrenia Spectrum and Psychotic Disorders" can only be diagnosed if symptoms last precisely 1–6 months.		
2	In these disorders, psychotic symptoms may not be fully defined and could require further diagnostic assessment.		
3	"Unspecified Psychotic Disorders" no longer exist in DSM-5.		
4	This diagnosis can be used when a key piece of information is missing to satisfy the criteria of a specific psychotic disorder.		
5	If psychotic symptoms are short but intense, they are always classified solely as Brief Psychotic Disorder.		
6	Use of this diagnostic category can be temporary, pending a more definitive diagnosis.		
7	This section includes atypical presentations that do not fit the classic criteria of the main psychotic disorders.		
8	If new clinical data emerge, the initial diagnosis cannot be changed.		
9	You must rule out substance-induced or medical causes to use this diagnosis.		
10	A clinician may use this category in an emergency department before having a complete picture.		

Matching Exercise

1. Atypical presentation [ ]
2. Incomplete information [ ]
3. Excluding organic or substance-induced causes [ ]
4. Follow-up re-evaluation [ ]
5. "Bridge" diagnosis [ ]
6. Uncertain onset [ ]

Descriptions:

- A. It is essential to gather medical and toxicological data to rule out substance use or physical conditions.
- B. When psychotic symptoms do not clearly fit into any defined DSM-5 disorders.
- C. The clinical picture may evolve, allowing a more accurate diagnosis later.
- D. Often, symptoms do not indicate whether it's Schizophrenia, Schizoaffective Disorder, or something else, so a general definition is chosen.
- E. The patient does not match the typical duration or core symptoms of the main disorders, leaving diagnostic questions unanswered.
- F. The clinician provides a provisional diagnosis while awaiting further exams and observation.

Case Study

A 20-year-old man presents to a psychiatric service with persecutory delusions and commanding auditory hallucinations that have been ongoing for about 3 weeks. There is no evidence of substance abuse, and preliminary medical tests show no organic pathology. However, the presentation does not fully meet the criteria for Brief Psychotic Disorder (the symptoms might persist), nor has it yet reached the 6-month timeframe required for Schizophrenia. There are also no affective symptoms suggesting Schizoaffective Disorder. The clinician decides to monitor symptom progression.

1. Which diagnostic category might be most appropriate at this stage?
   - A. Schizophrenia
   - B. Brief Psychotic Disorder
   - C. Other (Unspecified) Schizophrenia Spectrum and Psychotic Disorder
   - D. Bipolar Disorder with Psychotic Features
2. Why is Schizophrenia not diagnosable at this point?
   - A. Because the patient is depressed
   - B. Because the symptom duration is still too short
   - C. Because a co-occurring Mood Disorder is required
   - D. Because there are no negative symptoms
3. Which action is most suitable in the diagnostic process?
   - A. Concluding that this is just an acute stress episode
   - B. Recording the diagnosis as final, without further evaluation
   - C. Recommending follow-up and observation to clarify how the presentation evolves
   - D. Immediately prescribing tricyclic antidepressants only

Answers

Multiple Choice Questions

1. B
2. C
3. B
4. A
5. B
6. C
7. B

True/False Questions

1. False
2. True
3. False
4. True
5. False
6. True
7. True
8. False
9. True
10. True

Matching Exercise

1. B
2. E
3. A
4. C
5. D
6. F

Case Study Answers and Explanations

1. C – Explanation: Since the psychotic symptoms do not meet the duration criteria for Schizophrenia, nor do they fully conform to Brief Psychotic Disorder or Schizoaffective Disorder, it is best to place them in the category "Other (Unspecified) Schizophrenia Spectrum and Psychotic Disorder" until more is known.
2. B – Explanation: To diagnose Schizophrenia, symptoms must persist for at least 6 months (including prodromal, active, and/or residual phases). Here, only 3 weeks have elapsed.
3. C – Explanation: Ongoing monitoring allows the collection of further information, ultimately leading to a more precise diagnosis. In the meantime, a provisional diagnosis from this section can be used.

Bipolar and Related Disorders

This category includes disorders where mood changes take center stage, featuring periods of elevated mood (mania or hypomania) and periods of lowered mood (depression). These disorders can appear in different forms, depending on how long episodes last, how intense they are, and how symptoms combine over time.

Bipolar I Disorder, for example, requires at least one manic episode, which may be preceded or followed by hypomanic or depressive episodes. A manic episode often involves a markedly high or irritable mood, increased energy, reduced need for sleep, accelerated mental and physical activity, rapid speech, and sometimes impulsive behavior with limited awareness of potential consequences (such as excessive spending or unrealistic ventures). In more severe cases, delusions or hallucinations may occur. A manic episode typically lasts a minimum of one week (or less if hospitalization is needed), whereas a hypomanic episode has similar traits but is less intense and lasts at least four days. Unlike mania, hypomania generally doesn't lead to severe functional impairment or hospital admission.

Bipolar II Disorder does not include full-blown mania; instead, individuals experience hypomanic phases alternating with clearly identifiable depressive episodes. These depressive phases are marked by low mood, a loss of interest in most activities, feelings of guilt or worthlessness, changes in appetite or sleep, fatigue, and concentration difficulties. Suicidal thoughts can also arise. Even without manic episodes, Bipolar II Disorder can be just as serious, since its depressive phases can be deep and long-lasting.

Another type of mood fluctuation is Cyclothymic Disorder, where milder hypomanic and depressive symptoms persist for extended periods (at least two years in adults, or one year in younger individuals), without more than two consecutive months free from symptoms. Although often underestimated, these ongoing ups and downs can still influence overall well-being and daily life.

From a diagnostic standpoint, it's important to distinguish these disorders from other conditions, such as Depressive Disorders or psychotic disorders. Substances or certain medications can mimic or worsen bipolar symptoms, and some medical conditions may have similar effects. Any evaluation should explore possible endocrine or neurological factors, as well as lifestyle habits (for instance, alcohol or stimulant use). Genetic and familial influences are also significant, as there is often a hereditary component.

Treatment often involves mood stabilizers or antipsychotics, combined with specific psychological support. Collaborating with the individual and, when possible, their family is a key part of recognizing early warning signs of relapse and intervening with appropriate strategies. Successful management can reduce how frequently and severely episodes occur, helping improve quality of life for those affected.

Bipolar I Disorder

Multiple Choice Questions

1. Which characteristic defines a Manic Episode in Bipolar I Disorder?
    - A. A distinctly depressed mood lasting at least 2 weeks
    - B. Absence of psychotic symptoms during the episode
    - C. A period of persistently elevated, expansive, or irritable mood lasting at least 1 week, or any duration if hospitalization is required
    - D. Only anxiety-related symptoms
2. Which of the following is a typical symptom that can occur during a Manic Episode?
    - A. Loss of interest in all activities
    - B. Psychomotor retardation
    - C. Inflated self-esteem or grandiosity
    - D. Persistent feelings of guilt and worthlessness
3. According to the DSM-5, to diagnose Bipolar I Disorder it is necessary that:
    - A. At least one Manic Episode has occurred in the patient's lifetime, regardless of history of Depressive Episodes
    - B. There is only one Major Depressive Episode, with no other episodes
    - C. At least 6 months of depressive symptoms have passed before the onset of a hypomanic episode
    - D. It always includes a Major Depressive Episode
4. Which of the following factors may increase the risk of a Manic Episode in a patient with Bipolar I Disorder?
    - A. Using certain antidepressants without the coverage of a mood stabilizer
    - B. Low stress levels and a strong support system
    - C. A regular lifestyle with no stressful events
    - D. Complete abstinence from alcohol and substance use
5. Which of the following symptoms, if present, might suggest hospitalization is needed during a Manic Episode?
    - A. Minimal impairment of social functioning
    - B. Ability to manage daily activities independently
    - C. Severe disinhibited or risky behaviors
    - D. Absence of interpersonal conflicts
6. What is the key difference between a Manic Episode and a Hypomanic Episode?
    - A. A hypomanic episode always lasts fewer than 2 days
    - B. A Manic Episode involves more severe functional impairment and/or may require hospitalization, whereas a Hypomanic Episode generally does not
    - C. Hypomanic episodes always involve psychotic symptoms
    - D. A hypomanic episode never includes an elevated mood
7. A patient diagnosed with Bipolar I Disorder may present with:
    - A. Only hypomanic episodes
    - B. Both manic and depressive episodes, where the manic episode is central to the diagnosis
    - C. Exclusively repeated depressive episodes over time
    - D. Only anxiety symptoms, without ever developing mania or hypomania

True/False Questions

		T	F
1	A single Hypomanic Episode is sufficient for a Bipolar I Disorder diagnosis.		
2	A Manic Episode can include psychotic symptoms.		
3	Mood stabilizers, such as lithium, can help prevent relapses.		
4	Bipolar I Disorder always requires a Major Depressive Episode for diagnosis.		
5	A manic state may require hospitalization for the safety of the patient or others.		
6	Bipolar I Disorder has no genetic or biological basis whatsoever.		
7	Stressful events, such as sleep deprivation, can trigger a Manic Episode.		
8	A Manic Episode in Bipolar I Disorder can last fewer than 7 days if hospitalization is required.		
9	A "Mixed Bipolar Episode" no longer exists as a category in DSM-5.		
10	Effective psychotherapy, such as CBT, can be a useful adjunct to medication in treating Bipolar I Disorder.		

Matching Exercise

1. Manic Episode [ ]
2. Major Depressive Episode [ ]
3. Risk of Relapse [ ]
4. Mood Stabilizers [ ]
5. Triggering Factors [ ]
6. Need for Hospitalization [ ]

Descriptions:

- A. Caused by factors such as changes in routine, reduced sleep, or significant stress
- B. Elevated or irritable mood, increased energy or activity, potentially severe functional impairment
- C. A clinical picture of depressed mood, loss of pleasure, cognitive and physical symptoms lasting at least 2 weeks
- D. Medications like lithium, valproic acid, or certain atypical antipsychotics used to prevent mood fluctuations
- E. May be necessary if the patient shows severe disinhibition, dangerous behaviors, or is unable to receive proper care at home
- F. The likelihood that a new Manic or Depressive Episode will recur in the future

Case Study

A 28-year-old man arrives at the Emergency Department displaying extreme agitation and grandiose ideas, claiming he has discovered a "revolutionary technology" and can contact heads of state to promote it. He reports not having slept for at least 4 days without feeling tired, and exhibits a marked increase in activity, jumping from one project to another without finishing any. His mood is irritable when anyone contradicts him, alternating between euphoria and bursts of anger. He has had at least two similar episodes in the past, one of which required hospitalization. He does not report a clear Depressive Episode. Currently, he appears disinhibited and has little awareness of the potential consequences of his actions.

1. Which clinical aspect is most indicative of a Manic Episode?
    - A. Marked depression with suicidal thoughts
    - B. Reduced need for sleep and increased energy with grandiose ideas, along with poor insight into risks
    - C. Predominantly generalized anxiety without mood changes
    - D. Exclusively paranoid delusions rather than grandiose ones
2. Why does this presentation meet the criteria for Bipolar I Disorder rather than a Hypomanic Episode?
    - A. Because there is no prior depressive episode
    - B. Because the patient does not have anxious symptoms
    - C. Because the severity of the condition and a history of hospitalizations point to significant functional impairment
    - D. Because it has lasted fewer than 4 days
3. Which treatment might be a priority given the risk of disinhibited and dangerous behaviors?
    - A. Supportive psychotherapy only
    - B. Mood stabilizers (such as lithium or valproate) and/or atypical antipsychotics, with possible hospitalization for safety
    - C. Anxiolytics alone for a short period
    - D. No pharmacological intervention, waiting for spontaneous remission

Answers

Multiple Choice Questions
1. C
2. C
3. A
4. A
5. C
6. B
7. B

True/False Questions
1. False
2. True
3. True
4. False
5. True
6. False
7. True
8. True
9. False
10. True

Matching Exercise
1. B
2. C
3. F
4. D
5. A
6. E

Case Study Answers and Explanations
1. B – Explanation: The increased energy, grandiose thinking, reduced need for sleep, and lack of insight into risks all point to a Manic Episode.
2. C – Explanation: A Manic Episode causes marked functional impairment, often requiring hospitalization, whereas a hypomanic episode generally involves milder impairment.
3. B – Explanation: In severe mania with disinhibition, mood stabilizers or antipsychotics should be considered. Hospitalization is often needed to ensure safety.

Bipolar II Disorder

Multiple Choice Questions

1. What is the defining characteristic of Bipolar II Disorder?
    - A. The presence of at least one full-blown Manic Episode
    - B. The presence of Hypomanic Episodes and at least one Major Depressive Episode
    - C. The absence of any Depressive Episodes
    - D. Exclusively manic episodes accompanied by psychotic symptoms
2. Which statement correctly describes a Hypomanic Episode?
    - A. A period of elevated or irritable mood lasting at least 1 week, with severe functional impairment
    - B. A period of elevated or irritable mood lasting at least 4 days, without marked functional impairment and with no need for hospitalization
    - C. A depressive phase lasting at least 2 weeks
    - D. A minimal restlessness that does not affect daily activities
3. Which factor most clearly distinguishes Bipolar II Disorder from Bipolar I Disorder?
    - A. The severity of depressive phases
    - B. The presence of psychotic mania in both disorders
    - C. Bipolar II never includes a full Manic Episode
    - D. The absence of any genetic factors in Bipolar II
4. In a Major Depressive Episode, which symptom is commonly observed?
    - A. Reduced need for sleep along with euphoria
    - B. Loss of pleasure (anhedonia) in nearly all activities
    - C. Elevated mood and hyperactivity
    - D. Racing thoughts and flight of ideas
5. Which scenario could be a potential trigger for a Hypomanic Episode in Bipolar II Disorder?
    - A. A regular sleep schedule and lack of stressful events
    - B. Taking antidepressants without an adequate mood stabilizer
    - C. Perfectly preserved social functioning
    - D. Gradual and well-managed discontinuation of stabilizing medication
6. Which of the following statements addresses the need for hospitalization during a Hypomanic Episode in Bipolar II Disorder?
    - A. Hypomania never requires hospitalization because it does not impair functioning
    - B. Hospitalization may be required only if it escalates into full mania or if the risk is too high
    - C. All Hypomanic Episodes demand mandatory hospitalization
    - D. Hospitalization is necessary only if comorbid with a psychotic disorder
7. Why are euthymic periods (when there are no symptoms) clinically significant in Bipolar II Disorder?
    - A. They never occur; the patient constantly cycles between hypomania and depression
    - B. They can represent inter-episode stability, during which the individual functions normally
    - C. They always coincide with low energy and low mood, though not reaching the threshold for depression
    - D. They are periods of moderate euphoria that inevitably lead to the next hypomanic episode

True/False Questions

		T	F
1	In Bipolar II Disorder, a full Manic Episode may never occur.		
2	A Hypomanic Episode in Bipolar II always causes severe functional impairment.		
3	Major Depressive Episodes in Bipolar II can be quite intense and may include suicidal ideation.		
4	Inappropriate antidepressant use can trigger a Hypomanic Episode in predisposed individuals.		
5	Hypomania typically lasts at least 2 weeks.		
6	In Bipolar II Disorder, the patient never experiences any period of wellness between episodes.		
7	A single Major Depressive Episode in one's lifetime, combined with one Hypomanic Episode, is enough to diagnose Bipolar II Disorder.		
8	Distinguishing Bipolar II from Major Depressive Disorder requires confirming the presence or absence of hypomanic episodes.		
9	Bipolar II Disorder never involves psychotic symptoms, neither in the hypomanic nor in the depressive phase.		
10	Family history can provide useful information to confirm a Bipolar II diagnosis.		

Matching Exercise

1. Hypomanic Episode
2. Major Depressive Episode
3. Euthymia
4. Reactivity to Antidepressants
5. Differentiation from Bipolar I
6. Degree of Functional Impairment

Descriptions:

- A. A phase characterized by elevated or irritable mood and increased energy, yet without severe impairment or need for hospitalization
- B. A period when the individual has no significant symptoms of mania/hypomania or depression
- C. When an antidepressant can precipitate a hypomanic phase in a predisposed individual
- D. Particularly important in Bipolar II, since "true mania" is not present
- E. Includes sadness, loss of interest or pleasure, along with possible sleep/appetite changes or suicidal thoughts
- F. Typically less severe in hypomania compared to mania, yet can be substantial during severe depressive episodes

Case Study

A 32-year-old woman reports a recent episode of elevated mood and high energy that lasted about 5 days. During that time, she felt more energetic, slept only 3 hours per night without feeling tired, started multiple creative projects, and was more social and talkative than usual. However, her family notes that while they recognized a change in her mood, she did not engage in behaviors extreme enough to require hospitalization. In the past, she experienced at least two Major Depressive Episodes marked by profound sadness and difficulty carrying out daily tasks. Her current psychiatric exam finds her mood back to normal (euthymic). No evidence of substance use or medical conditions explains her symptoms.

1. Which aspect primarily indicates that this recent episode is Hypomanic rather than Manic?
   - A. It lasted fewer than 3 days
   - B. There was no change whatsoever from her usual behavior
   - C. There was no severe impairment or need for hospitalization
   - D. She experienced delusions and hallucinations
2. Based on her clinical history, why is Bipolar II Disorder a likely consideration?
   - A. She has at least one Hypomanic Episode plus one or more Major Depressive Episodes
   - B. She only had one Depressive Episode without hypomania
   - C. She previously needed hospitalization for mania
   - D. She has never experienced any period of wellness
3. Which treatment strategy might be indicated, considering her history of Depressive Episodes and a Hypomanic Episode?
   - A. High-dose antidepressants alone
   - B. Mood stabilizers (e.g., lithium, valproate) and possibly an antidepressant with caution
   - C. Pure psychoanalysis without any pharmacological support
   - D. High-dose typical antipsychotics, regardless of her symptoms

Answers

Multiple Choice Questions

1. B
2. B
3. C
4. B
5. B
6. B
7. B

True/False Questions

1. True
2. False
3. True
4. True
5. False
6. False
7. True
8. True
9. False
10. True

Matching Exercise

1. A
2. E
3. B
4. C
5. D
6. F

Case Study Answers and Explanations

1. C – Explanation: The absence of marked functional impairment and no need for hospitalization distinguish a Hypomanic Episode from a Manic one.
2. A – Explanation: Bipolar II Disorder requires at least one Hypomanic Episode and one (or more) Major Depressive Episodes.
3. B – Explanation: In Bipolar II Disorder, treatment often involves mood stabilizers, sometimes accompanied by antidepressants, but with caution to avoid triggering hypomania or mania.

Cyclothymic Disorder

Multiple Choice Questions

1. **What is the main feature of Cyclothymic Disorder?**
    - A. Alternation between manic and depressive episodes
    - B. At least 2 years of mild hypomanic and depressive symptoms not meeting full criteria
    - C. Complete absence of mood issues
    - D. A single brief Hypomanic Episode
2. **What distinguishes Cyclothymic Disorder from Bipolar I and II?**
    - A. No anxiety symptoms
    - B. Psychotic mania
    - C. Chronic mild symptoms never meeting full criteria
    - D. Onset only after age 60
3. **When would you suspect Cyclothymic Disorder?**
    - A. Severe Manic Episode followed by Depression
    - B. 2 years of frequent mood swings, not meeting criteria for Hypomania or Depression
    - C. One Major Depressive Episode lasting 6 months
    - D. Psychosis with severe mania
4. **What rules out Cyclothymic Disorder?**
    - A. 2 months of complete wellness
    - B. Symptoms below criteria for Major Depression
    - C. Symptoms starting in adolescence and continuing
    - D. Symptoms only due to substance abuse
5. **What is a common complication of Cyclothymic Disorder?**
    - A. No depressive or anxious symptoms
    - B. Higher risk of Bipolar I or II
    - C. Optimal social and emotional function
    - D. Strong stress-coping skills
6. **What is the minimum symptom duration for Cyclothymic Disorder (adults)?**
    - A. 6 months
    - B. 1 year
    - C. 2 years
    - D. 5 years
7. **What helps patients with mild Cyclothymic symptoms?**
    - A. Ignoring the condition
    - B. Psychoeducation, therapy, and mood stabilizers if needed
    - C. Only prescribing anxiolytics
    - D. High-dose antipsychotics preventively

True/False Questions

Mark each statement as True (✓) or False (X).

		T	F
1	Cyclothymic Disorder implies the presence of regular manic episodes.		
2	In Cyclothymic Disorder, symptoms are constant with no relatively stable mood periods.		
3	A minimum duration of 2 years (1 year in minors) is necessary for a Cyclothymic Disorder diagnosis.		
4	In Cyclothymic Disorder, hypomanic and depressive symptoms never fully meet the criteria for a Hypomanic or Major Depressive Episode.		
5	Individuals with Cyclothymic Disorder always have extremely impaired social functioning.		
6	Cyclothymic Disorder can sometimes progress to Bipolar I or II Disorder.		
7	Substance or alcohol abuse can complicate the diagnosis of Cyclothymic Disorder.		
8	In some cases, Cyclothymic Disorder may include brief euthymic periods, though they are usually very short.		
9	Having mixed episodes with mania and psychosis rules out Cyclothymic Disorder.		
10	Cyclothymic Disorder categorically excludes any subthreshold depressive symptoms.		

Matching Exercise

1. Chronic course [ ]
2. Subthreshold [ ]
3. Psychoeducation [ ]
4. Possible progression to Bipolar [ ]
5. Exclusion criterion [ ]
6. Periods of wellness [ ]

Descriptions:

- A. One of the primary risks in Cyclothymic Disorder is that symptoms may intensify and lead to a full Bipolar Disorder
- B. Hypomanic and depressive symptoms never reach the full criteria for a complete episode
- C. An important tool to help the patient recognize early mood fluctuations and prevent worsening
- D. Refers to the fact that patients can experience symptom-free intervals but never longer than 2 consecutive months
- E. Cyclothymic Disorder persists for at least 2 years in adults (1 year in children and adolescents)
- F. Substance abuse may better explain the mood swings; if that alone accounts for the symptoms, it rules out a primary Cyclothymic Disorder

Case Study

A 40-year-old man describes having frequent mood fluctuations for about 3 years. Sometimes he feels more energetic, talkative, and confident, though not enough to impair his functioning or require hospitalization. During these "up" periods, he sleeps very little but continues to perform adequately at work. Other times, he feels down, has trouble getting out of bed, and experiences mild pessimism, though he still manages his responsibilities. He has never had a full Major Depressive Episode or a true manic/hypomanic phase. He reports no period of complete mood stability lasting longer than a month. There is no evidence of substance abuse or a medical condition that could explain these mood swings.

1. Which detail points most strongly to Cyclothymic Disorder?
    - A. The presence of a severe manic episode with psychosis
    - B. At least 3 years of ongoing mood swings, never intense enough to meet criteria for mania/hypomania or major depression
    - C. A single Major Depressive Episode lasting six months
    - D. The absence of any depressive symptoms
2. Why is substance abuse considered an exclusion criterion if it's the sole explanation for mood swings?
    - A. Because substance use can never affect mood
    - B. Because Cyclothymic Disorder always includes psychotic mania
    - C. Because mood fluctuations resulting solely from substance use do not qualify as a primary mood disorder
    - D. Because substance-induced symptoms never include high-energy phases
3. Which therapeutic approach might be suitable for this patient?
    - A. No intervention, given the subthreshold symptoms
    - B. Psychoeducation and possible mood stabilizers (e.g., lithium) if symptoms worsen
    - C. Immediate hospitalization
    - D. High-dose typical antipsychotics only

Answers

Multiple Choice Questions

1. B
2. C
3. B
4. D
5. B
6. C
7. B

True/False Questions

1. False
2. False
3. True
4. True
5. False
6. True
7. True
8. True
9. True
10. False

Matching Exercise

1. E
2. B
3. C
4. A
5. F
6. D

Case Study Answers and Explanations

1. B – Explanation: Cyclothymic Disorder involves at least 2 years (3 in this example) of ongoing, subthreshold mood swings, never meeting the full criteria for Major Depression or full-blown Hypomania/Mania.
2. C – Explanation: If substance use alone accounts for the mood fluctuations, it is not a primary mood disorder. This must be ruled out before diagnosing Cyclothymic Disorder.
3. B – Explanation: Psychoeducation helps manage symptoms and detect warning signs of escalation. If symptoms intensify, mood stabilizers may be indicated.

Other Bipolar and Related Disorders

Multiple Choice Questions

1. Which of the following could fit under DSM-5's "Other Bipolar and Related Disorders"?
    - A. A purely depressive disorder with no mania/hypomania
    - B. Bipolar-like mood changes that don't meet full criteria for Bipolar I, II, or Cyclothymic Disorder
    - C. A Major Depressive Episode with slight irritability but no energy changes
    - D. Any mixed state with psychosis
2. An "Other Specified Bipolar and Related Disorder" is diagnosed when:
    - A. Bipolar I or II criteria are fully met
    - B. The term "bipolar" is used as a synonym for "major depression"
    - C. Bipolar I/II criteria are not met, but mood changes (e.g., brief hypomania, partial mixed features) are clinically significant
    - D. No mood episodes ever occurred
3. Which example might suggest an "Unspecified Bipolar and Related Disorder"?
    - A. A single 2-month Manic Episode followed by major depression
    - B. Episodes hinting at mania/hypomania but not meeting duration/intensity, yet causing distress
    - C. A classic Cyclothymic Disorder with required timeframes met
    - D. One mild irritability spell and nothing else
4. When do we use "Bipolar Disorder with Mixed Features"?
    - A. A depressive episode with some manic signs (e.g., high energy, racing thoughts)
    - B. A purely manic episode with no depression
    - C. A simple Major Depressive Episode without agitation
    - D. Manic and depressive episodes appearing at separate times
5. Why is "Other Bipolar and Related Disorders" useful?
    - A. It covers mild schizophrenia
    - B. It classifies all mood disorders as "bipolar"
    - C. It captures partial bipolar features that don't meet full criteria
    - D. It has no practical use
6. In "Other Specified Bipolar..." with "Short (2–3 day) Hypomanic Episodes and Major Depression":
    - A. It's Bipolar II, since depression is present
    - B. Hypomanic episodes are too short for Bipolar II but are still significant
    - C. It's a depressive disorder with irritability
    - D. Must be Cyclothymic Disorder
7. A patient has a Depressive Episode with some manic-like features (e.g., agitation, fast thoughts) but no full mania/hypomania. This is:
    - A. Classic Bipolar I
    - B. Major Depression with anxiety
    - C. Bipolar with Mixed Features (subthreshold mania)
    - D. Schizoaffective Disorder

True/False Questions

		T	F
1	The diagnostic classification "Other Specified Bipolar Disorder" is exclusively temporary and cannot progress to a diagnosis of Bipolar I or II.		
2	The terms "specified" and "unspecified" are utilized when primary criteria for bipolar disorders are not entirely satisfied, but the clinical presentation retains characteristics of a bipolar spectrum condition.		
3	The DSM-5 strictly prohibits the concurrent manifestation of manic and depressive symptoms within a single episode.		
4	A diagnosis of "Bipolar Disorder with Mixed Features" may pertain to a predominantly depressive episode that exhibits certain manic symptoms.		
5	"Unspecified Bipolar Disorder" is employed when insufficient clinical data (e.g., in an emergency room setting) precludes differentiation between Bipolar I and Bipolar II.		
6	A hypomanic episode lasting only two days may be classified as "Other Specified Bipolar Disorder" due to its failure to meet the duration threshold for Bipolar II.		
7	The category "Bipolar Disorder with Mixed Features" does not exist; it is not possible for manic and depressive symptoms to co-occur.		
8	Even atypical presentations of bipolar disorders are capable of inducing substantial psychological distress and impairment.		
9	The DSM-5 excludes the recognition of residual forms of bipolar disorder.		
10	The "specified" designation enables the clinician to specify the reasons why full diagnostic criteria are not fulfilled (e.g., brief hypomanic episodes or the presence of mixed symptoms).		

Matching Exercise

1. Other Specified Bipolar [ ]
2. Unspecified Bipolar [ ]
3. Mixed Features [ ]
4. Brief Hypomania [ ]
5. Depression + partial hypomanic signs [ ]
6. Clinical utility of "Other Bipolar and Related Disorders" [ ]

Descriptions:

- A. Lack of full info or unclear criteria but bipolar is suspected
- B. Both mania/hypomania and depression signs appear together, not fully meeting either set
- C. A category to classify partial/atypical bipolar forms
- D. Used if relevant bipolar traits are present but a criterion is missing (e.g., short hypomania)
- E. Example: 2–3 day hypomania still has clinical impact
- F. A "mixed" depressive episode with agitation, racing thoughts, low need for sleep

Case Study

A 35-year-old has been depressed for ~3 weeks but also reports agitation, racing thoughts, and reduced sleep (3–4 hours). No true euphoria of mania/hypomania. Similar episodes in the past never met full mania or hypomania but included some manic-like signs. Doesn't qualify for Bipolar I/II, and current episode isn't a full mixed episode. Still, the distress is significant.

1. Best diagnostic fit?
   - A. Bipolar I, Manic Episode with anxiety
   - B. Major Depression, no specifiers
   - C. Other Specified Bipolar... (e.g., Subthreshold Mixed Features)
   - D. Bipolar II, Hypomanic Episode
2. Why not Bipolar II?
   - A. Current mania is too severe
   - B. No typical Major Depression was ever found
   - C. No fully defined hypomania meeting duration/intensity
   - D. Mania must last at least 2 months
3. Which approach helps when bipolar symptoms are incomplete?
   - A. No diagnosis, wait for clearer episodes
   - B. Use "Other Specified Bipolar..." to note partial/mixed traits
   - C. Just label it Bipolar I for safety
   - D. Ignore mixed signs, give only anxiolytics

Answers

Multiple Choice

1. B
2. C
3. C
4. A
5. C
6. B
7. C

True/False

1. False
2. True
3. False
4. True
5. True
6. True
7. False
8. True
9. False
10. True

Matching

1. D
2. A
3. B
4. E
5. F
6. C

Case Study

1. C – Depressive episode with some manic-like signs, not full mania/hypomania → "Other Specified"
2. C – No hypomanic episode meeting 4-day minimum
3. B – "Other Specified" captures partial bipolar features, aiding treatment planning

Depressive Disorders

This group includes conditions where a persistently low mood or an inability to experience pleasure in usual activities is the main concern. It's not just a matter of feeling sad or discouraged for a brief period. Instead, the depressive symptoms—such as loss of interest, feelings of worthlessness, constant fatigue, difficulty concentrating, changes in appetite or sleep—are so intense and prolonged that they significantly affect day-to-day functioning and relationships.

Among the most recognized disorders in this category is Major Depressive Disorder, characterized by episodes of depressed mood and related symptoms lasting at least two weeks. When these episodes recur, individuals may go through periods of remission followed by relapses. Another important condition is Persistent Depressive Disorder (formerly Dysthymia), in which depressive symptoms are less acute but more chronic, persisting for at least two years in adults (one year in younger people) without lengthy intervals of full remission.

Disruptive Mood Dysregulation Disorder is diagnosed in childhood or adolescence and involves excessive irritability and intense anger outbursts disproportionate to the situation, both at home and at school. This diagnosis was introduced for children who show severe mood instability but do not meet the criteria for Bipolar Disorder.

Premenstrual Dysphoric Disorder occurs in some women during the late phase of the menstrual cycle, with symptoms easing in the days following menstruation. It is marked by emotional swings, pronounced sadness, irritability, and a sense of feeling overwhelmed, potentially impacting social and occupational functioning.

In clinical assessment, it is important to differentiate Depressive Disorders from other circumstances that might share similar features, such as complicated grief or stress-related reactions. Medical conditions (for instance, hypothyroidism or nutritional deficiencies) and substance use can also mimic depressive episodes. Assessment should thoroughly investigate any signs of psychosis, anxiety, or personality disorders that could overlap and complicate the overall picture.

Treatment typically combines pharmacological options—antidepressants and, at times, other specific medications—with structured psychological approaches such as cognitive-behavioral therapy or interpersonal therapy. In more severe situations, especially in the presence of suicidal ideation or intense depressive symptoms, a multidisciplinary strategy with regular follow-up and family or caregiver involvement may be indicated. The ultimate goal is to alleviate symptoms, support the resumption of everyday activities, and prevent relapses, providing continuous assistance so the individual can regain psychological and physical well-being.

Disruptive Mood Dysregulation Disorder (DMDD)

Multiple Choice Questions

1. What is the main feature of Disruptive Mood Dysregulation Disorder according to the DSM-5?
    - A. Manic episodes marked by euphoria and high energy
    - B. Chronic irritability and frequent outbursts of anger disproportionate to the situation
    - C. Depressive phases with constant suicidal ideation
    - D. Regular alternation between mania and major depression
2. In which age group can DMDD be diagnosed?
    - A. From early childhood up to age 5
    - B. Between 6 and 18 years, with onset before age 10
    - C. Only in adulthood (over 18)
    - D. Exclusively in adolescence (12 to 17)
3. How often must "temper outbursts" occur for DMDD criteria to be met, according to the DSM-5?
    - A. At least once a day
    - B. Sporadically, without a defined frequency
    - C. At least 3 times per week
    - D. Only during particularly stressful events
4. What criterion makes these outbursts clinically relevant for DMDD?
    - A. They must always target peers and never adults
    - B. They occur solely in one setting (home or school)
    - C. The anger reaction is excessive relative to the trigger, in intensity or duration
    - D. They must coincide with full-blown manic or hypomanic episodes
5. To differentiate DMDD from pediatric Bipolar Disorder, a key consideration is:
    - A. Whether full manic/hypomanic episodes are present
    - B. Whether the child shows only sadness without irritability
    - C. Whether onset occurs after age 18
    - D. Whether there are no self-control problems
6. Which common outcome might be seen if DMDD is neither identified nor addressed?
    - A. Rapid progression to schizophrenia
    - B. Growing social isolation, academic problems, and possible later development of mood or anxiety disorders
    - C. Complete spontaneous resolution within a few weeks
    - D. Very severe manic episodes with psychosis
7. Which of the following factors would exclude the diagnosis of DMDD?
    - A. Onset of temper outbursts after age 10
    - B. A history of manic or hypomanic episodes suggesting Bipolar Disorder
    - C. Presence of irritability in only one specific environment
    - D. Frequent episodes of aggression lasting fewer than 3 months

True/False Questions

		T	F
1	DMDD cannot be diagnosed if the child has ever had manic or hypomanic episodes.		
2	Temper outbursts in DMDD must involve an exaggerated response to situational provocation rather than being premeditated and intentional.		
3	Irritability between outbursts is a defining and persistent characteristic of DMDD.		
4	DMDD symptoms must persist for at least one year, in at least two distinct settings such as home and school.		
5	DMDD cannot be diagnosed if there is evidence of clearly defined manic episodes.		
6	DMDD symptoms must necessarily have an onset before age 10 and not after.		
7	If untreated, DMDD can profoundly impair academic performance, interpersonal relationships, and social functioning.		
8	Chronic irritability, extending beyond temper outbursts, is a common feature among children with DMDD.		
9	DMDD cannot be diagnosed if the symptoms are more adequately explained by another mood or anxiety disorder.		
10	Oppositional Defiant Disorder (ODD) may coexist with DMDD only when irritability and outbursts do not entirely account for the symptoms of both disorders.		

Matching Exercise

1. Chronic irritability [ ]
2. Disproportionate anger outbursts [ ]
3. Multiple settings [ ]
4. Difference from Bipolar Disorder [ ]
5. Minimum duration [ ]
6. Possible consequences [ ]

Descriptions:

- A. At least 12 months with no lengthy symptom-free periods (≥3 months)
- B. Intense anger reactions exceeding the stimulus
- C. Must occur in at least two contexts (e.g., home/school), with greater severity in at least one
- D. Between outbursts, the child's baseline mood remains irritable or angry
- E. No true manic/hypomanic episodes, rather chronic irritability and frequent "tantrums"
- F. Increased risk of social isolation, poor academic performance, and eventual mood/anxiety disorders

Case Study

An 8-year-old has shown intense anger outbursts for about a year, occurring at least 3–4 times per week. These episodes involve yelling and throwing objects over relatively minor triggers (e.g., mild scolding). Outside these episodes, the child remains chronically irritable, often argues with classmates and siblings. Parents report that these behaviors occur both at home and at school. No signs of mania (e.g., euphoria or abnormally high energy) have been observed. Academic performance is declining, and peers tend to exclude him.

1. Which feature most strongly suggests a DMDD diagnosis?
   - A. A hypomanic episode of at least 4 days
   - B. Frequent, disproportionate anger outbursts plus constant irritability
   - C. Rare anger (once a month) with mostly neutral mood
   - D. No difficulty adapting at school
2. Why is it not Bipolar Disorder?
   - A. There are no mania/hypomania episodes
   - B. The child is too young for Bipolar Disorder
   - C. The child sleeps regularly
   - D. The outbursts are not linked to periods of intense euphoria
3. Which initial intervention is indicated?
   - A. High-dose antipsychotics
   - B. Psychoeducation, parent training, and anger management strategies
   - C. Immediate psychiatric hospitalization
   - D. No intervention, just "normal tantrums"

Answers

Multiple Choice Questions

1. B
2. B
3. C
4. C
5. A
6. B
7. B

True/False Questions

1. True
2. False
3. True
4. True
5. False
6. False
7. True
8. True
9. True
10. True

Matching Exercise

1. D
2. B
3. C
4. E
5. A
6. F

Case Study Answers and Explanations

1. B – Constant irritability and frequent, excessive outbursts are hallmarks of DMDD.
2. A – Bipolar Disorder requires true manic/hypomanic episodes, which are absent here.
3. B – Initial steps often involve psychoeducation, training for parents, and anger regulation techniques.

Major Depressive Disorder (MDD)

Multiple Choice Questions

1. Which of the following criteria is key for diagnosing a Major Depressive Episode according to the DSM-5?
    - A. Having had at least one Hypomanic or Manic Episode in the past
    - B. Persistently elevated or euphoric mood with reduced need for sleep
    - C. Depressed mood or loss of interest/pleasure in most activities for at least 2 weeks
    - D. Shifts in mood between irritability and euphoria with no periods of normal mood
2. Which symptom is not typically associated with a Major Depressive Episode?
    - A. Deep and persistent sadness
    - B. Marked decrease or increase in appetite
    - C. Intense euphoria with high energy
    - D. Psychomotor agitation or retardation
3. For a diagnosis of Major Depressive Disorder, the symptoms:
    - A. Must last at least 2 consecutive days
    - B. May appear only once in a lifetime, without any further episodes
    - C. Must cause clinically significant distress or impairment in social, occupational, or other important areas of functioning
    - D. Can never be associated with thoughts of death or suicidal ideation
4. Which of the following factors can raise the risk of developing a Major Depressive Episode?
    - A. A highly regular, stress-free life
    - B. Absence of childhood trauma
    - C. Family history of mood disorders and/or significant adverse events
    - D. Strong social and family support
5. A Major Depressive Episode with psychotic features differs from a non-psychotic one in that it:
    - A. Involves delusions or hallucinations, whether mood-congruent or not
    - B. Lasts less time than a standard depressive episode
    - C. Excludes guilt or self-devaluation
    - D. Excludes psychomotor retardation
6. "Major Depressive Disorder, Single Episode" refers to:
    - A. Symptom onset after age 60
    - B. Only one Major Depressive Episode in the patient's lifetime, with no recurrences
    - C. At least two depressive episodes occurring in quick succession
    - D. An episode lasting only 1 week
7. Which of the following might complicate the diagnosis of Major Depressive Disorder?
    - A. The co-occurrence of a full Manic Episode
    - B. The presence of hypersomnia or loss of appetite
    - C. The fact that the episode lasts more than 2 weeks
    - D. The patient experiencing suicidal thoughts

True/False Questions

		T	F
1	In Major Depressive Disorder, "mixed features" requires at least three manic/hypomanic symptoms.		
2	Suicidal ideation in Major Depressive Disorder includes thoughts of death, specific plans, or attempts.		
3	Psychotic symptoms in Major Depression must be evaluated for mood congruence.		
4	Fatigue and low energy must occur nearly every day and impair functioning in MDD.		
5	A Major Depressive Episode must last at least 2 weeks, with depressed mood or loss of interest as key symptoms.		
6	Major Depressive Disorder episodes can recur, especially with multiple prior episodes or stressors.		
7	Hypersomnia can be part of Major Depression, especially in atypical presentations.		
8	Severe MDD with psychotic features involves mood-congruent delusions or hallucinations.		
9	In adolescents, MDD may manifest as irritability rather than pervasive sadness.		
10	Postpartum depression is classified as MDD with peripartum onset, not a separate disorder.		

Matching Exercise

1. Depressed Mood [ ]
2. Loss of Interest (Anhedonia) [ ]
3. Changes in Appetite [ ]
4. Psychomotor Agitation or Retardation [ ]
5. Suicidal Ideation [ ]
6. Recurrent Major Depressive Disorder [ ]

Descriptions:

- A. May involve low appetite or, conversely, overeating
- B. Repeated depressive episodes separated by periods of remission
- C. Recurrent thoughts of death, plans, or suicide attempts
- D. The individual reports sadness, emptiness, or hopelessness most of the day
- E. Slowed movements and speech, or conversely, restlessness
- F. Loss of pleasure in activities once found enjoyable, including decreased sexual desire

Case Study

A 30-year-old woman has, for the past two months, felt persistently sad, low-energy, and uninterested in previously enjoyable activities (spending time with friends, watching movies, gardening). She has noticed a marked decrease in appetite and has lost 5 kg. She frequently feels guilty "for no apparent reason" and has trouble concentrating at work. Mornings are especially hard, and she feels fatigued throughout the day. At times, she's had thoughts like "maybe it would be better not to wake up," though she hasn't formed a specific suicidal plan. There is no history of manic or hypomanic moods. Her social and occupational functioning has worsened.

1. Which factor most strongly points to a Major Depressive Episode?
   - A. A marked decrease in the need for sleep
   - B. Alternation of euphoria and sadness
   - C. Persistently depressed mood, loss of pleasure, low energy, and guilt for at least 2 weeks
   - D. Brief angry outbursts
2. Why is this not a bipolar picture?
   - A. Because she sleeps very little
   - B. She has no history or current signs of mania/hypomania
   - C. The duration of symptoms is too short
   - D. There is no family history of mood disorders
3. What could be an initial treatment approach?
   - A. No therapy, as it will resolve spontaneously in a few days
   - B. Starting an antidepressant and considering psychotherapy (e.g., cognitive behavioral therapy)
   - C. Only prescribing anxiolytics as needed
   - D. Advising against any physical activity and waiting for spontaneous improvement

Answers

Multiple Choice Questions
1. C
2. C
3. C
4. C
5. A
6. B
7. A

True/False Questions
1. False
2. True
3. True
4. True
5. True
6. True
7. True
8. True
9. True
10. False

Matching Exercise
1. D
2. F
3. A
4. E
5. C
6. B

Case Study Answers and Explanations
1. C – A depressed mood, anhedonia, fatigue, and guilt for at least 2 weeks are key indicators of a Major Depressive Episode.
2. B – There are no signs of mania or hypomania, which are required to consider a bipolar spectrum disorder.
3. B – Commonly, an antidepressant plus psychotherapy (especially CBT) is recommended as a first step.

Persistent Depressive Disorder (Dysthymia)

Multiple Choice Questions

1. Which key feature distinguishes Persistent Depressive Disorder (Dysthymia) from Major Depressive Disorder according to the DSM-5?
   - A. The presence of hallucinations and delusions
   - B. A prolonged duration of depressive symptoms (at least 2 years in adults) with often subthreshold intensity
   - C. Alternation between marked euphoria and brief depressive episodes
   - D. Absence of any anxiety symptoms during the depressed periods
2. Compared to Major Depressive Disorder, how is mood typically characterized in Dysthymia?
   - A. Profoundly euphoric for most of the day
   - B. Constantly shifting between irritability and anger
   - C. Chronically depressed, often described as a "constant sadness"
   - D. Normal, with only rare fluctuations
3. For diagnosing Persistent Depressive Disorder in children and adolescents, symptoms must be present for at least:
   - A. 6 months
   - B. 1 year
   - C. 2 years
   - D. 3 months
4. Which of the following symptoms may accompany Dysthymia, even if typically less intense than in a Major Depressive Episode?
   - A. Euphoric mood with hints of mania
   - B. Changes in appetite (decreased or increased), sleep problems, low self-esteem, and trouble concentrating
   - C. Total loss of interest in every activity and absolute social withdrawal
   - D. Constant delusions of guilt and persecution
5. Can a patient with Dysthymia also develop Major Depressive Episodes?
   - A. No, it is incompatible with Persistent Depressive Disorder
   - B. Yes, a chronic dysthymic condition can sometimes be overlaid by a Major Depressive Episode (double depression)
   - C. Yes, but it immediately transforms into Bipolar Disorder
   - D. No, because Dysthymia rules out any form of Major Depressive Episode
6. According to the DSM-5, for Persistent Depressive Disorder (Dysthymia) in adults, depressive symptoms must not be absent for longer than:
   - A. Two consecutive months
   - B. Six consecutive months
   - C. One consecutive month
   - D. Two consecutive weeks
7. Which of the following factors can complicate the diagnosis of Dysthymia?
   - A. Late onset (after age 60) with no anxiety symptoms
   - B. Co-occurrence of anxiety disorders or other affective disorders that mask chronic symptoms
   - C. Brief hypomanic episodes featuring strong euphoria
   - D. Absence of depressive symptoms before age 30

True/False Questions

		T	F
1	In Persistent Depressive Disorder, symptom intensity can fluctuate but generally remains milder than Major Depressive Disorder.		
2	Dysthymia often begins during childhood or adolescence and may persist for many years.		
3	Individuals with Dysthymia may experience Major Depressive Episodes, leading to a "double depression" diagnosis.		
4	Two years of persistent depressive symptoms are required to diagnose Dysthymia in adults.		
5	Low self-esteem, poor concentration, and reduced energy are key features of Persistent Depressive Disorder.		
6	Symptom-free periods in Persistent Depressive Disorder cannot exceed two months within the diagnostic timeframe.		
7	Persistent Depressive Disorder is often labeled as chronic depression due to its prolonged duration and consistent symptoms.		
8	Major Depressive Episodes can occur alongside Dysthymia, complicating the clinical presentation.		
9	Day-to-day variations in mood are possible in Dysthymia, even though the overall pattern is chronic.		
10	Early-onset Dysthymia is associated with greater severity, higher comorbidity, and poorer treatment response.		

Matching Exercise

1. Chronically depressed mood [ ]
2. Double Depression [ ]
3. Minimum duration in adults [ ]
4. Minimum duration in childhood/adolescence [ ]
5. Low self-esteem [ ]
6. Persistent Depressive Disorder (Dysthymia) [ ]

Descriptions:

- A. Chronic depressive symptoms lasting at least 2 years in adults
- B. An overlap of a Major Depressive Episode on top of a dysthymic condition
- C. Constant sadness, a "down" mood most of the day
- D. At least 1 year of symptoms if onset occurs before age 18
- E. Often related to feelings of inadequacy and low self-confidence
- F. The DSM-5 name for what was previously known as "Dysthymia"

Case Study

A 40-year-old man describes feeling a "background" of sadness most days for many years, going back to his teenage years. He cannot recall periods longer than a few weeks without feeling "down." He also reports reduced appetite, sleep disturbances, low self-esteem, and ongoing demotivation. While he has never had a depressive episode so severe as to stop him from functioning entirely, in recent months these symptoms have worsened to the point that they now resemble a Major Depressive Episode. He has no history of mania or hypomania.

1. Which element suggests this is Persistent Depressive Disorder?
   - A. Noticeable euphoria alternating with low moods
   - B. Long-term depressed mood, subthreshold for years, now exacerbated
   - C. Absence of depressive symptoms during adolescence
   - D. Presence of past hypomanic episodes
2. How do we describe the current worsening of symptoms, where they approximate a Major Depressive Episode on top of chronic Dysthymia?
   - A. Automatic transition to Bipolar Disorder
   - B. Double Depression (Major Depressive Episode overlapping Dysthymia)
   - C. Spontaneous remission
   - D. A psychotic episode tied to mood
3. What might be an initial therapeutic approach?
   - A. No intervention, since Dysthymia does not respond to specific treatments
   - B. Start an antidepressant and/or psychotherapy (e.g., Cognitive Behavioral or Interpersonal Therapy), considering any recent triggers
   - C. Only short-term anxiolytics
   - D. Immediate ECT

Answers

Multiple Choice Questions

1. B
2. C
3. B
4. B
5. B
6. A
7. B

True/False Questions

1. False
2. True
3. True
4. True
5. True
6. True
7. True
8. True
9. False
10. True

Matching Exercise

1. C
2. B
3. A
4. D
5. E
6. F

Case Study Answers and Explanations

1. B – A chronically depressed mood over many years at a subthreshold level, now intensified, is typical of Dysthymia (Persistent Depressive Disorder).
2. B – When a Major Depressive Episode is superimposed on a dysthymic background, this is referred to as "Double Depression."
3. B – Treatment often involves antidepressant medication and psychotherapeutic support, exploring potential triggers that may have led to the exacerbation.

Premenstrual Dysphoric Disorder (PMDD)

Multiple Choice Questions

1. Which of the following is the main feature of Premenstrual Dysphoric Disorder (PMDD) according to the DSM-5?
    - A. Manic episodes exclusively in the premenstrual phase
    - B. Emotional and physical symptoms occurring during most menstrual cycles, causing significant functional impairment
    - C. A single depressive episode in adolescence
    - D. Absence of anxious or irritable symptoms
2. During which phase of the menstrual cycle do PMDD symptoms typically intensify?
    - A. The ovulatory phase
    - B. The early follicular phase
    - C. The week before menstruation, subsiding in the first few days of flow
    - D. Post-menopausal period
3. Which of the following symptoms is commonly associated with PMDD?
    - A. Persistent euphoria with hyperactivity
    - B. Deep sadness, marked irritability, anxiety, and emotional lability
    - C. Complete amnesia and derealization
    - D. Stable delusions of grandeur throughout the cycle
4. To diagnose PMDD, symptoms must be:
    - A. Always mild and not affect functioning
    - B. Present every single day of the month
    - C. Severe enough to interfere with daily activities, work, school, or relationships
    - D. Totally absent right after ovulation
5. Which feature helps distinguish PMDD from Major Depressive Disorder?
    - A. PMDD is only seen in males, with atypical symptoms
    - B. PMDD follows a cyclical pattern linked to the luteal phase, with partial or complete remission at other times
    - C. Major Depressive Disorder occurs only in the postpartum period
    - D. PMDD includes constant paranoid delusions
6. Which of the following factors might increase the likelihood of developing PMDD?
    - A. No genetic or hormonal predisposition
    - B. A stress-free lifestyle with no challenges
    - C. Family history of mood disorders, hormonal imbalances, and/or chronic stress
    - D. A single situational anxiety episode in childhood
7. Which treatment is often indicated for PMDD in moderately to severely affected individuals?
    - A. Passive monitoring without any intervention
    - B. Regressive psychoanalysis plus typical antipsychotics
    - C. Antidepressants (SSRIs) during symptomatic phases and/or hormonal therapy, alongside supportive interventions (psychotherapy, lifestyle changes)
    - D. Immediate electroconvulsive therapy (ECT)

True/False Questions

		T	F
1	PMDD symptoms appear exclusively during ovulation and disappear entirely after it.		
2	Irritability, mood swings, and anxiety are typical emotional symptoms of PMDD.		
3	By definition, PMDD does not affect social or occupational functioning.		
4	For a PMDD diagnosis, observing symptoms for just one month is sufficient; repeated cycles are not required.		
5	Some women with PMDD may benefit from SSRIs taken only during the luteal phase of the cycle.		
6	PMDD can present physical symptoms such as breast tenderness, headaches, and bloating.		
7	Men can develop PMDD if they have a family history of mood disorders.		
8	Lifestyle changes, such as diet and exercise, may help relieve some PMDD symptoms.		
9	PMDD is always characterized by severe depressive episodes lasting the entire menstrual cycle.		
10	The use of hormonal contraceptives can sometimes alleviate PMDD symptoms but does not guarantee complete remission.		

Matching Exercise

1. Luteal phase [ ]
2. Emotional lability [ ]
3. Overlap with Major Depressive Disorder [ ]
4. Physical symptoms [ ]
5. Intermittent SSRI treatment [ ]
6. Impact on functioning [ ]

Descriptions:

- A. Rapidly shifting mood (e.g., irritability, sadness, anxiety)
- B. Significantly undermines quality of life and relationships if untreated
- C. Cycle phase in which PMDD symptoms typically appear and worsen
- D. Taking medication only during the critical phase of the cycle rather than continuously
- E. May coexist, but PMDD follows a monthly cyclical pattern
- F. Bloating, breast tenderness, headaches

Case Study

A 28-year-old woman has, for at least one year, experienced a marked worsening of mood, anxiety, and irritability about a week before her period, with a gradual lessening in the first few days of flow. She reports relationship and work difficulties during that time, including sudden crying spells and pronounced emotional instability. She also experiences physical symptoms such as abdominal bloating and breast tenderness. Once her period starts, symptoms nearly disappear. She has no manic or hypomanic episodes at any other time of the month. Her occupational and social functioning suffer in these "critical" days.

1. Which factor supports a PMDD diagnosis in this woman?
   - A. True mania limited to a two-day window
   - B. Cyclical emotional and physical symptoms that arise in the premenstrual phase and subside during or shortly after flow
   - C. Absence of anxiety
   - D. Persistent low mood without fluctuation throughout the month
2. How is this cyclical pattern, which worsens in the luteal phase and improves after menstrual onset, defined?
   - A. Menstrual-related cyclothymia
   - B. Episodic course of Major Depressive Disorder
   - C. Typical course of PMDD
   - D. Psychotic episode associated with the cycle
3. Which treatment approach might be considered?
   - A. None, since symptoms resolve spontaneously
   - B. SSRIs taken luteally or continuously, possibly plus stress management techniques
   - C. Typical antipsychotics at high doses
   - D. Pre-menstrual electroconvulsive therapy

Answers

Multiple Choice Questions

1. B
2. C
3. C
4. C
5. B
6. C
7. C

True/False Questions (8 total)

1. False
2. True
3. False
4. False
5. True
6. True
7. False
8. True
9. False
10. True

Matching Exercise

1. C
2. A
3. E
4. F
5. D
6. B

Case Study Answers and Explanations

1. B – Her cyclical emotional and physical symptoms in the premenstrual phase, with near-total relief during menstruation, align with PMDD.
2. C – This cyclical pattern is characteristic of PMDD.
3. B – SSRIs taken luteally or continuously, plus stress-management techniques, are often recommended.

Prolonged Grief Disorder

Multiple Choice Questions

1. Which of the following is a diagnostic criterion for Prolonged Grief Disorder according to the DSM-5-TR?
   - A. Persistent inability to accept the loss for at least 6 months
   - B. Intense yearning or longing for the deceased lasting at least 12 months
   - C. Recurrent episodes of anger in response to the loss
   - D. Physical symptoms related to grief emerging within 1 month of the loss
2. Which of the following is **not** a typical symptom of Prolonged Grief Disorder?
   - A. Persistent difficulty resuming daily life
   - B. Loss of interest in routine activities
   - C. Excessive fear of physical illness
   - D. Persistent sense of emotional emptiness
3. Which of the following differential diagnoses is essential to consider in Prolonged Grief Disorder?
   - A. Major Depressive Disorder
   - B. Generalized Anxiety Disorder
   - C. Post-Traumatic Stress Disorder
   - D. All of the above
4. According to the DSM-5-TR, how much time must pass after the loss to diagnose Prolonged Grief Disorder in adults?
   - A. 6 months
   - B. 12 months
   - C. 18 months
   - D. 24 months
5. Which of the following treatment approaches is most commonly recommended for Prolonged Grief Disorder?
   - A. Pharmacological treatment with SSRIs
   - B. Grief-focused therapy
   - C. Group therapy for anxiety management
   - D. Dialectical Behavior Therapy (DBT)
6. Which of the following risk factors increases the likelihood of developing Prolonged Grief Disorder?
   - A. Sudden or traumatic loss
   - B. Family history of complicated grief
   - C. Lack of adequate social support
   - D. All of the above
7. What distinguishes Prolonged Grief Disorder from other psychiatric conditions?
   - A. Excessive focus on the specific loss
   - B. Absence of physical symptoms
   - C. Symptoms exclusively related to anxiety
   - D. Duration limited to 6 months

True/False Questions

		T	F
1	Prolonged Grief Disorder can only be diagnosed after 6 months from the loss.		
2	The prevalence of Prolonged Grief Disorder is consistent across all cultures.		
3	Pharmacological therapy is always the first-line treatment for Prolonged Grief Disorder.		
4	Diagnosis requires the presence of functional impairments that significantly interfere with daily life.		
5	Individuals with a strong social support network are less likely to develop Prolonged Grief Disorder.		
6	The DSM-5-TR includes a specific section to differentiate normal grief from Prolonged Grief Disorder.		
7	Children can develop Prolonged Grief Disorder, but diagnostic criteria differ from adults.		
8	Cognitive Behavioral Therapy is ineffective in treating this disorder.		
9	Prolonged Grief Disorder completely overlaps with Major Depressive Disorder.		
10	Losing a pet cannot result in Prolonged Grief Disorder according to the DSM-5-TR.		

Matching Exercise

1. Inability to accept the loss [ ]
2. Intense yearning for the deceased [ ]
3. Persistent sense of emptiness or worthlessness [ ]
4. Difficulty reinvesting in relationships or activities [ ]
5. Sudden loss as a risk factor [ ]
6. Grief-focused therapy [ ]

Descriptions:

- A. A psychotherapeutic treatment that helps individuals process the loss and adjust.
- B. A core symptom of Prolonged Grief Disorder that involves excessive focus on the loss.
- C. A central feeling characterizing Prolonged Grief Disorder.
- D. Predisposing factor linked to traumatic or unexpected events.
- E. Functional impairment interfering with the ability to form new relationships.
- F. Persistent longing and desire for the loved one.

Case Study

Jessica, a 42-year-old woman, lost her husband 18 months ago in a sudden car accident. Since then, she reports a persistent inability to accept the loss, intense yearning for her husband, and a pervasive sense of emptiness. She struggles to return to work and avoids social activities. Despite having family support, she feels unable to imagine a life without her husband. She has no prior history of psychiatric conditions.

1. Which treatment would be most appropriate for Jessica?
   - A. Grief-focused therapy
   - B. Pharmacological treatment with antipsychotics
   - C. Group therapy for social anxiety
   - D. No treatment, as her symptoms are normal
2. Which symptom distinguishes Jessica's case as Prolonged Grief Disorder?
   - A. Loss of appetite
   - B. Persistent inability to accept the loss
   - C. Episodes of anger
   - D. Sleep disturbances
3. Which differential diagnosis should be considered?
   - A. Post-Traumatic Stress Disorder
   - B. Obsessive-Compulsive Disorder
   - C. Social Anxiety Disorder
   - D. Borderline Personality Disorder

Answers

Multiple Choice Questions:

1. B
2. C
3. D
4. B
5. B
6. D
7. A

True/False Questions:

1. False
2. False
3. False
4. True
5. True
6. True
7. True
8. False
9. False
10. False

Matching Exercise:

1. B
2. F
3. C
4. E
5. D
6. A

Case Study Answers and Explanations:

1. A – Explanation: Grief-focused therapy is the most effective approach to help Jessica process the loss and rebuild her life.
2. B – Explanation: Persistent inability to accept the loss is a hallmark symptom of Prolonged Grief Disorder.
3. A – Explanation: Post-Traumatic Stress Disorder is a relevant differential diagnosis given the sudden nature of the loss.

Other Depressive Disorders

Multiple Choice Questions

1. Which of the following typically falls under the DSM-5 category "Other Depressive Disorders"?
    - A. A complete Major Depression with hallucinations
    - B. Hypomanic episodes alternating with manic episodes
    - C. Depressive presentations whose symptoms do not fully meet the criteria for Major Depressive Disorder, Dysthymia, or PMDD, yet are still clinically significant
    - D. A purely anxiety-related disorder without mood components
2. When do you use the diagnosis "Specified Depressive Disorder" versus "Unspecified Depressive Disorder"?
    - A. "Specified" when bipolar symptoms overlap; "Unspecified" if symptoms are purely anxious
    - B. "Specified" when you want to clarify why the full criteria are not met (e.g., insufficient duration); "Unspecified" when there is insufficient information for a more precise diagnosis
    - C. "Specified" is synonymous with atypical Major Depression; "Unspecified" is psychotic Major Depression
    - D. There is no difference: they are identical designations
3. In which scenario might one diagnose a "Specified Depressive Disorder"?
    - A. A single 4-day hypomanic episode without depressed mood
    - B. A depressive symptomatology lasting 1 week, causing significant impairment but not meeting the 2-week minimum for Major Depression
    - C. A Major Depressive Episode meeting all criteria fully
    - D. A condition purely tied to psychotic disorders with no depressive features
4. Which of the following clinical presentations might be labeled "Unspecified Depressive Disorder"?
    - A. A patient with a clear manic episode
    - B. Someone about whom very little is known (e.g., briefly seen in an ER), presenting with poorly investigated depressive symptoms
    - C. A Bipolar II pattern with rapid cycles
    - D. A person who develops secondary OCD
5. Which factor makes the "Other Depressive Disorders" category useful?
    - A. It classifies every form of Depression as "untreatable"
    - B. It helps capture atypical or incomplete depressive situations, ensuring important clinical data are not lost
    - C. It disallows the use of other diagnostic specifiers
    - D. It is exclusively for seasonal depression
6. Why might one opt for the label "Other Depressive Disorders" in a clinical setting (e.g., ER)?
    - A. Because recognizing any mood disorder is impossible
    - B. To confirm the patient does not have an anxiety condition
    - C. Because there is insufficient information to diagnose Major Depression or another more specific disorder, yet the presentation appears depressive in nature
    - D. To simplify searching for an underlying bipolar condition
7. Which option describes a "Specified Depressive Disorder" with subthreshold duration and intensity?
    - A. A single day of sadness without a clear cause
    - B. Episodes of depressed mood lasting about 10 days, recurring cyclically, but never reaching the 14-day minimum for Major Depression
    - C. Dysthymia persisting for over 2 years
    - D. A mild euphoric period following bereavement

True/False Questions

		T	F
1	The “Specified” and “Unspecified” categories are reserved exclusively for depressive disorders with atypical presentations.		
2	“Specified Depressive Disorder” clarifies why the full criteria of a depressive disorder are unmet, such as insufficient symptom duration or frequency.		
3	An “Unspecified Depressive Disorder” is used when the clinician cannot determine whether symptoms align with a specific depressive category due to limited information.		
4	A “Specified Depressive Disorder” cannot be diagnosed if a past hypomanic episode has occurred and the current symptoms suggest Bipolar II Disorder.		
5	The “Specified” and “Unspecified” categories provide flexibility for noting depressive features that deviate from standard criteria, like atypical symptom patterns.		
6	The “Specified” and “Unspecified” categories should not be used in emergency settings, even if a depressive disorder is suspected.		
7	A “Specified Depressive Disorder” may include depressive episodes lasting less than two weeks but with severe functional impairment.		
8	These categories (Specified/Unspecified) are inappropriate for replacing Major Depressive Disorder diagnoses unless the duration of symptoms is below diagnostic thresholds.		
9	It is permissible to use “Specified Depressive Disorder” for depressive episodes that fail to meet the minimum two-week duration for MDD.		
10	“Unspecified Depressive Disorder” can be applied even if there is strong clinical suspicion of Bipolar Disorder but insufficient evidence to confirm it.		

Matching Exercise

1. Subthreshold presentations [ ]
2. Unclear reason (little info) [ ]
3. “Short duration” specifier [ ]
4. Save time in the ER [ ]
5. Depressive presentation [ ]
6. Need for additional data [ ]

Descriptions:

- A. Used in emergencies when it’s impossible to define MDD or another disorder precisely
- B. Early stages of a depressive picture, with insufficient duration or intensity for MDD
- C. The patient shows signs of depression, but the minimum duration is not met
- D. Designed to avoid diagnostic confusion and to avoid losing atypical depressive cases
- E. When a Depressive Disorder is suspected, but there is not enough evidence to confirm it
- F. A scenario in which it is clear the picture is depressive, but it doesn’t meet the full criteria for MDD, Dysthymia, or PMDD

Case Study

A 25-year-old man arrives at the ER with depressive symptoms (marked sadness, guilt, low energy, poor concentration) for about 10 days. It's unclear whether he has had any past manic episodes or recent bereavement. He reports significant distress affecting his work and relationships, but he does not fully meet the criteria for a Major Depressive Episode (requiring at least 2 weeks). Moreover, information is lacking to rule out a more defined mood disorder (like Dysthymia or PMDD). This appears to be a depressive condition needing further data before a more precise diagnosis can be made.

1. Which diagnosis might be most fitting here, given the short duration and limited information?
   - A. Specified Depressive Disorder (Brief Episode)
   - B. Unspecified Depressive Disorder
   - C. Major Depressive Disorder with Psychotic Features
   - D. Rapid-cycling Bipolar Disorder
2. Which strategy would recognize the depressive dimension without forcing a complete diagnosis?
   - A. Admitting the patient into a schizophrenia protocol
   - B. Using "Other Depressive Disorders" (Specified or Unspecified) and indicating missing criteria
   - C. Recording no diagnosis until mania appears
   - D. Labeling it Major Depressive Disorder even though the duration is insufficient
3. What initial therapeutic and diagnostic step would be advisable?
   - A. No intervention, given the short duration
   - B. Gathering more information (history, possible tests), assessing the need for psychological or pharmacological support depending on severity
   - C. Prescribing high-dose typical antipsychotics
   - D. Immediate electroconvulsive therapy

Answers

Multiple Choice Questions

1. C
2. B
3. B
4. B
5. B
6. C
7. B

True/False Questions

1. False
2. True
3. True
4. True
5. True
6. False
7. True
8. False
9. True
10. False

Matching Exercise

1. B
2. A
3. C
4. D
5. F
6. E

Case Study Answers and Explanation

1. B – Unspecified Depressive Disorder may be more appropriate, given the limited info and sub-2-week duration.
2. B – Labeling the presentation as "Other Depressive Disorder" (Specified or Unspecified) highlights the depressive element without forcing a standard MDD label.
3. B – Collect more details, evaluate severity, and consider psychological or pharmacological intervention if needed.

Anxiety Disorders

This category includes conditions where excessive worry or intense fear extends beyond what might be considered a helpful response to danger or a motivator for improved performance. These disorders involve cognitive, emotional, and physical symptoms such as recurring alarm thoughts, muscle tension, restlessness, palpitations, sweating, and difficulty concentrating. Such symptoms may significantly affect everyday life, limiting social activities, job performance, or school achievement.

Among Anxiety Disorders, Generalized Anxiety Disorder (GAD) is marked by persistent, hard-to-control worry about various areas of life (health, work, relationships) coupled with restlessness, irritability, and fatigue. Panic Disorder involves sudden, severe episodes of anxiety (panic attacks), often followed by fear of future attacks or life changes made to avoid them. Agoraphobia centers on the fear of being in places or situations where escape might be hard, or where help might not be available if a panic attack occurs—crowded places, open spaces, or public transportation, for example.

Some forms of anxiety relate to specific triggers: Specific Phobia refers to a persistent, irrational fear of objects or situations (such as spiders, flying, or heights), so intense that the person systematically avoids the feared object or situation. Social Anxiety Disorder (Social Phobia) centers on interactions in which one feels judged by others (speaking in public, meeting new people), to the point of disrupting daily life. Selective Mutism usually appears in childhood, where a child capable of speaking freely at home remains silent in social settings perceived as anxious.

From a diagnostic standpoint, it's important to rule out medical conditions (such as cardiac issues or hyperthyroidism) or the influence of stimulants that can mimic these symptoms. Clinicians should also distinguish between different anxiety disorders, as they sometimes coexist with other issues like depression or obsessive-compulsive disorders.

Regarding treatment, cognitive-behavioral therapy is often considered particularly effective, incorporating relaxation techniques, gradual exposure to the feared stimulus, and cognitive restructuring of unhelpful beliefs. In some cases, psychiatrists may prescribe anti-anxiety or antidepressant medications, especially if symptoms are very disabling or accompany other mental health challenges. Coordination among professionals (psychologists, psychiatrists, primary care physicians) and the active participation of the individual with anxiety are key to establishing an effective treatment plan.

Separation Anxiety Disorder

Multiple Choice Questions

1. Which of the following is a primary diagnostic criterion for Separation Anxiety Disorder?
    - A. Excessive fear of meeting new people.
    - B. Marked anxiety when separated from an attachment figure.
    - C. Repetitive behaviors aimed at reducing anxiety.
    - D. Episodes of elevated mood and impulsive behaviors.
2. Which symptom is commonly associated with Separation Anxiety Disorder in children?
    - A. Social withdrawal and lack of friends.
    - B. Vocal or physical protests when separating from a caregiver.
    - C. Motor disturbances such as tremors or tics.
    - D. Obsessive behaviors related to cleanliness.
3. Separation Anxiety Disorder can be diagnosed in which age group?
    - A. Only in children under 12 years old.
    - B. Exclusively in adolescents.
    - C. Both in children and adults.
    - D. Only in adults over 18 years old.
4. How long must symptoms persist for a diagnosis of Separation Anxiety Disorder?
    - A. At least two weeks.
    - B. At least one month in children, six months in adults.
    - C. At least three months.
    - D. At least one year.
5. Which differential diagnosis is most important to rule out when considering Separation Anxiety Disorder?
    - A. Major Depressive Disorder.
    - B. Obsessive-Compulsive Disorder.
    - C. Agoraphobia.
    - D. Post-Traumatic Stress Disorder.
6. A child with Separation Anxiety Disorder is most likely to display:
    - A. Excessive risk-taking behaviors.
    - B. Crying or tantrums during separations.
    - C. Aggressive behavior toward strangers.
    - D. A marked interest in solitary activities.
7. Which treatment is commonly considered effective for Separation Anxiety Disorder?
    - A. Cognitive-behavioral therapy.
    - B. Electroconvulsive therapy.
    - C. Pharmacological treatment alone.
    - D. Minimal psychosocial interventions.

True/False Questions

		T	F
1	Separation Anxiety Disorder is limited to children.		
2	Symptoms of Separation Anxiety Disorder include excessive worry about the well-being of attachment figures.		
3	The most effective treatment for Separation Anxiety Disorder is always pharmacological.		
4	Adults can develop Separation Anxiety Disorder in response to stressful events.		
5	Separation Anxiety Disorder is a type of specific phobia.		
6	A diagnostic criterion is the inability to sleep away from home without an attachment figure.		
7	Individuals with this disorder may experience physical symptoms such as headaches or nausea during separations.		
8	Symptoms must cause clinically significant distress or impairment in social, academic, or occupational areas.		
9	Experiencing separations during early childhood prevents the development of this disorder.		
10	Exposure therapy is a useful technique in treating Separation Anxiety Disorder.		

Matching Exercise

1. Early separation from attachment figures. [ ]
2. Cognitive-behavioral therapy. [ ]
3. Minimum duration of symptoms for adults. [ ]
4. Physical symptoms related to anxiety. [ ]
5. Onset of the disorder. [ ]
6. Related differential diagnosis. [ ]

Descriptions:

- A. A therapeutic method aimed at altering dysfunctional thoughts.
- B. Six months of persistent symptoms.
- C. Headaches, nausea, abdominal pain.
- D. Common in childhood but may also emerge in adulthood.
- E. Trauma from separation or loss.
- F. Agoraphobia.

Case Study

Anna, an 8-year-old girl, displays excessive crying when she has to go to school, accompanied by abdominal pain and nausea. She fears that something might happen to her mother while they are apart. She refuses to sleep away from home and avoids school trips. The family does not report specific traumas but mentions that the mother is often very anxious.

1. What is the most prominent symptom supporting a diagnosis of Separation Anxiety Disorder?
   - A. Abdominal pain.
   - B. Anxiety about being separated from her mother.
   - C. Fear of school.
   - D. Refusal to attend school trips.
2. Which treatment would be most appropriate for Anna?
   - A. Cognitive-behavioral therapy.
   - B. Pharmacological treatment only.
   - C. Parent psychoeducation without direct therapy for Anna.
   - D. Intensive residential treatment.
3. Which of the following differential diagnoses should be ruled out?
   - A. Obsessive-Compulsive Disorder.
   - B. Major Depressive Disorder.
   - C. Panic Disorder.
   - D. Agoraphobia.

Answers

Multiple Choice Questions:
1. B
2. B
3. C
4. B
5. C
6. B
7. A

True/False Questions:
1. False
2. True
3. False
4. True
5. False
6. True
7. True
8. True
9. False
10. True

Matching Exercise:
1. E
2. A
3. B
4. C
5. D
6. F

Case Study Answers and Explanations:
1. B. Explanation: Anxiety about being separated from her mother is central to Separation Anxiety Disorder.
2. A. Explanation: Cognitive-behavioral therapy is the first-line treatment for this disorder.
3. D. Explanation: Agoraphobia shares some characteristics but has distinct diagnostic criteria.

Selective Mutism

Multiple Choice Questions

1. Which of the following is a hallmark feature of Selective Mutism?
   - A. Lack of interest in social interaction.
   - B. Consistent failure to speak in specific social situations despite speaking in others.
   - C. Repetitive motor behaviors during anxiety-provoking situations.
   - D. Language delay unrelated to social settings.
2. What is a common setting where symptoms of Selective Mutism are most noticeable?
   - A. At home with family.
   - B. During one-on-one conversations with peers.
   - C. In structured settings like school or public gatherings.
   - D. When engaging in physical activities.
3. How long must the inability to speak in specific social contexts persist to meet diagnostic criteria for Selective Mutism?
   - A. At least one week.
   - B. At least one month.
   - C. At least three months.
   - D. At least six months.
4. Selective Mutism is most commonly comorbid with which of the following conditions?
   - A. Specific Learning Disorder.
   - B. Social Anxiety Disorder.
   - C. Autism Spectrum Disorder.
   - D. Attention-Deficit/Hyperactivity Disorder (ADHD).
5. Which of the following must be ruled out before diagnosing Selective Mutism?
   - A. Hearing impairment or language disorder.
   - B. Sleep disturbances.
   - C. Developmental coordination disorder.
   - D. Oppositional Defiant Disorder.
6. A key feature distinguishing Selective Mutism from Social Anxiety Disorder is:
   - A. Presence of physical symptoms such as sweating.
   - B. A consistent failure to speak in specific social contexts.
   - C. Preference for solitary activities.
   - D. Avoidance of speaking in all situations, including at home.
7. Which of the following treatments has shown the most efficacy for Selective Mutism?
   - A. Intensive psychoanalysis.
   - B. Pharmacological treatment as the sole intervention.
   - C. Behavioral interventions focusing on gradual exposure and positive reinforcement.
   - D. Group therapy with minimal individual attention.

True/False Questions

		T	F
1	Selective Mutism is diagnosed only if the individual does not speak in any context—including both home and school or other social settings.		
2	Adults can be diagnosed with Selective Mutism, though it is more commonly identified in children, and may co-occur with conditions such as Social Anxiety Disorder.		
3	A key feature of Selective Mutism is that it significantly interferes with one's educational or occupational functioning, or with normal social communication.		
4	For a DSM-5 diagnosis of Selective Mutism, the individual must show a complete lack of speech in every social context for at least three consecutive months.		
5	According to the DSM-5, symptoms of Selective Mutism must persist for at least one month and cannot be limited solely to the first month of school.		
6	Selective Mutism cannot be better explained by simple unfamiliarity with or discomfort in using a specific language in the social context.		
7	A diagnosis of Selective Mutism requires that the reluctance to speak is not attributable to a primary communication disorder (e.g., stuttering) and does not occur exclusively during an Autism Spectrum Disorder.		
8	Selective Mutism is most commonly identified for the first time in adolescence and is rarely recognized in children under age six.		
9	In the DSM-5, Selective Mutism is classified among the Anxiety Disorders, alongside conditions such as Social Anxiety Disorder (Social Phobia).		
10	Individuals with Selective Mutism may still communicate via nonverbal methods—such as gestures or writing—in settings where they remain verbally silent.		

Matching Exercise

1. Consistent inability to speak in specific social settings. [ ]
2. Comorbidity commonly observed with Selective Mutism. [ ]
3. Duration required for a diagnosis. [ ]
4. Primary age of onset. [ ]
5. Common treatment approach. [ ]
6. Differential condition to be ruled out. [ ]

Descriptions:

- A. Social Anxiety Disorder.
- B. One month.
- C. Gradual exposure with positive reinforcement.
- D. Hearing impairment or language disorder.
- E. Early childhood (typically before age 5).
- F. Failure to speak despite ability in other settings.

Case Study

A 7-year-old girl, Mia, is referred to a psychologist because she has never spoken in school, despite being able to speak fluently at home. Her teachers describe her as cooperative but silent, even when prompted to respond in class. Her parents mention that she becomes visibly anxious around unfamiliar adults. Mia does not show signs of a language delay or any hearing impairment.

1. What is the most likely diagnosis for Mia?
    - A. Social Anxiety Disorder.
    - B. Selective Mutism.
    - C. Autism Spectrum Disorder.
    - D. Speech Sound Disorder.
2. Which of the following would be the most appropriate initial intervention for Mia?
    - A. Immediate initiation of medication.
    - B. Behavioral therapy with gradual exposure to speaking tasks.
    - C. Family therapy focusing on parental anxiety.
    - D. Group therapy for children with speech delays.
3. Which differential diagnosis must be ruled out in Mia's case?
    - A. Attention-Deficit/Hyperactivity Disorder (ADHD).
    - B. Specific Learning Disorder.
    - C. Hearing impairment or language disorder.
    - D. Oppositional Defiant Disorder.

Answers

Multiple Choice Questions:

1. B
2. C
3. B
4. B
5. A
6. B
7. C

True/False Questions:

1. False
2. True
3. True
4. False
5. True
6. True
7. True
8. False
9. True
10. True

Matching Exercise:

1. F
2. A
3. B
4. E
5. C
6. D

Case Study Answers and Explanations:

1. B. Explanation: Mia's symptoms align with the diagnostic criteria for Selective Mutism, particularly her inability to speak in specific contexts despite being able to do so in others.
2. B. Explanation: Gradual exposure and positive reinforcement are evidence-based approaches for Selective Mutism.
3. C. Explanation: Hearing impairment or language disorder must be excluded before confirming the diagnosis.

Specific Phobia

Multiple Choice Questions

1. Which of the following distinguishes Specific Phobia from Social Anxiety Disorder?
   - A. The focus of fear is on performance or social scrutiny in Social Anxiety Disorder, whereas Specific Phobia is tied to a specific object or situation.
   - B. Both disorders involve persistent fear of specific triggers, so they are clinically identical.
   - C. Social Anxiety Disorder does not involve physical symptoms, while Specific Phobia does.
   - D. Specific Phobia is limited to childhood, while Social Anxiety Disorder can occur at any age.
2. A person with Specific Phobia, blood-injection-injury subtype, might differ physiologically from other phobia subtypes in that they:
   - A. Experience an increased heart rate and hyperventilation only.
   - B. Are less likely to faint during exposure to the feared stimulus.
   - C. Show an initial increase in heart rate followed by a vasovagal response causing fainting.
   - D. Do not experience physiological symptoms like other phobia subtypes.
3. In Specific Phobia, avoidance behaviors:
   - A. Are always absent because the person chooses to confront the feared stimulus.
   - B. Serve to temporarily reduce anxiety but reinforce the fear over time.
   - C. Are not a diagnostic requirement according to the DSM-5.
   - D. Must occur in all contexts to qualify for a diagnosis.
4. When treating Specific Phobia, which of the following interventions is considered most effective?
   - A. Gradual exposure therapy combined with relaxation techniques.
   - B. Long-term pharmacotherapy with anxiolytics.
   - C. Hypnosis to explore unconscious fears.
   - D. Avoiding the feared stimulus altogether to reduce distress.
5. What is an important factor to rule out when diagnosing Specific Phobia?
   - A. The person's acknowledgment that their fear is excessive.
   - B. The fear's association with a traumatic event.
   - C. That the fear is better explained by another mental disorder, such as Panic Disorder or PTSD.
   - D. The presence of a physical disability limiting exposure to the stimulus.
6. Which of the following is unique to the blood-injection-injury subtype compared to other phobia subtypes?
   - A. The absence of any physical symptoms.
   - B. The necessity for pharmacological treatment.
   - C. The risk of fainting due to a distinct vasovagal response.
   - D. The fear developing exclusively in early childhood.
7. Which scenario would most likely result in a diagnosis of Specific Phobia?
   - A. A person avoids elevators because they have a recurring fear of being trapped.
   - B. A person avoids social events due to a fear of being judged.
   - C. A person avoids public transportation due to fear of panic attacks.
   - D. A person fears leaving their home due to worries about safety in multiple locations.

True/False Questions

		T	F
1	According to the DSM-5, it is not necessary for the phobic stimulus to immediately trigger anxiety or fear when diagnosing Specific Phobia.		
2	Specific Phobias may include objects or situations such as flying, heights, animals, or injections, and they often involve persistent avoidance of the feared stimulus.		
3	A key criterion for Specific Phobia is that the fear or anxiety is out of proportion to the actual danger, taking the person's cultural context into account.		
4	The DSM-5 requires that symptoms of a Specific Phobia persist for at least 6 months in both adults and children.		
5	According to the DSM-5, Specific Phobias can occur with or without situational panic attacks, as long as there is intense and persistent anxiety related to the feared stimulus.		
6	Comorbidity between Specific Phobias and other anxiety disorders—such as Social Anxiety Disorder or Agoraphobia—is relatively common.		
7	The DSM-5 includes the need for clinically significant impairment, but does not require active avoidance of the phobic stimulus.		
8	For a diagnosis of Specific Phobia, symptoms must occur exclusively in the context of Post-Traumatic Stress Disorder (PTSD) or Obsessive-Compulsive Disorder (OCD).		
9	In the DSM-5, Specific Phobias may be further classified into subtypes (e.g., blood-injection-injury, situational, animal, natural environment, etc.).		
10	In the DSM-5, Specific Phobia and Social Anxiety Disorder (Social Phobia) are considered the same diagnosis, distinguished only by a specifier.		

Matching Exercise

1. Physiological response in blood-injection-injury subtype. [ ]
2. Effective intervention for treating Specific Phobia. [ ]
3. Key feature of avoidance behaviors in Specific Phobia. [ ]
4. Duration required for diagnosis. [ ]
5. Differentiating feature from Panic Disorder. [ ]
6. Common comorbid condition with Specific Phobia. [ ]

Descriptions:

- A. Systematic desensitization with gradual exposure.
- B. Six months or longer.
- C. Temporary relief from anxiety but reinforcement of fear.
- D. Triggered by specific stimuli, not unexpected attacks.
- E. Vasovagal response leading to fainting.
- F. Social Anxiety Disorder.

Case Study

James, a 30-year-old man, avoids flying due to an intense fear of being in enclosed spaces. Despite knowing air travel is statistically safe, he experiences rapid heartbeat, sweating, and dizziness at the thought of boarding a plane. He once booked a flight but canceled it at the last minute, opting to drive 12 hours to avoid the anxiety of flying. He has no history of traumatic events related to flying, and his fear does not generalize to other forms of transportation.

1. Based on James's symptoms, what feature of Specific Phobia is most relevant to his case?
    - A. The fear is triggered by a specific situation rather than multiple settings.
    - B. The fear generalizes to all forms of transportation.
    - C. The fear involves concerns about public scrutiny.
    - D. The fear is reinforced by repeated traumatic experiences.
2. Which treatment method is most likely to be effective for James?
    - A. Avoidance strategies to reduce immediate distress.
    - B. Gradual exposure therapy targeting flying-related stimuli.
    - C. Long-term pharmacological intervention with benzodiazepines.
    - D. Psychoanalysis to uncover repressed fears.
3. Which differential diagnosis should be ruled out in James's case?
    - A. Panic Disorder.
    - B. Agoraphobia.
    - C. Social Anxiety Disorder.
    - D. Generalized Anxiety Disorder.

Answers

Multiple Choice Questions:
1. A
2. C
3. B
4. A
5. C
6. C
7. A

True/False Questions:
1. False
2. True
3. True
4. True
5. True
6. True
7. False
8. False
9. True
10. False

Matching Exercise:
1. E
2. A
3. C
4. B
5. D
6. F

Case Study Answers and Explanations:
1. A. Explanation: James's fear is specific to flying, making this a classic case of situational Specific Phobia.
2. B. Explanation: Gradual exposure therapy is evidence-based and effective for reducing fear responses.
3. B. Explanation: Agoraphobia involves fear across multiple settings, unlike James's specific fear of flying.

Social Anxiety Disorder (Social Phobia)

Multiple Choice Questions

1. Which of the following is a core feature of Social Anxiety Disorder (SAD)?
    - A. Persistent fear of being judged or humiliated in social situations.
    - B. Avoidance of specific objects or animals.
    - C. Excessive worry about multiple life domains.
    - D. Recurrent and unexpected panic attacks in various settings.
2. In Social Anxiety Disorder, which of the following situations is most likely to provoke fear?
    - A. Being in an open space like a park.
    - B. Speaking in front of an audience.
    - C. Driving alone at night.
    - D. Traveling on an airplane.
3. Which subtype of Social Anxiety Disorder focuses on a single specific situation?
    - A. Generalized.
    - B. Non-specific.
    - C. Situational.
    - D. Performance.
4. Which of the following statements differentiates Social Anxiety Disorder from Avoidant Personality Disorder?
    - A. Social Anxiety Disorder is characterized by fear of rejection in all interpersonal relationships.
    - B. Avoidant Personality Disorder involves pervasive avoidance across all domains, while Social Anxiety Disorder is often limited to specific social settings.
    - C. Social Anxiety Disorder does not involve fear of rejection.
    - D. Avoidant Personality Disorder is typically treated with exposure therapy alone.
5. What is a common comorbidity in individuals with Social Anxiety Disorder?
    - A. Generalized Anxiety Disorder.
    - B. Schizophrenia.
    - C. Conduct Disorder.
    - D. Obsessive-Compulsive Personality Disorder.
6. Which intervention is considered first-line treatment for Social Anxiety Disorder?
    - A. Long-term use of benzodiazepines.
    - B. Cognitive-behavioral therapy focused on exposure and cognitive restructuring.
    - C. Psychodynamic therapy exploring early childhood conflicts.
    - D. Hypnosis aimed at uncovering unconscious fears.
7. Which of the following physical symptoms is commonly associated with Social Anxiety Disorder?
    - A. Frequent fainting episodes.
    - B. Sweating, trembling, and blushing.
    - C. Recurrent vomiting in social settings.
    - D. Severe headaches unrelated to anxiety-provoking situations.

True/False Questions

		T	F
1	In the DSM-5, there is a "performance only" specifier for Social Anxiety Disorder, in which fear is restricted to performance situations.		
2	Social Anxiety Disorder necessarily requires the presence of panic attacks in every feared social situation.		
3	According to the DSM-5, the fear of engaging in informal conversations can meet the diagnostic criteria for Social Anxiety Disorder.		
4	A diagnosis of Social Anxiety Disorder can still be made even if the individual's social impairment is fully attributable to an Autism Spectrum Disorder.		
5	A minimum duration of 6 months for symptoms is a key factor distinguishing Social Anxiety Disorder from more transient periods of shyness.		
6	If an individual with Social Anxiety Disorder appears merely shy, the clinical diagnosis can be disregarded.		
7	In the DSM-5, if a person experiences anxiety only in the presence of unfamiliar people—but not with family members or close friends—Social Anxiety Disorder is automatically ruled out.		
8	Sociocultural context plays a critical role in determining whether the individual's fear is out of proportion to the actual threat.		
9	According to the DSM-5, Social Anxiety Disorder precludes the simultaneous diagnosis of other anxiety disorders.		
10	Social Anxiety Disorder can be generalized or limited to performance situations, and in both cases, the individual may experience substantial impairment.		

Matching Exercise

1. Fear of public speaking or performing. [ ]
2. A common physical symptom in Social Anxiety Disorder. [ ]
3. Duration required for diagnosis of Social Anxiety Disorder. [ ]
4. Common comorbidity with Social Anxiety Disorder. [ ]
5. Effective treatment for Social Anxiety Disorder. [ ]
6. A differentiating feature of Avoidant Personality Disorder. [ ]

Descriptions:

- A. Six months or longer.
- B. Sweating, blushing, or trembling.
- C. Cognitive-behavioral therapy.
- D. Generalized Anxiety Disorder.
- E. Pervasive avoidance across all interpersonal relationships.
- F. Performance-only subtype.

Case Study

Emma, a 24-year-old graduate student, reports intense fear and anxiety during classroom presentations and group discussions. She avoids socializing with peers, fearing that they will judge her as incompetent. Emma often blushes and trembles during public speaking, which further reinforces her fear. Despite excelling academically, she feels her social anxiety is preventing her from networking and advancing in her career. She denies any traumatic social experiences in the past and is otherwise healthy.

1. Which diagnostic criterion is most relevant in Emma's case?
    - A. Excessive worry about multiple domains of life.
    - B. Persistent fear of being negatively evaluated in social situations.
    - C. Avoidance of all social interactions, including family gatherings.
    - D. Physical symptoms unrelated to social situations.
2. What would be the most effective initial treatment for Emma?
    - A. Long-term pharmacological treatment with sedatives.
    - B. Cognitive-behavioral therapy focusing on exposure and cognitive restructuring.
    - C. Psychoanalysis to explore past traumatic events.
    - D. Group therapy for general anxiety management.
3. Which of the following must be ruled out before confirming a diagnosis of Social Anxiety Disorder?
    - A. Generalized Anxiety Disorder.
    - B. Schizophrenia.
    - C. Specific Phobia.
    - D. Avoidant Personality Disorder.

Answers

Multiple Choice Questions:

1. A
2. B
3. D
4. B
5. A
6. B
7. B

True/False Questions:

1. True
2. False
3. True
4. False
5. True
6. False
7. False
8. True
9. False
10. True

Matching Exercise:

1. F
2. B
3. A
4. D
5. C
6. E

Case Study Answers and Explanations:

1. B. Explanation: Emma's persistent fear of negative evaluation in academic settings is a hallmark feature of Social Anxiety Disorder.
2. B. Explanation: Cognitive-behavioral therapy is evidence-based and effective, particularly for addressing avoidance and cognitive distortions.
3. D. Explanation: Avoidant Personality Disorder shares overlapping features but involves pervasive avoidance across all interpersonal domains.

Panic Disorder

Multiple Choice Questions

1. Which of the following is a hallmark feature of Panic Disorder?
   - A. Persistent and excessive worry about various life events.
   - B. Recurrent and unexpected panic attacks accompanied by concern about future attacks.
   - C. Avoidance of specific objects or situations triggering fear.
   - D. Constant fear of being embarrassed in social situations.
2. For a diagnosis of Panic Disorder, panic attacks must:
   - A. Occur exclusively in response to specific phobic stimuli.
   - B. Be predictable and occur at regular intervals.
   - C. Be unexpected and involve intense fear or discomfort.
   - D. Be triggered by physical activity or exertion.
3. Which of the following symptoms is most characteristic of a panic attack?
   - A. Persistent low mood and lack of energy.
   - B. Palpitations, chest pain, dizziness, and fear of dying.
   - C. Obsessive thoughts and compulsive behaviors.
   - D. Fear of leaving home and interacting with others.
4. Which feature differentiates Panic Disorder from Agoraphobia?
   - A. Panic Disorder involves fear of specific places.
   - B. Agoraphobia involves fear of being unable to escape or find help during a panic attack.
   - C. Agoraphobia is not associated with panic attacks.
   - D. Panic Disorder always involves fear of public spaces.
5. Which of the following comorbid conditions is most commonly associated with Panic Disorder?
   - A. Major Depressive Disorder.
   - B. Bipolar Disorder.
   - C. Schizophrenia.
   - D. Autism Spectrum Disorder.
6. Which treatment approach is considered first-line for Panic Disorder?
   - A. Exposure therapy alone.
   - B. Long-term benzodiazepine use without therapy.
   - C. Cognitive-behavioral therapy (CBT) focusing on interoceptive exposure.
   - D. Psychoanalysis to uncover unconscious fears.
7. What is the role of pharmacotherapy in treating Panic Disorder?
   - A. It is the sole treatment approach for most cases.
   - B. It is used to manage acute symptoms or as an adjunct to therapy.
   - C. It is primarily focused on antipsychotic medications.
   - D. It is not recommended in the management of Panic Disorder.

True/False Questions

		T	F
1	Panic attacks in Panic Disorder can solely be attributed to the direct physiological effects of a substance or a general medical condition.		
2	Panic Disorder requires that panic attacks are confined to a single specific type of situation or context.		
3	A hallmark of Panic Disorder is the persistent fear of additional panic attacks or their consequences.		
4	Somatic symptoms like palpitations, sweating, and trembling are typical of panic attacks and may contribute to the vicious cycle of fear.		
5	The diagnosis of Panic Disorder can be made even in the presence of a medical condition that fully explains the symptoms of panic attacks.		
6	Comorbidity with other anxiety disorders, such as agoraphobia, is not considered relevant for Panic Disorder in the DSM-5.		
7	Diagnostic criteria require a significant change in behavior related to panic attacks, such as avoiding specific places or situations.		
8	Panic attacks must occur daily for at least one month to meet the temporal criterion for Panic Disorder.		
9	Panic Disorder is considered more common in women than in men, according to epidemiological data.		
10	Panic Disorder may onset in adulthood, with symptoms that can appear suddenly without an apparent cause.		

Matching Exercise

1. Physical symptom often reported during a panic attack. [ ]
2. Key differentiating feature of Panic Disorder. [ ]
3. Common comorbidity with Panic Disorder. [ ]
4. A core component of CBT for Panic Disorder. [ ]
5. Duration required for concern about panic attacks to meet diagnostic criteria. [ ]
6. A condition that may be confused with Panic Disorder due to overlapping symptoms. [ ]

Descriptions:

- A. Interoceptive exposure.
- B. Fear of future attacks and behavioral changes lasting one month or longer.
- C. Palpitations or dizziness.
- D. Major Depressive Disorder.
- E. Agoraphobia.
- F. Recurrent and unexpected panic attacks.

Case Study

Alex, a 28-year-old office worker, presents with recurrent episodes of intense fear accompanied by chest pain, sweating, dizziness, and a feeling of losing control. These episodes occur unpredictably, even while relaxing at home. Alex now avoids situations like driving or being far from home, fearing another attack. He describes constant worry about when the next episode might occur and feels increasingly restricted in his daily activities.

1. Which feature in Alex's case is critical for diagnosing Panic Disorder?
    - A. Recurrent episodes of chest pain unrelated to fear.
    - B. Predictable panic attacks triggered by specific phobic stimuli.
    - C. Recurrent, unexpected panic attacks and avoidance behaviors.
    - D. Fear of public spaces and crowded areas.
2. What would be the most effective treatment approach for Alex?
    - A. Exposure therapy without addressing the panic symptoms.
    - B. Cognitive-behavioral therapy focusing on interoceptive exposure and cognitive restructuring.
    - C. Long-term use of sedative medications to manage anxiety.
    - D. Psychoanalysis to address underlying childhood conflicts.
3. Which of the following conditions should be ruled out before diagnosing Panic Disorder?
    - A. Specific Phobia.
    - B. Generalized Anxiety Disorder.
    - C. Cardiovascular or other medical conditions.
    - D. Schizophrenia.

Answers

Multiple Choice Questions:

1. B
2. C
3. B
4. B
5. A
6. C
7. B

True/False Questions:

1. True
2. False
3. True
4. True
5. False
6. False
7. True
8. False
9. True
10. True

Matching Exercise:

1. C
2. F
3. D
4. A
5. B
6. E

Case Study Answers and Explanations:

1. C. Explanation: Alex's symptoms include recurrent, unexpected panic attacks and significant behavioral changes due to fear of future attacks, aligning with Panic Disorder.
2. B. Explanation: Cognitive-behavioral therapy, including interoceptive exposure, is the gold standard for addressing both the physical and cognitive aspects of Panic Disorder.
3. C. Explanation: Medical conditions, particularly cardiovascular issues, must be ruled out to ensure symptoms are not caused by a physical condition.

Agoraphobia

Multiple Choice Questions

1. Which of the following scenarios is most characteristic of Agoraphobia?
   - A. Fear of specific social scrutiny during public speaking.
   - B. Avoidance of crowded places, open spaces, or traveling alone due to fear of being unable to escape or find help if panic-like symptoms occur.
   - C. Persistent fear of a specific object, such as spiders or heights.
   - D. Excessive worry about multiple aspects of daily life, including health and finances.
2. For a diagnosis of Agoraphobia, which of the following is required?
   - A. The fear must be limited to one specific setting, such as elevators or airplanes.
   - B. The person must experience significant distress in at least two different types of situations, such as open spaces and public transportation.
   - C. The fear must result from past trauma in a specific setting.
   - D. Symptoms must be directly caused by substance use or a medical condition.
3. Which of the following distinguishes Agoraphobia from Panic Disorder?
   - A. Agoraphobia does not involve avoidance behaviors.
   - B. Panic Disorder includes unexpected panic attacks, while Agoraphobia centers on fear of specific environments where escape might be difficult.
   - C. Agoraphobia requires a history of traumatic experiences in public spaces.
   - D. Panic Disorder always involves fear of public embarrassment.
4. Which of the following comorbid conditions is most commonly associated with Agoraphobia?
   - A. Schizophrenia.
   - B. Post-Traumatic Stress Disorder (PTSD).
   - C. Panic Disorder.
   - D. Obsessive-Compulsive Disorder (OCD).
5. What is the minimum number of situations that must provoke fear or anxiety for an Agoraphobia diagnosis according to the DSM-5?
   - A. One.
   - B. Two.
   - C. Three.
   - D. Four.
6. Which of the following is a common misconception about Agoraphobia?
   - A. It involves fear of open spaces only.
   - B. It can coexist with Panic Disorder.
   - C. Symptoms include distress in situations where escape is difficult.
   - D. Cognitive-behavioral therapy is an effective treatment.
7. Which treatment approach is considered most effective for Agoraphobia?
   - A. Psychoanalysis to address unconscious conflicts.
   - B. Cognitive-behavioral therapy focusing on gradual exposure to feared situations.
   - C. Pharmacological treatment without psychotherapy.
   - D. Avoidance of all anxiety-provoking situations.

True/False Questions

		T	F
1	Agoraphobia requires that symptoms are exclusively related to the fear of crowded places, such as markets or squares.		
2	A central feature of agoraphobia is the fear or anxiety about situations where escape might be difficult or help might not be available in the event of panic symptoms or embarrassment.		
3	To diagnose agoraphobia, symptoms must be present for at least six consecutive months but can vary in intensity.		
4	Active avoidance of feared situations is considered a diagnostic criterion for agoraphobia in the DSM-5.		
5	Agoraphobia can be diagnosed in the absence of other anxiety disorders, provided the criteria are met.		
6	Fear associated with agoraphobia is often disproportionate to the actual danger posed by the feared situations, according to diagnostic criteria.		
7	Agoraphobia typically manifests only in social contexts and not in physically isolated situations.		
8	The diagnosis of agoraphobia requires that symptoms are directly attributable to the physiological effects of a substance or general medical condition.		
9	Agoraphobia can onset in both adolescence and adulthood, with variations in symptom severity.		
10	Treatment for agoraphobia often includes both cognitive-behavioral therapy and, when necessary, anxiolytic or antidepressant medications.		

Matching Exercise

1. Fear of being in a crowd or queue. [ ]
2. Minimum duration required for diagnosis. [ ]
3. Effective treatment approach. [ ]
4. A key differentiating feature from Panic Disorder. [ ]
5. Common comorbid condition. [ ]
6. A situation that may provoke fear in Agoraphobia. [ ]

Descriptions:

- A. Fear of being unable to escape.
- B. Six months.
- C. Cognitive-behavioral therapy with exposure.
- D. Panic Disorder.
- E. Public transportation or open spaces.
- F. Crowded places like malls or stadiums.

Case Study

Lisa, a 34-year-old woman, reports intense fear and avoidance of traveling on buses and trains, shopping in crowded malls, and walking alone in open spaces. She worries about experiencing dizziness or losing control in these situations and feels trapped. Her fear began after a panic attack on a train two years ago. Lisa's symptoms have progressively worsened, and she now avoids leaving her home unless accompanied by her husband.

1. Which aspect of Lisa's case is most critical for diagnosing Agoraphobia?
    - A. The presence of fear in specific social settings like public speaking.
    - B. Avoidance of multiple environments due to fear of being unable to escape.
    - C. A history of trauma unrelated to public spaces.
    - D. The absence of panic-like symptoms in triggering situations.
2. What treatment would be most effective for Lisa?
    - A. Gradual exposure therapy targeting her feared situations.
    - B. Psychoanalysis to explore childhood experiences.
    - C. Long-term pharmacological treatment without therapy.
    - D. Avoiding all anxiety-provoking situations to reduce immediate distress.
3. Which differential diagnosis should be considered and ruled out in Lisa's case?
    - A. Social Anxiety Disorder.
    - B. Major Depressive Disorder.
    - C. Panic Disorder.
    - D. Specific Phobia.

Answers

Multiple Choice Questions:

1. B
2. B
3. B
4. C
5. B
6. A
7. B

True/False Questions:

1. False
2. True
3. False
4. True
5. False
6. True
7. False
8. False
9. True
10. True

Matching Exercise:

1. F
2. B
3. C
4. A
5. D
6. E

Case Study Answers and Explanations:

1. B. Explanation: Lisa's fear of multiple environments due to the perceived inability to escape or find help is a hallmark feature of Agoraphobia.
2. A. Explanation: Gradual exposure therapy is evidence-based and effective for reducing avoidance behaviors and fear responses.
3. C. Explanation: Panic Disorder must be ruled out because Lisa's symptoms began after a panic attack, which could indicate a comorbid condition.

Generalized Anxiety Disorder (GAD)

Multiple Choice Questions

1. Which of the following is a defining feature of Generalized Anxiety Disorder (GAD)?
    - A. Recurrent panic attacks triggered by specific situations.
    - B. Persistent and excessive worry about multiple areas of life, such as work, health, and finances.
    - C. Avoidance of specific objects or places due to fear of harm.
    - D. Obsessional thoughts paired with compulsive behaviors.
2. For a diagnosis of GAD, how long must excessive worry and anxiety persist?
    - A. At least two weeks.
    - B. At least one month.
    - C. At least three months.
    - D. At least six months.
3. Which of the following physical symptoms is most commonly associated with GAD?
    - A. Chest pain and fear of dying.
    - B. Restlessness, muscle tension, and sleep disturbances.
    - C. Fainting and dizziness.
    - D. Repetitive behaviors like hand washing.
4. How does GAD differ from Major Depressive Disorder (MDD)?
    - A. GAD includes pervasive worry, while MDD is characterized by low mood and loss of interest or pleasure.
    - B. MDD involves physical symptoms, while GAD does not.
    - C. GAD always involves panic attacks, while MDD does not.
    - D. MDD is associated with worry about the future, while GAD is not.
5. Which of the following statements best describes the course of GAD?
    - A. It is always acute and self-limiting.
    - B. It tends to be chronic and fluctuates in severity.
    - C. It is episodic and linked to specific triggers.
    - D. It resolves without treatment within a few weeks.
6. Which of the following treatments has the strongest evidence base for GAD?
    - A. Cognitive-behavioral therapy focusing on cognitive restructuring and relaxation techniques.
    - B. Psychoanalysis targeting unconscious fears.
    - C. Hypnotherapy to address underlying trauma.
    - D. Lifestyle changes without psychotherapy or pharmacological intervention.
7. What is an important differential diagnosis to rule out before diagnosing GAD?
    - A. Obsessive-Compulsive Disorder.
    - B. Specific Phobia.
    - C. Hyperthyroidism or other medical conditions.
    - D. Autism Spectrum Disorder.

True/False Questions

		T	F
1	Generalized anxiety in Generalized Anxiety Disorder (GAD) is restricted to specific situations or life events.		
2	A diagnostic feature of GAD is the difficulty in controlling persistent worry.		
3	Physical symptoms such as muscle tension and sleep disturbances are common diagnostic criteria for GAD.		
4	GAD is diagnosable only when anxiety is accompanied by recurrent panic attacks.		
5	Anxiety in GAD must be present for at least six months and pertain to a variety of events or activities.		
6	Comorbidity with other psychiatric disorders, such as major depressive disorder, is common in GAD.		
7	GAD is considered a rare disorder according to DSM-5 epidemiological data.		
8	Symptoms of GAD may include irritability, difficulty concentrating, and chronic fatigue.		
9	The diagnosis of GAD requires that symptoms are solely attributable to the physiological effects of a substance or a medical condition.		
10	Therapeutic interventions for GAD include approaches such as cognitive-behavioral therapy and, in some cases, pharmacological treatment.		

Matching Exercise

1. Excessive worry about multiple areas of life. [ ]
2. Duration required for diagnosis. [ ]
3. Common physical symptoms in GAD. [ ]
4. Effective treatment approach. [ ]
5. Differential diagnosis to rule out. [ ]
6. Key differentiating feature from Panic Disorder. [ ]

Descriptions:

- A. Six months or longer.
- B. Restlessness, muscle tension, and fatigue.
- C. Cognitive-behavioral therapy.
- D. Hyperthyroidism or other medical conditions.
- E. Persistent worry, not limited to specific panic attacks.
- F. Pervasive worry about work, finances, or health.

Case Study

Tom, a 40-year-old accountant, reports constant worry about his job performance, health, and finances. He describes feeling restless and tense, having trouble concentrating, and experiencing fatigue despite sleeping for eight hours. His symptoms have persisted for over a year, and he feels they are interfering with his ability to enjoy life. Tom has no history of panic attacks, and his physical examination and lab tests are normal.

1. What feature in Tom's case is critical for diagnosing GAD?
   - A. Persistent and excessive worry across multiple domains of life.
   - B. Recurrent panic attacks and avoidance of public spaces.
   - C. Physical symptoms exclusively related to cardiovascular issues.
   - D. Short-term symptoms triggered by a recent stressful event.
2. Which treatment would likely be most effective for Tom?
   - A. Cognitive-behavioral therapy focusing on relaxation techniques and addressing cognitive distortions.
   - B. Psychoanalysis to uncover unconscious conflicts.
   - C. Lifestyle changes, such as exercise and diet, without psychotherapy.
   - D. Hypnotherapy to address underlying fears.
3. Which differential diagnosis should be ruled out before confirming GAD?
   - A. Specific Phobia.
   - B. Major Depressive Disorder.
   - C. Hyperthyroidism or other medical conditions.
   - D. Social Anxiety Disorder.

Answers

Multiple Choice Questions:
1. B
2. D
3. B
4. A
5. B
6. A
7. C

True/False Questions:
1. False
2. True
3. True
4. False
5. True
6. True
7. False
8. True
9. False
10. True

Matching Exercise:
1. F
2. A
3. B
4. C
5. D
6. E

Case Study Answers and Explanations:
1. A. Explanation: Tom's pervasive and excessive worry across multiple domains, coupled with physical symptoms, aligns with the diagnostic criteria for GAD.
2. A. Explanation: Cognitive-behavioral therapy is evidence-based and effective, focusing on relaxation techniques and addressing cognitive distortions.
3. C. Explanation: Medical conditions, such as hyperthyroidism, must be ruled out to ensure the symptoms are not caused by a physical illness.

Other Anxiety Disorders

Multiple Choice Questions

1. What characterizes Other Specified Anxiety Disorder?
    - A. Anxiety symptoms that cause distress but do not fully meet criteria for any specific anxiety disorder.
    - B. Symptoms exclusively caused by substance use or a medical condition.
    - C. Anxiety symptoms triggered by a single, identifiable phobia.
    - D. Symptoms limited to a traumatic event.
2. Which is an example of Other Specified Anxiety Disorder?
    - A. Subthreshold panic attacks causing distress but not meeting full Panic Disorder criteria.
    - B. Persistent fear of spiders meeting criteria for Specific Phobia.
    - C. Social avoidance due to fear of judgment meeting criteria for Social Anxiety Disorder.
    - D. Recurrent, unexpected panic attacks.
3. What differentiates "Other Specified Anxiety Disorder" from "Unspecified Anxiety Disorder"?
    - A. "Other Specified" allows the clinician to explain why full criteria are not met, while "Unspecified" does not.
    - B. "Unspecified" is used only in medical settings.
    - C. "Other Specified" refers only to culturally specific fears.
    - D. There is no difference between the two terms.
4. Which treatment approach is commonly effective for Other Specified Anxiety Disorder?
    - A. Cognitive-behavioral therapy focusing on specific symptoms.
    - B. Avoidance strategies to reduce immediate distress.
    - C. Pharmacotherapy alone without psychotherapy.
    - D. Hypnotherapy as the primary intervention.
5. Which of the following is a valid clinical presentation of Other Specified Anxiety Disorder?
    - A. Cultural-specific fears that do not align with standard DSM-5 anxiety categories.
    - B. Anxiety episodes lasting less than one minute without functional impairment.
    - C. Specific Phobia diagnosed based on fear of animals.
    - D. Full criteria met for Social Anxiety Disorder.
6. What should clinicians rule out before diagnosing Other Specified Anxiety Disorder?
    - A. Underlying medical conditions or substance use.
    - B. Past traumatic experiences causing the symptoms.
    - C. Fear responses linked to physical disabilities.
    - D. Specific triggers leading to predictable anxiety.
7. Which of the following is a key component of diagnosing Other Specified Anxiety Disorder?
    - A. Symptoms must cause significant distress or functional impairment.
    - B. The anxiety must persist for more than a year.
    - C. Avoidance behaviors must be a dominant feature.
    - D. The anxiety must involve physical symptoms only.

True/False Questions

		T	F
1	A diagnosis of Unspecified Anxiety Disorder requires at least six months of persistent symptoms.		
2	The main difference between Specified and Unspecified Anxiety Disorders lies in whether or not a clear justification is provided for why full criteria are unmet.		
3	An example of Specified Anxiety Disorder could be situational anxiety related exclusively to a specific social event, without meeting criteria for social phobia.		
4	The diagnosis of Specified Anxiety Disorder cannot be applied to pediatric patients.		
5	The Unspecified category is frequently used in emergency settings where complete clinical information may not be available.		
6	A Specified Anxiety Disorder may include less common symptoms, such as generalized anxiety lasting less than six months, if justified by the clinician.		
7	The presence of comorbidity, such as major depressive disorder, automatically excludes the use of Specified or Unspecified Anxiety Disorder categories.		
8	Unspecified Anxiety Disorders always include symptoms of panic attacks, regardless of the clinical context.		
9	The choice between Specified and Unspecified depends on the level of detail the clinician wants to document in the diagnostic report.		
10	An Unspecified Anxiety Disorder is a valid option if the symptoms are atypical but significantly impair daily functioning.		

Matching Exercise

1. Subthreshold panic attacks. [ ]
2. Requirement for diagnosis of Other Specified Anxiety Disorder. [ ]
3. Difference from Unspecified Anxiety Disorder. [ ]
4. Cultural influence on anxiety presentation. [ ]
5. Common treatment approach. [ ]
6. Functional impact of symptoms. [ ]

Descriptions:

- A. Symptoms must cause distress or impairment in daily life.
- B. Allows the clinician to specify why full diagnostic criteria are not met.
- C. Limited-symptom panic attacks causing distress but not meeting Panic Disorder criteria.
- D. Targeted therapy, including CBT and relaxation techniques.
- E. Anxiety related to culturally specific fears or rituals.
- F. No medical or substance-related explanation for symptoms.

Case Study

Sofia, a 26-year-old college student, reports experiencing anxiety episodes that include mild heart palpitations, sweating, and dizziness, but these do not meet the intensity or frequency required for Panic Disorder. These episodes primarily occur during exam periods and cause her significant distress, making it difficult to concentrate. Despite the anxiety, Sofia does not avoid exams or other academic activities. Her symptoms have persisted for more than six months.

1. What feature in Sofia's case supports a diagnosis of Other Specified Anxiety Disorder?
   - A. Anxiety episodes that fully meet the criteria for Panic Disorder.
   - B. Limited-symptom panic attacks that cause distress but do not meet the full diagnostic criteria for Panic Disorder.
   - C. Avoidance of anxiety-provoking situations.
   - D. Symptoms lasting less than three months.
2. Which treatment would be most appropriate for Sofia?
   - A. Psychoanalysis focusing on past childhood conflicts.
   - B. Cognitive-behavioral therapy targeting her stress management and anxiety symptoms.
   - C. Pharmacotherapy without addressing her situational triggers.
   - D. Avoidance strategies to reduce immediate distress.
3. Which differential diagnosis should be ruled out in Sofia's case?
   - A. Social Anxiety Disorder.
   - B. Major Depressive Disorder.
   - C. Generalized Anxiety Disorder.
   - D. Medical causes, such as thyroid dysfunction.

Answers

Multiple Choice Questions:
1. B
2. C
3. A
4. A
5. A
6. A
7. B

True/False Questions:
1. True
2. True
3. True
4. False
5. False
6. True
7. False
8. True
9. True
10. True

Matching Exercise:
1. C
2. A
3. B
4. E
5. D
6. F

Case Study Answers and Explanations:
1. B. Explanation: Sofia's symptoms align with the category of limited-symptom panic attacks, which are part of Other Specified Anxiety Disorder.
2. B. Explanation: Cognitive-behavioral therapy is evidence-based and effective for addressing situational anxiety and improving stress management.
3. D. Explanation: Medical causes, such as thyroid dysfunction, must be excluded to confirm the diagnosis.

Obsessive-Compulsive and Related Disorders

This diagnostic category includes various conditions marked by unwanted thoughts, impulses, or images (obsessions) that cause anxiety or distress, and by repetitive behaviors or mental acts (compulsions) aimed at reducing the discomfort triggered by these obsessions. In Obsessive-Compulsive Disorder (OCD), these rituals and thoughts become so intertwined that they interfere with daily activities, creating a cycle that the individual struggles to break. Common obsessions often involve contamination, order, or fear of harming oneself or others. Typical compulsions include repeated hand-washing, checking locks or stoves, or mentally counting certain sequences.

Body Dysmorphic Disorder focuses on perceived physical flaws (sometimes nonexistent or barely noticeable) that produce significant distress and lead a person to repeatedly check or attempt to alter the "imperfect" body part. Hoarding Disorder involves difficulty discarding possessions, even those with little or no value, due to fear of losing something important or strong emotional attachment. This behavior can create extremely cluttered living spaces that become hard to inhabit.

Other conditions in this category include Trichotillomania, which involves pulling out one's own hair, and Excoriation Disorder, characterized by persistent picking at the skin (often the face, but also other areas), sometimes causing lesions. Both behaviors can bring temporary relief but may lead to physical complications and social discomfort.

From a diagnostic perspective, it is essential to differentiate these disorders from other anxiety conditions and from medical or neurological issues that might explain the symptoms (for example, dermatological problems or motor-control disorders). Cultural factors must also be taken into account, as certain rituals or customs might resemble compulsive behaviors but serve a recognized symbolic purpose within their context.

Treatment for Obsessive-Compulsive and Related Disorders often combines medication (especially SSRIs) with cognitive-behavioral therapy, which typically includes exposure and response prevention techniques. In more complex cases, a multidisciplinary strategy may be appropriate, involving different healthcare professionals and, when indicated, support from relatives or others close to the person. The goal is to disrupt the cycle of obsessions and compulsions by offering strategies to handle negative thoughts and emotions in a more balanced way.

Obsessive-Compulsive Disorder (OCD)

Multiple Choice Questions

1. A key diagnostic feature of Obsessive-Compulsive Disorder (OCD) is:
   - A. Recurrent, intrusive thoughts or urges that are not resisted.
   - B. Persistent worries about daily life that do not involve specific rituals.
   - C. Recurrent obsessions or compulsions that are time-consuming or cause significant distress.
   - D. Avoidance of specific situations to prevent anxiety.
2. Which of the following would most likely be classified as an obsession in OCD?
   - A. A person is preoccupied with fears of contamination despite evidence to the contrary.
   - B. A person repeatedly checks if the door is locked before leaving.
   - C. A person avoids public transportation due to fear of germs.
   - D. A person experiences situational panic attacks in crowded spaces.
3. Compulsions in OCD are primarily aimed at:
   - A. Avoiding feared objects or places.
   - B. Preventing or reducing anxiety associated with obsessions.
   - C. Improving social interactions.
   - D. Addressing underlying medical concerns.
4. Which subtype of OCD is characterized by intrusive, distressing thoughts without overt compulsions?
   - A. Contamination subtype.
   - B. Pure obsessional OCD ("Pure O").
   - C. Hoarding disorder.
   - D. Checking subtype.
5. What distinguishes OCD from Generalized Anxiety Disorder (GAD)?
   - A. OCD involves specific, intrusive thoughts or rituals, while GAD is characterized by pervasive worry about various life events.
   - B. OCD is not associated with avoidance behaviors.
   - C. GAD involves compulsions to manage worry.
   - D. GAD symptoms are always more severe than OCD symptoms.
6. Which of the following is a recommended first-line treatment for OCD?
   - A. Long-term use of benzodiazepines.
   - B. Exposure and response prevention (ERP) therapy.
   - C. Hypnotherapy to address unconscious fears.
   - D. Group therapy as the sole intervention.
7. A clinician suspects OCD in a patient who spends hours each day organizing items "perfectly." What question might the clinician ask to clarify the diagnosis?
   - A. "Do you feel a sense of satisfaction after organizing?"
   - B. "Do these behaviors help you avoid interactions with others?"
   - C. "Do you feel distressed if you cannot perform these behaviors?"
   - D. "Have you experienced these symptoms for more than six months?"

True/False Questions

		T	F
1	Obsessions in Obsessive-Compulsive Disorder (OCD) are always related to contamination fears.		
2	Diagnostic criteria for OCD include repetitive compulsions that the individual feels driven to perform to reduce anxiety associated with obsessions.		
3	Compulsions can include both observable behaviors and mental acts, such as counting or repeating phrases.		
4	OCD requires that obsessions or compulsions are present every day for at least six months.		
5	Obsessions are intrusive thoughts, images, or impulses that cause significant distress.		
6	A diagnosis of OCD can be made even when the individual is aware that the obsessions or compulsions are irrational or excessive.		
7	OCD is diagnosable only in the absence of comorbidities with other psychiatric disorders, such as generalized anxiety disorder.		
8	OCD symptoms can significantly interfere with social, occupational, or other important areas of an individual's life.		
9	Compulsions in OCD are always directly related to the content of the obsessions.		
10	Treatment for OCD does not include pharmacological interventions but exclusively cognitive-behavioral therapy.		

Matching Exercise

1. Intrusive, unwanted thoughts. [ ]
2. Time-consuming behaviors aimed at reducing anxiety. [ ]
3. Effective therapy for OCD. [ ]
4. Subtype without visible compulsions. [ ]
5. A treatment often combined with ERP. [ ]
6. A key differentiating feature from GAD. [ ]

Descriptions:

- A. Exposure and response prevention (ERP).
- B. Pure obsessional OCD ("Pure O").
- C. Selective serotonin reuptake inhibitors (SSRIs).
- D. Obsessions.
- E. Compulsions.
- F. Ritualistic behaviors tied to specific, intrusive thoughts.

Case Study

David, a 35-year-old accountant, spends several hours each evening checking his appliances to ensure they are turned off. He describes intrusive thoughts of causing a house fire and reports feeling compelled to check multiple times before going to bed. These behaviors are impacting his sleep and ability to perform at work. David acknowledges that his fears are excessive but feels unable to stop.

1. Which feature in David's case is most critical for diagnosing OCD?
    - A. Excessive time spent checking appliances despite no actual danger.
    - B. Avoidance of public spaces.
    - C. Sleep disturbances unrelated to compulsive behaviors.
    - D. Recurrent panic attacks triggered by specific settings.
2. Which treatment would be most effective for David?
    - A. Cognitive-behavioral therapy with exposure and response prevention (ERP).
    - B. Hypnotherapy to explore underlying fears.
    - C. Long-term use of sedative medications.
    - D. Psychoanalysis to uncover unconscious conflicts.
3. Which differential diagnosis should be considered and ruled out?
    - A. Generalized Anxiety Disorder.
    - B. Major Depressive Disorder.
    - C. Schizophrenia.
    - D. Hoarding disorder.

Answers

Multiple Choice Questions:

1. C
2. A
3. B
4. B
5. A
6. B
7. C

True/False Questions:

1. False
2. True
3. True
4. False
5. True
6. True
7. False
8. True
9. False
10. False

Matching Exercise:

1. D
2. E
3. A
4. B
5. C
6. F

Case Study Answers and Explanations:

1. A. Explanation: David's excessive and time-consuming checking behaviors align with compulsions in OCD, driven by intrusive thoughts of harm.
2. A. Explanation: Exposure and response prevention (ERP) is evidence-based and highly effective for reducing compulsions and distress.
3. A. Explanation: Generalized Anxiety Disorder must be ruled out, as it involves pervasive worry but lacks the intrusive thoughts and ritualistic behaviors seen in OCD.

Body Dysmorphic Disorder (BDD)

Multiple Choice Questions

1. Which of the following is a defining characteristic of Body Dysmorphic Disorder (BDD)?
    - A. Persistent worry about body weight despite being within a healthy range.
    - B. Preoccupation with one or more perceived physical flaws that are not observable or appear slight to others.
    - C. Recurrent urges to perform rituals to prevent imagined harm.
    - D. Avoidance of social interactions due to generalized anxiety.
2. Which behavior is most commonly associated with BDD?
    - A. Excessive grooming or mirror-checking.
    - B. Persistent refusal to eat in social settings.
    - C. Avoidance of public spaces due to fear of panic attacks.
    - D. Ritualistic hand-washing to reduce contamination fears.
3. What distinguishes BDD from an eating disorder?
    - A. BDD focuses on specific physical features, while eating disorders focus on weight and body shape.
    - B. Eating disorders do not involve body image concerns.
    - C. BDD involves fear of food-related contamination.
    - D. Both conditions always involve excessive exercise as a primary symptom.
4. A person with BDD is most likely to:
    - A. Seek reassurance about their appearance from others.
    - B. Experience a fear of losing control in public spaces.
    - C. Engage in compulsive rituals unrelated to physical appearance.
    - D. Avoid any attempts to alter their physical appearance.
5. Which of the following treatments is considered most effective for BDD?
    - A. Psychodynamic therapy focusing on childhood conflicts.
    - B. Cognitive-behavioral therapy (CBT) with a focus on cognitive restructuring and exposure therapy.
    - C. Long-term use of benzodiazepines without psychotherapy.
    - D. Hypnotherapy targeting unconscious fears.
6. Which population is at higher risk for developing BDD?
    - A. Individuals with a history of trauma or bullying related to their appearance.
    - B. People with no history of mental health issues.
    - C. Individuals with purely medical conditions.
    - D. People exclusively in high socioeconomic groups.
7. Which of the following differential diagnoses must be considered when evaluating for BDD?
    - A. Social Anxiety Disorder.
    - B. Panic Disorder.
    - C. Generalized Anxiety Disorder.
    - D. Obsessive-Compulsive Disorder.

True/False Questions

		T	F
1	Concerns in BDD can involve any body part, including microscopic details like skin pores.		
2	A diagnosis of BDD can only be made if the patient is aware that their concerns are irrational.		
3	Repeated mirror checking or seeking reassurance are behaviors associated with BDD according to the DSM-5.		
4	BDD is closely linked to eating disorders and requires that concerns focus on weight or body shape.		
5	Cosmetic surgery often fails to resolve BDD symptoms and can sometimes worsen the condition.		
6	BDD is frequently comorbid with obsessive-compulsive disorder and social anxiety disorder.		
7	According to the DSM-5, BDD does not require that concerns interfere with social or occupational functioning to be diagnosed.		
8	BDD concerns can include invisible flaws to others, such as the shape of ears or the size of hands.		
9	BDD symptoms must be present for at least six months to qualify for a diagnosis.		
10	Treatment for BDD includes cognitive-behavioral therapy, often combined with medications like SSRIs.		

Matching Exercise

1. Persistent preoccupation with perceived physical flaws. [ ]
2. Excessive behaviors related to appearance, such as grooming. [ ]
3. Effective treatment approach for BDD. [ ]
4. A differentiating factor between BDD and Social Anxiety Disorder. [ ]
5. Common consequence of untreated BDD. [ ]
6. Population at higher risk for BDD. [ ]

Descriptions:

- A. Cognitive-behavioral therapy.
- B. Flaws that are not observable or appear slight to others.
- C. Avoidance of social or occupational activities due to distress.
- D. Specific focus on appearance-related preoccupations.
- E. Individuals with a history of bullying about their looks.
- F. Reassurance-seeking or mirror-checking.

Case Study

Elena, a 25-year-old artist, spends hours each day examining her skin in the mirror, convinced that her pores are abnormally large. She frequently avoids social gatherings, fearing others will notice her "defect." Despite reassurance from family and friends, she continues to feel distressed about her appearance and has considered cosmetic procedures to "fix" her skin. Her preoccupation is interfering with her ability to meet deadlines and attend gallery events.

1. What feature of Elena's case supports a diagnosis of BDD?
    - A. Generalized anxiety about various life events.
    - B. Preoccupation with a perceived flaw that is not apparent to others.
    - C. Avoidance of public spaces unrelated to appearance.
    - D. Ritualistic behaviors unrelated to body image.
2. What treatment would likely be most effective for Elena?
    - A. Cognitive-behavioral therapy focusing on exposure and cognitive restructuring.
    - B. Psychoanalysis to uncover childhood trauma.
    - C. Pharmacotherapy with antipsychotics alone.
    - D. Avoidance of social interactions to reduce immediate distress.
3. Which differential diagnosis should be ruled out in Elena's case?
    - A. Panic Disorder.
    - B. Obsessive-Compulsive Disorder.
    - C. Generalized Anxiety Disorder.
    - D. Major Depressive Disorder.

Answers

Multiple Choice Questions:
1. B
2. A
3. A
4. A
5. B
6. A
7. D

True/False Questions:
1. True
2. False
3. False
4. True
5. False
6. True
7. True
8. True
9. True
10. False

Matching Exercise:
1. B
2. F
3. A
4. D
5. C
6. E

Case Study Answers and Explanations:
1. B. Explanation: Elena's excessive preoccupation with her pores, which are not objectively noticeable to others, aligns with the diagnostic criteria for BDD.
2. A. Explanation: Cognitive-behavioral therapy, particularly exposure and cognitive restructuring, is an evidence-based treatment for reducing distress and dysfunctional beliefs in BDD.
3. B. Explanation: OCD must be ruled out, as it shares similar repetitive thoughts and behaviors but is not limited to appearance-related concerns.

Hoarding Disorder

Multiple Choice Questions

1. Which of the following scenarios best illustrates Hoarding Disorder?
    - A. A person avoids public spaces due to fear of embarrassment.
    - B. A person accumulates items to the point that their home becomes unusable but resists discarding them due to perceived emotional or practical value.
    - C. A person compulsively cleans their house to prevent contamination.
    - D. A person purchases items in bulk but uses them systematically.
2. What is a key distinction between Hoarding Disorder and collecting?
    - A. Collecting involves accumulating items without displaying them.
    - B. Hoarding Disorder is characterized by distress and impaired functioning, while collecting is typically organized and purposeful.
    - C. Hoarding involves only low-value items, while collecting focuses on valuable objects.
    - D. Collecting does not involve any emotional attachment to items.
3. A hallmark feature of Hoarding Disorder is:
    - A. Difficulty organizing and deciding which possessions to keep or discard.
    - B. Fear of germs leading to repetitive cleaning.
    - C. Obsessive thoughts about symmetry and order.
    - D. Avoidance of specific social situations due to anxiety.
4. What emotional response is most commonly reported by individuals with Hoarding Disorder when asked to discard items?
    - A. Indifference or lack of emotion.
    - B. Relief and a sense of accomplishment.
    - C. Anxiety or distress at the thought of losing possessions.
    - D. Excitement about acquiring new items to replace discarded ones.
5. Which of the following therapeutic approaches is most effective for treating Hoarding Disorder?
    - A. Cognitive-behavioral therapy focusing on decluttering and decision-making skills.
    - B. Hypnosis to uncover unconscious fears.
    - C. Pharmacotherapy as a standalone treatment.
    - D. Psychoanalysis targeting early childhood experiences.
6. How does insight typically present in individuals with Hoarding Disorder?
    - A. Most individuals have high insight and actively seek help.
    - B. Insight can vary, with many individuals believing their behaviors are justified despite significant impairment.
    - C. Individuals with Hoarding Disorder always lack insight and believe their behaviors are rational.
    - D. Insight is irrelevant for the diagnosis of Hoarding Disorder.
7. Which question would be most helpful in assessing whether someone's behaviors meet criteria for Hoarding Disorder?
    - A. "Do you feel joy when acquiring new possessions?"
    - B. "Have you been collecting items for a long time?"
    - C. "Do your possessions make it difficult to use your living spaces effectively?"
    - D. "Do you feel physically attached to specific objects?"

True/False Questions

		T	F
1	Hoarding Disorder requires that hoarding behaviors necessarily compromise more than one room in the house.		
2	A diagnosis of Hoarding Disorder can be made even in the presence of very low or absent insight.		
3	Hoarding behaviors, according to the DSM-5, must be present for at least six months and cause significant distress or functional impairment.		
4	Pathological hoarding is always associated with compulsive acquisition of new items, regardless of their value.		
5	Hoarding Disorder can include the preservation of items with high sentimental value but low economic value.		
6	According to the DSM-5, a diagnosis of Hoarding Disorder does not require that the behavior interferes with the individual's or others' physical safety.		
7	Patients with Hoarding Disorder rarely require therapeutic interventions, as their condition is self-limiting.		
8	Difficulty discarding items is often motivated by the irrational belief that they might be useful in the future or have a unique value.		
9	Hoarding Disorder is frequently comorbid with other mental disorders, such as Obsessive-Compulsive Disorder and Major Depressive Disorder.		
10	Treatment for Hoarding Disorder focuses exclusively on cognitive-behavioral therapy, with limited results from medication use.		

Matching Exercise

1. Difficulty discarding items. [ ]
2. Emotional response to discarding possessions. [ ]
3. Effective treatment approach. [ ]
4. Distinction from OCD. [ ]
5. Common consequences of untreated Hoarding Disorder. [ ]
6. Insight in Hoarding Disorder. [ ]

Descriptions:

- A. Anxiety or distress at the thought of losing possessions.
- B. Impairment in social or home functioning due to clutter.
- C. Decision-making challenges related to possessions.
- D. Cognitive-behavioral therapy focusing on organization and behavior change.
- E. Lack of compulsive rituals aimed at reducing anxiety.
- F. Insight ranges from good to poor, with some believing their behaviors are justified.

Case Study

Martha, a 58-year-old librarian, lives in a house filled with stacks of newspapers, books, and old clothing. She insists that these items have sentimental value or could be useful in the future. Her family has repeatedly offered to help her clean, but Martha becomes visibly distressed at the suggestion. She cannot use her dining table for meals or her bedroom for sleeping due to the clutter, but she denies that it's a problem.

1. What aspect of Martha's case most strongly supports a diagnosis of Hoarding Disorder?
    - A. Her refusal to let family members clean her home.
    - B. Her inability to discard possessions, leading to significant functional impairment.
    - C. Her attachment to sentimental items.
    - D. Her profession as a librarian, which involves working with large quantities of books.
2. Which treatment approach would be most effective for Martha?
    - A. Cognitive-behavioral therapy focusing on decluttering and decision-making.
    - B. Psychoanalysis targeting unresolved conflicts.
    - C. Avoidance of intervention to respect Martha's autonomy.
    - D. Pharmacotherapy without psychotherapy.
3. Which differential diagnosis should be considered and ruled out?
    - A. Obsessive-Compulsive Disorder.
    - B. Body Dysmorphic Disorder.
    - C. Social Anxiety Disorder.
    - D. Specific Phobia.

Answers

Multiple Choice Questions:
1. B
2. B
3. A
4. C
5. A
6. B
7. C

True/False Questions:
1. False
2. True
3. True
4. True
5. False
6. False
7. False
8. False
9. True
10. True

Matching Exercise:
1. C
2. A
3. D
4. E
5. B
6. F

Case Study Answers and Explanations:
1. B. Explanation: Martha's inability to discard items and the resulting functional impairment align with the diagnostic criteria for Hoarding Disorder.
2. A. Explanation: Cognitive-behavioral therapy is the most effective treatment for Hoarding Disorder, addressing both decision-making and organizational skills.
3. A. Explanation: OCD must be ruled out, as it can share overlapping features but includes compulsive rituals aimed at reducing anxiety.

Trichotillomania (Hair-Pulling Disorder)

Multiple Choice Questions

1. Which of the following is a hallmark feature of Trichotillomania?
    - A. Persistent pulling of hair resulting in hair loss, accompanied by repeated attempts to stop.
    - B. Recurrent picking at the skin leading to sores or lesions.
    - C. Avoidance of public spaces due to fear of judgment.
    - D. Excessive grooming and styling of hair to achieve symmetry.
2. What distinguishes Trichotillomania from Obsessive-Compulsive Disorder (OCD)?
    - A. Trichotillomania involves rituals aimed at reducing anxiety.
    - B. Hair-pulling is often preceded by tension or triggered by boredom, without the intrusive thoughts typical of OCD.
    - C. Trichotillomania always involves compulsions to neutralize intrusive thoughts.
    - D. OCD is exclusively focused on contamination fears, while Trichotillomania is not.
3. Which of the following areas is most commonly affected in individuals with Trichotillomania?
    - A. Arms and legs.
    - B. Scalp, eyebrows, and eyelashes.
    - C. Hands and feet.
    - D. Chest and abdomen.
4. What emotional response often precedes hair-pulling episodes in Trichotillomania?
    - A. Excitement and euphoria.
    - B. Intense tension or anxiety that is relieved by pulling hair.
    - C. Indifference or lack of emotion.
    - D. Persistent sadness unrelated to the behavior.
5. Which treatment approach has shown the most efficacy in treating Trichotillomania?
    - A. Habit Reversal Training (HRT) combined with cognitive-behavioral therapy (CBT).
    - B. Pharmacotherapy with benzodiazepines alone.
    - C. Hypnotherapy focused on unconscious fears.
    - D. Long-term psychoanalysis exploring early childhood trauma.
6. Which of the following is a valid question to assess the functional impact of Trichotillomania?
    - A. "Do you avoid certain activities or interactions because of visible hair loss?"
    - B. "Do you perform rituals to reduce anxiety about germs?"
    - C. "Do you spend significant time organizing or cleaning your living space?"
    - D. "Do you experience relief when your hair regrows?"
7. Which of the following is a common comorbidity with Trichotillomania?
    - A. Generalized Anxiety Disorder.
    - B. Anorexia Nervosa.
    - C. Schizophrenia.
    - D. Conduct Disorder.

True/False Questions

		T	F
1	Hair-pulling disorder (trichotillomania) is diagnosable only if the behavior is associated with significant anxiety.		
2	Patients with trichotillomania are always aware of their hair-pulling behaviors.		
3	According to the DSM-5, trichotillomania involves a recurrent inability to resist the urge to pull out hair, resulting in noticeable hair loss.		
4	Hair-pulling behavior must be attributable to a general medical condition or the physiological effects of a substance to receive a diagnosis of trichotillomania.		
5	Trichotillomania can cause significant distress or impairment in social, occupational, or other areas of daily life.		
6	Hair-pulling episodes always occur during moments of full awareness by the patient.		
7	Areas affected by hair-pulling can include not only the scalp but also eyelashes, eyebrows, and other body areas with hair.		
8	Trichotillomania may be comorbid with other psychiatric disorders, such as Obsessive-Compulsive Disorder and Major Depression.		
9	Individuals with trichotillomania may adopt avoidance strategies, such as wearing hats or makeup to cover affected areas.		
10	Treatment for trichotillomania relies exclusively on pharmacological therapy, with behavioral therapies showing little efficacy.		

Matching Exercise

1. Commonly affected areas. [ ]
2. Emotional state preceding hair-pulling. [ ]
3. Effective treatment approach. [ ]
4. Functional impact of the behavior. [ ]
5. Common comorbid conditions. [ ]
6. Insight into the behavior. [ ]

Descriptions:

- A. Tension or anxiety relieved by hair-pulling.
- B. Habit Reversal Training combined with cognitive-behavioral therapy.
- C. Scalp, eyebrows, and eyelashes.
- D. Generalized Anxiety Disorder and skin-picking disorder.
- E. Avoidance of social interactions due to visible hair loss.
- F. Varies from good insight to denial of the problem's impact.

Case Study

Lila, a 17-year-old high school student, reports feeling a strong urge to pull out her eyelashes whenever she is stressed or bored. She describes feeling a sense of relief immediately after pulling but later regrets the behavior when she notices gaps in her eyelashes. Lila avoids eye contact with others and has started wearing makeup to hide the hair loss. Despite her efforts, her behaviors persist, and she feels unable to stop.

1. Which feature of Lila's case is most indicative of Trichotillomania?
   - A. Persistent worry about her appearance.
   - B. Recurrent pulling of hair with noticeable hair loss and failed attempts to stop.
   - C. Avoidance of social interactions unrelated to hair-pulling.
   - D. Feelings of sadness unrelated to stress or boredom.
2. Which treatment approach would be most effective for Lila?
   - A. Habit Reversal Training combined with CBT.
   - B. Psychoanalysis to explore unconscious fears.
   - C. Long-term use of antipsychotic medication.
   - D. Hypnotherapy to address underlying trauma.
3. Which differential diagnosis should be ruled out in Lila's case?
   - A. Body Dysmorphic Disorder.
   - B. Obsessive-Compulsive Disorder.
   - C. Social Anxiety Disorder.
   - D. Specific Phobia.

Answers

Multiple Choice Questions:

1. A
2. B
3. B
4. B
5. A
6. A
7. A

True/False Questions:

1. True
2. False
3. True
4. False
5. True
6. False
7. True
8. True
9. True
10. False

Matching Exercise:

1. C
2. A
3. B
4. E
5. D
6. F

Case Study Answers and Explanations:

1. B. Explanation: Lila's recurrent pulling of hair, resulting in noticeable hair loss, and her inability to stop despite distress align with the diagnostic criteria for Trichotillomania.
2. A. Explanation: Habit Reversal Training combined with CBT is an evidence-based approach for addressing repetitive behaviors in Trichotillomania.
3. B. Explanation: OCD must be ruled out due to overlapping repetitive behaviors but differing triggers and motivations.

Excoriation (Skin-Picking) Disorder

Multiple Choice Questions

1. Which of the following best describes the nature of Excoriation Disorder?
    - A. Recurrent picking at the skin, leading to lesions, despite repeated attempts to stop.
    - B. Persistent scratching due to allergic reactions or skin conditions.
    - C. A compulsive need to clean or disinfect the skin to avoid contamination.
    - D. Scratching behaviors exclusively triggered by external irritants like clothing.
2. A clinician is assessing a patient with skin-picking behaviors. Which feature would most strongly support a diagnosis of Excoriation Disorder rather than a dermatological condition?
    - A. The behavior occurs exclusively in response to visible acne or scabs.
    - B. The patient reports a sense of tension before picking and relief afterward.
    - C. The skin lesions are concentrated in areas exposed to sunlight.
    - D. The patient scratches only during allergic flare-ups.
3. Which of the following differentiates Excoriation Disorder from Body Dysmorphic Disorder (BDD)?
    - A. Excoriation Disorder involves attempts to conceal perceived defects.
    - B. Skin-picking in Excoriation Disorder is driven by tactile or emotional urges, rather than a focus on appearance.
    - C. BDD never involves behaviors targeting the skin.
    - D. Excoriation Disorder is always associated with anxiety about appearance.
4. Which question would be most useful to explore the functional impairment caused by Excoriation Disorder?
    - A. "Do you feel compelled to pick your skin when stressed?"
    - B. "Have you avoided work or social events due to visible lesions?"
    - C. "Do you feel a need to wash your hands after touching your skin?"
    - D. "Are you concerned about infections resulting from picking?"
5. Which of the following treatment components is essential for managing Excoriation Disorder?
    - A. Habit Reversal Training (HRT) to replace skin-picking with alternative behaviors.
    - B. Psychoanalysis to explore early childhood trauma.
    - C. Pharmacotherapy using antipsychotic medications.
    - D. Hypnotherapy to uncover unconscious conflicts.
6. In assessing Excoriation Disorder, why is it critical to rule out medical or dermatological conditions?
    - A. Medical conditions can mimic picking-related skin lesions.
    - B. Dermatological conditions are the primary cause of Excoriation Disorder.
    - C. The disorder cannot be diagnosed in the presence of any skin condition.
    - D. Skin-picking is always secondary to physical conditions.
7. Which of the following comorbid conditions is most frequently associated with Excoriation Disorder?
    - A. Bipolar Disorder.
    - B. Obsessive-Compulsive Disorder (OCD).
    - C. Schizophrenia.
    - D. Panic Disorder.

True/False Questions

		T	F
1	Excoriation disorder can be diagnosed even in the absence of visible skin lesions, as long as the behavior causes significant distress.		
2	According to the DSM-5, a diagnosis of excoriation disorder excludes behaviors that can be attributed to another psychiatric condition, such as Obsessive-Compulsive Disorder.		
3	Skin-picking behaviors are often automatic and not always accompanied by a conscious desire to pick at the skin.		
4	Excoriation disorder requires that the individual has made repeated attempts to reduce or stop the behavior without success.		
5	Trichotillomania and excoriation disorder share identical diagnostic criteria, differing only in the target (hair vs skin).		
6	A diagnosis of excoriation disorder can be made even if the behavior occurs exclusively in response to acute stress situations.		
7	Individuals with excoriation disorder rarely seek treatment, as they often consider the behavior an acceptable part of themselves.		
8	The most frequently affected areas in excoriation disorder are the scalp and nails, despite the common belief that it primarily involves the face.		
9	Excoriation disorder is more common in women than in men, with an estimated ratio of approximately 3:1.		
10	The most effective treatment for excoriation disorder is a combination of cognitive-behavioral therapy and selective serotonin reuptake inhibitors (SSRIs).		

Matching Exercise

1. Emotional states commonly linked to skin-picking episodes. [ ]
2. Common treatment method for Excoriation Disorder. [ ]
3. Differential diagnosis to rule out. [ ]
4. Physical consequences of Excoriation Disorder. [ ]
5. Functional impact of the disorder. [ ]
6. Behavioral patterns preceding skin-picking. [ ]

Descriptions:

- A. Tension or boredom often precedes picking episodes.
- B. Infections, scarring, and delayed healing of lesions.
- C. Avoidance of social or professional activities due to visible damage.
- D. Obsessive-Compulsive Disorder (OCD) or dermatological conditions.
- E. Habit Reversal Training and CBT techniques.
- F. Gratification or temporary relief following picking.

Case Study

Jenna, a 32-year-old retail manager, reports spending hours each evening picking at small imperfections on her arms and face. She feels a sense of relief after picking but becomes distressed when she notices scars forming. Her behaviors have led to repeated infections, and she avoids social situations to hide the lesions. Jenna acknowledges that she wants to stop but feels unable to resist the urge when she is bored or stressed.

1. Which feature of Jenna's case strongly supports a diagnosis of Excoriation Disorder?
   - A. Avoidance of social events unrelated to her appearance.
   - B. Picking behaviors that result in noticeable scarring and distress despite attempts to stop.
   - C. Obsessive focus on perceived skin defects and attempts to conceal them.
   - D. The presence of skin infections requiring medical treatment.
2. Which intervention would be most effective for Jenna?
   - A. Habit Reversal Training combined with cognitive-behavioral therapy.
   - B. Psychoanalysis to uncover unconscious motivations.
   - C. Long-term use of sedatives to manage urges.
   - D. Cosmetic treatments to reduce scarring and improve appearance.
3. Which differential diagnosis should be ruled out before confirming Excoriation Disorder?
   - A. Body Dysmorphic Disorder.
   - B. Panic Disorder.
   - C. Generalized Anxiety Disorder.
   - D. Post-Traumatic Stress Disorder.

Answers

Multiple Choice Questions:
1. A
2. B
3. B
4. B
5. A
6. A
7. B

True/False Questions:
1. True
2. True
3. False
4. True
5. False
6. True
7. False
8. False
9. True
10. False

Matching Exercise:
1. A
2. E
3. D
4. B
5. C
6. F

Case Study Answers and Explanations:
1. B. Explanation: Jenna's behaviors align with the diagnostic criteria for Excoriation Disorder, particularly her inability to stop picking despite distress and scarring.
2. A. Explanation: Habit Reversal Training and CBT are evidence-based interventions that address the behavioral and cognitive components of the disorder.
3. A. Explanation: Body Dysmorphic Disorder must be ruled out, as it can involve picking behaviors driven by appearance-related concerns.

OCD Related Disorders

Multiple Choice Questions

1. Which of the following is a feature of Body-Focused Repetitive Behaviors (BFRBs), such as hair-pulling or nail-biting?
    - A. The behaviors are intentional and always planned in response to intrusive thoughts.
    - B. The behaviors are often automatic, occurring during periods of boredom or relaxation.
    - C. The behaviors are performed exclusively to reduce anxiety about contamination.
    - D. The behaviors are driven by the desire for physical perfection.
2. A patient spends significant time re-checking the alignment of objects on their desk. They report that failing to do so causes discomfort but does not involve intrusive thoughts about harm. This presentation is most consistent with:
    - A. OCD with a focus on contamination.
    - B. Hoarding Disorder.
    - C. Obsessive-Compulsive Personality Disorder (OCPD).
    - D. Body Dysmorphic Disorder (BDD).
3. A clinician is evaluating a patient with repetitive behaviors. Which of the following questions would best differentiate OCD from OCPD?
    - A. "Do you feel your behaviors are excessive or irrational?"
    - B. "Are you preoccupied with physical appearance?"
    - C. "Do you avoid situations where anxiety might arise?"
    - D. "Are you experiencing distress due to unwanted intrusive thoughts?"
4. Why might an individual be diagnosed with "Other Specified Obsessive-Compulsive and Related Disorders" instead of OCD?
    - A. The compulsions are minimal and do not cause significant impairment.
    - B. The obsessions are limited to specific phobias.
    - C. The individual experiences compulsions but denies any associated distress.
    - D. The behaviors are directly caused by a medical condition.
5. What distinguishes Body Dysmorphic Disorder (BDD) from Excoriation Disorder?
    - A. BDD involves preoccupation with perceived appearance flaws, while Excoriation Disorder involves behaviors unrelated to appearance concerns.
    - B. BDD behaviors are typically automatic, while Excoriation Disorder is deliberate.
    - C. Excoriation Disorder involves avoidance of social situations due to physical scars.
    - D. BDD symptoms always include skin-picking as a primary behavior.
6. Which of the following is a critical component in the treatment of Body-Focused Repetitive Behaviors?
    - A. Habit Reversal Training (HRT).
    - B. Exposure and Response Prevention (ERP) therapy.
    - C. Psychoanalysis focused on early childhood conflicts.
    - D. Exclusive use of pharmacotherapy.
7. A patient presents with repetitive handwashing to relieve anxiety about contamination, but denies other compulsions. Which differential diagnosis should be considered?
    - A. Hoarding Disorder.
    - B. Social Anxiety Disorder.
    - C. Generalized Anxiety Disorder (GAD).
    - D. Specific Phobia.

True/False Questions

		T	F
1	OCD-related disorders necessarily include visible behavioral compulsions, as mental acts do not meet diagnostic criteria.		
2	Trichotillomania and excoriation disorder share diagnostic similarities with OCD but do not necessarily require obsessions as a prerequisite.		
3	To diagnose Body Dysmorphic Disorder (BDD), the patient must always exhibit repetitive behaviors such as mirror checking or skin touching.		
4	Hoarding Disorder was included in OCD-related disorders in the DSM-5 due to its frequent comorbidity with Obsessive-Compulsive Disorder.		
5	In OCD-related disorders, symptom severity is always proportional to the patient's level of insight into their behavior.		
6	Pharmacological treatment for OCD-related disorders is limited to selective serotonin reuptake inhibitors (SSRIs), as other drugs have no proven efficacy.		
7	Diagnostic criteria for excoriation disorder require that skin lesions are always accompanied by significant distress perceived by the patient.		
8	Compulsive behaviors in OCD-related disorders must always be tied to the reduction of a specific anxiety to meet DSM-5 criteria.		
9	Hoarding Disorder can include compulsive acquisition behaviors, but these are not mandatory to meet diagnostic criteria.		
10	Body Dysmorphic Disorder is classified as an anxiety disorder in the DSM-5 because		

Matching Exercise

1. Emotional states commonly linked to repetitive behaviors. [ ]
2. Common treatment method for repetitive behaviors. [ ]
3. Differential diagnosis to rule out. [ ]
4. Functional impact of the behaviors. [ ]
5. Physical consequences of certain obsessive-compulsive behaviors. [ ]
6. Behavioral patterns distinguishing compulsions from other repetitive behaviors. [ ]

Descriptions:

- A. Tension or boredom often precedes repetitive behaviors.
- B. Habit Reversal Training (HRT) and CBT techniques.
- C. Avoidance of social or professional activities due to visible damage.
- D. Obsessive-Compulsive Disorder (OCD) or dermatological conditions.
- E. Infections, scarring, or delayed healing of lesions.
- F. Gratification or temporary relief following the behavior.

Case Study

Adrian, a 35-year-old architect, begins avoiding social gatherings after his coworkers comment on his frequent lateness to meetings. Adrian explains that he often needs to spend 30–60 minutes before leaving home checking electrical appliances to ensure they are off. He insists these rituals are necessary for his safety, even though he has never experienced any real harm. While Adrian acknowledges that these behaviors are interfering with his life, he feels powerless to stop them.

1. Which element of Adrian's case strongly indicates OCD rather than another obsessive-compulsive-related disorder?
   - A. His awareness that his behaviors interfere with his daily life.
   - B. His repetitive checking rituals, driven by irrational fears.
   - C. His belief that his behaviors are necessary for safety.
   - D. His avoidance of social gatherings.
2. What treatment is most appropriate for Adrian?
   - A. Exposure and Response Prevention (ERP) therapy targeting his checking behaviors.
   - B. Psychoanalysis to uncover subconscious fears related to safety.
   - C. Habit Reversal Training to reduce ritualistic behaviors.
   - D. Pharmacotherapy with benzodiazepines alone.
3. Which differential diagnosis should be ruled out in Adrian's case?
   - A. Hoarding Disorder.
   - B. Obsessive-Compulsive Personality Disorder (OCPD).
   - C. Generalized Anxiety Disorder (GAD).
   - D. Body Dysmorphic Disorder (BDD).

Answers

Multiple Choice Questions:

1. B
2. C
3. A
4. A
5. A
6. A
7. C

True/False Questions:

1. False
2. True
3. False
4. False
5. True
6. False
7. True
8. True
9. False
10. True

Matching Exercise:

1. A
2. B
3. D
4. C
5. E
6. F

Case Study Answers and Explanations:

1. B. Explanation: The repetitive nature of his checking behaviors, driven by irrational fears, is characteristic of OCD.
2. A. Explanation: ERP therapy is the most effective treatment for OCD, as it focuses on reducing compulsions and managing anxiety.
3. B. Explanation: OCPD must be ruled out, as it shares features like orderliness but lacks distress related to rituals.

Trauma- and Stressor-Related Disorders

This section covers conditions that emerge following traumatic events or highly stressful situations. Their manifestations can range from avoidance and hyperarousal to deeper changes in behavior and emotions. A well-known example is Posttraumatic Stress Disorder (PTSD), which can develop after life-threatening or extremely distressing experiences such as severe accidents, violence, or natural disasters. Common symptoms include intrusive memories (flashbacks or nightmares), avoidance of places or situations tied to the event, a persistent state of alertness, and intense emotional reactions even in the absence of actual danger.

Another related condition is Acute Stress Disorder, which presents symptoms similar to PTSD but limited to the first four weeks following the event. Should these signs continue beyond that period, or recur periodically, it may be appropriate to consider a diagnosis of PTSD. In both scenarios, the onset of anxiety, distress, or feelings of emotional numbness often disrupts daily functioning, relationships, and work.

This category also includes Adjustment Disorders, which appear when stressful life changes—such as losing a job, ending a relationship, or moving—overwhelm an individual's usual coping mechanisms, leading to responses that are out of proportion to the trigger. These may involve deep sadness, heightened anxiety, or problematic behaviors, without meeting the criteria for other mood or anxiety disorders.

In children exposed to neglect or abuse, Reactive Attachment Disorder and Disinhibited Social Engagement Disorder illustrate two possible outcomes of adverse early experiences. The former is marked by difficulty seeking and maintaining emotional bonds with caregivers, while the latter features overly friendly behavior toward unfamiliar adults, reflecting disrupted attachment processes.

From a diagnostic standpoint, it is important to identify the nature of the traumatic or stressful event and consider the timeframe between the event and the onset of symptoms. Clinicians also examine protective factors, such as social support, and risk factors, which may include preexisting psychological or physical conditions. Treatment often involves cognitive-behavioral strategies to help process the trauma and reduce avoidance, along with relaxation techniques and, if needed, anti-anxiety or antidepressant medications. Psychological support and the creation of a safe environment play a central role in helping individuals regain control, gradually reducing the intensity of distressing memories and reactions.

Reactive Attachment Disorder

Multiple Choice Questions

1. Which of the following is a key diagnostic criterion for reactive attachment disorder (RAD) as per the DSM-5?
    - A. Repeated episodes of unprovoked aggressive behavior
    - B. Lack of attachment behaviors toward caregivers
    - C. Excessive desire for social isolation
    - D. Displaying hyperactive behaviors
2. Which condition is most commonly associated with the development of RAD?
    - A. Multiple adoptions at an older age
    - B. Overly protective caregiving
    - C. Traumatic experiences with consistent caregivers
    - D. Early placement in a stable family environment
3. In what age range can RAD be diagnosed?
    - A. Infants up to 6 months
    - B. Between 9 months and 5 years
    - C. From 6 to 12 years old
    - D. Adolescents over 12 years old
4. Which of the following is a common behavior in children with RAD?
    - A. Inappropriate affectionate responses to strangers
    - B. Inability to smile in social situations
    - C. Lack of emotional responsiveness toward primary caregivers
    - D. Persistent requests for physical contact from caregivers
5. The onset of RAD must occur:
    - A. Before 9 months of age
    - B. Before 5 years of age
    - C. During adolescence
    - D. At any point in life
6. Which of the following is *not* a characteristic of RAD?
    - A. Emotionally withdrawn or inhibited behaviors
    - B. Substance abuse
    - C. Failure to seek comfort in stressful situations
    - D. Lack of selective attachment to a caregiver
7. The primary treatment approach for RAD focuses on:
    - A. Pharmacological therapy
    - B. Establishing a stable and nurturing environment
    - C. Cognitive-behavioral therapy
    - D. Reducing contact with strangers

True/False

		T	F
1	Reactive Attachment Disorder is more common in children who experienced severe neglect during their early years.		
2	According to the DSM-5, RAD can manifest in children raised in stable family settings but lacking adequate emotional stimulation.		
3	Children with RAD may develop overly disinhibited social behaviors, such as indiscriminately approaching strangers for comfort.		
4	A diagnosis of RAD requires that the child shows clear signs of social avoidance in at least two different contexts.		
5	RAD is never diagnosed in children older than 5 years, even if symptoms persist.		
6	A diagnosis of RAD is associated with difficulties in forming reciprocal emotional relationships with caregivers or peers.		
7	RAD behaviors, such as social withdrawal, are often attributed to a combination of genetic and environmental factors.		
8	Physical neglect is considered a primary requirement for a diagnosis of RAD, regardless of the presence of emotional abuse.		
9	Treatment for RAD requires a multidisciplinary approach, including interventions directed at both the child and the family context.		
10	Clinical manifestations of RAD are easily distinguishable from those of autism spectrum disorder based solely on social behavior.		

Matching Exercise

1. Withdrawn behavior toward caregivers. [ ]
2. Lack of selective attachment. [ ]
3. Experiences of early neglect. [ ]
4. Age of onset for diagnosis. [ ]
5. Primary treatment. [ ]
6. Inhibited emotional responses. [ ]

Descriptions:

- A. Between 9 months and 5 years
- B. Establishing a stable and nurturing environment
- C. Inhibited emotional responses toward caregivers
- D. Absence of a bond with a specific caregiver
- E. Neglect or abuse in early childhood
- F. Detached behavior from caregivers

Case Study

A 3-year-old child, adopted six months ago, shows minimal interaction with their adoptive parents. The child does not seek comfort when distressed and does not respond affectionately to their caregivers. Before adoption, the child lived in an orphanage with inadequate care. There are no aggressive behaviors, but the child is emotionally withdrawn.

1. What is the most appropriate intervention for this child?
   - A. Pharmacological therapy to improve mood
   - B. Enrollment in a specialized school
   - C. Establishing a stable and nurturing environment
   - D. Cognitive-behavioral therapy
2. Which clinical feature supports the diagnosis of RAD?
   - A. Aggressive behaviors toward adoptive parents
   - B. Absence of selective attachment to a caregiver
   - C. Excessive affectionate responses toward strangers
   - D. High levels of hyperactivity
3. What is a likely cause of the disorder?
   - A. Prenatal trauma
   - B. Neglect during early childhood
   - C. Genetic problems
   - D. Overprotective family environment

Answers

Multiple Choice Questions:

1. B
2. A
3. B
4. C
5. B
6. B
7. B

True/False Questions:

1. False
2. True
3. False
4. True
5. False
6. True
7. False
8. True
9. False
10. True

Matching Exercise:

1. F
2. D
3. E
4. A
5. B
6. C

Case Study Answers and Explanations:

1. C Explanation: Establishing a stable and nurturing environment is the primary treatment for promoting secure attachment.
2. B Explanation: Lack of selective attachment to a caregiver is a key diagnostic feature of RAD.
3. B Explanation: Early neglect is one of the primary causes of RAD.

Disinhibited Social Engagement Disorder, DSED

Multiple Choice Questions

1. Which of the following is a hallmark feature of DSED?
    - A. Lack of responsiveness to social interactions
    - B. Overly familiar behavior with unfamiliar adults
    - C. Persistent avoidance of social interactions
    - D. Emotional withdrawal from caregivers
2. What type of caregiving environment is most commonly linked to the development of DSED?
    - A. Overprotective caregiving
    - B. Stable and supportive family environment
    - C. Severe neglect or frequent changes in caregivers
    - D. Highly structured institutional care
3. At what age range can DSED first be observed?
    - A. Infancy (birth to 12 months)
    - B. Toddlerhood (1–3 years)
    - C. Middle childhood (6–12 years)
    - D. Adolescence (13 years and older)
4. Which of the following behaviors is **not** characteristic of DSED?
    - A. Actively approaching unfamiliar adults without hesitation
    - B. Diminished or absent checking back with caregivers in unfamiliar settings
    - C. Excessive shyness when interacting with peers
    - D. Willingness to go off with strangers
5. DSED is most strongly associated with:
    - A. Prenatal exposure to drugs or alcohol
    - B. Lack of consistent emotional support in early life
    - C. Genetic predisposition to disinhibited behaviors
    - D. Presence of co-occurring developmental disabilities
6. Which intervention is most beneficial for a child with DSED?
    - A. Medication to reduce impulsive behavior
    - B. Therapy to develop structured routines and boundaries
    - C. Limiting exposure to unfamiliar adults
    - D. Cognitive-behavioral therapy targeting attachment issues
7. What is a distinguishing factor between DSED and RAD?
    - A. DSED involves inhibited behaviors, while RAD involves disinhibited behaviors
    - B. RAD typically occurs in adolescents, while DSED occurs in children under 10
    - C. DSED involves over-familiarity with strangers, while RAD involves emotional withdrawal
    - D. RAD and DSED are indistinguishable and represent the same condition

True/False

		T	F
1	Disinhibited Social Engagement Disorder (DSED) manifests as disinhibited social behaviors, such as indiscriminately approaching strangers.		
2	DSED symptoms require that the child has a clear inability to form secure attachments with primary caregivers.		
3	To diagnose DSED, the DSM-5 requires a history of social neglect or early maltreatment.		
4	Children with DSED may display overly familiar behaviors with adults, regardless of their level of familiarity.		
5	DSED is diagnosable only in children who have experienced severe physical neglect, excluding other forms of emotional abuse or neglect.		
6	A diagnosis of DSED requires that disinhibited behavior is present across all social contexts, not just in specific situations.		
7	Treatment for DSED includes interventions aimed at improving the child's ability to recognize appropriate social boundaries.		
8	Symptoms of DSED are easily confused with those of Oppositional Defiant Disorder, due to the presence of impulsive behaviors.		
9	DSED is considered a rare disorder, primarily occurring in children raised in institutional settings or with frequent caregiver changes.		
10	Children with DSED do not necessarily show behaviors of avoidance or social withdrawal, unlike Reactive Attachment Disorder (RAD).		

Matching Exercise

1. Overly familiar behavior with strangers. [ ]
2. Risk factor for DSED. [ ]
3. Distinction between DSED and RAD. [ ]
4. Lack of checking back with caregivers in unfamiliar situations. [ ]
5. Primary treatment focus. [ ]
6. Age range for observable symptoms. [ ]

Descriptions:

- A. Severe neglect or frequent caregiver changes
- B. Consistent caregiving relationships
- C. Over-familiarity with unfamiliar adults
- D. Emotional withdrawal versus over-familiarity
- E. Toddlerhood to middle childhood
- F. Reduced or absent checking behavior

Case Study

A 4-year-old boy has been in foster care since birth and has experienced frequent changes in caregivers. He displays overly familiar behavior, such as hugging strangers and sitting on their laps without hesitation. In unfamiliar settings, he does not look back to check for his current caregiver and shows no signs of distress when separated from them.

1. Which behavior most strongly supports a diagnosis of DSED?
    - A. Hesitancy to interact with peers
    - B. Lack of checking back with caregivers in new situations
    - C. Preference for solitary play
    - D. Frequent temper tantrums when routines change
2. What is the most appropriate intervention for this child?
    - A. Cognitive-behavioral therapy to reduce anxiety
    - B. Therapy focused on developing structured routines and consistent caregiving
    - C. Medication to address impulsive behaviors
    - D. Enrollment in a preschool for social development
3. Which factor is the most likely contributor to this child's behaviors?
    - A. Early and consistent neglect
    - B. Overexposure to peers in foster care
    - C. Inherited impulsive tendencies
    - D. Overprotective caregiving environments

Answers

Multiple Choice Questions:

1. B
2. C
3. B
4. C
5. B
6. B
7. C

True/False Questions:

1. True
2. False
3. True
4. True
5. False
6. False
7. True
8. False
9. True
10. True

Matching Exercise:

1. C
2. A
3. D
4. F
5. B
6. E

Case Study Answers and Explanations:

1. B Explanation: Failure to check back with caregivers in unfamiliar settings is a key feature of DSED.
2. B Explanation: Establishing consistent caregiving relationships is the cornerstone of treatment for DSED.
3. A Explanation: Frequent caregiver changes and early neglect are strongly associated with the development of DSED.

Post-Traumatic Stress Disorder, PTSD

Multiple Choice Questions

1. Which of the following is a required diagnostic criterion for PTSD?
    - A. Persistent delusions or hallucinations
    - B. Direct exposure to a traumatic event
    - C. Symptoms of mania following a traumatic experience
    - D. Chronic low mood lasting more than two weeks
2. Which symptom cluster is NOT part of the diagnostic criteria for PTSD?
    - A. Intrusion symptoms
    - B. Avoidance symptoms
    - C. Negative alterations in cognition and mood
    - D. Psychomotor retardation
3. How long must PTSD symptoms persist to meet diagnostic criteria?
    - A. One week
    - B. One month
    - C. Three months
    - D. Six months
4. Which of the following is an example of an intrusion symptom in PTSD?
    - A. Avoiding reminders of the trauma
    - B. Persistent negative beliefs about oneself
    - C. Recurrent, distressing dreams related to the trauma
    - D. Difficulty falling asleep
5. PTSD is associated with which type of arousal and reactivity symptoms?
    - A. Reduced startle response
    - B. Emotional numbness
    - C. Hypervigilance and exaggerated startle response
    - D. Excessive optimism
6. In children under 6 years old, PTSD symptoms may manifest as:
    - A. Recurrent aggression toward peers
    - B. Play reenactment of the traumatic event
    - C. Chronic low self-esteem
    - D. Persistent hyperactivity
7. The most effective evidence-based therapy for PTSD includes:
    - A. Long-term use of benzodiazepines
    - B. Cognitive Processing Therapy or Prolonged Exposure Therapy
    - C. Group therapy without trauma focus
    - D. Psychoanalysis

True/False

		T	F
1	PTSD can only be diagnosed in the presence of a traumatic event directly experienced by the individual.		
2	One of the diagnostic criteria for PTSD is the presence of intrusive symptoms such as flashbacks, distressing memories, or recurring dreams.		
3	PTSD may include dissociative symptoms, such as depersonalization and derealization, in a specific subtype of the disorder.		
4	According to the DSM-5, PTSD requires symptoms to be present for at least six months after the traumatic event.		
5	Persistent avoidance of stimuli associated with the trauma is a mandatory diagnostic criterion for PTSD.		
6	Children with PTSD may exhibit symptoms through repetitive play reflecting themes or aspects of the traumatic event.		
7	A diagnosis of PTSD requires that symptoms cause clinically significant distress or impairment in important areas of life.		
8	Symptoms of PTSD must be exclusively attributable to the traumatic event without the presence of other psychological or medical factors.		
9	PTSD can only be diagnosed in adults, while children and adolescents fall into a separate diagnostic category.		
10	Treatment for PTSD may include approaches such as trauma-focused cognitive-behavioral therapy and EMDR (Eye Movement Desensitization and Reprocessing).		

Matching Exercise

1. Intrusion symptom. [ ]
2. Avoidance behavior. [ ]
3. Negative alteration in mood. [ ]
4. Arousal and reactivity symptom. [ ]
5. Therapy commonly used for PTSD. [ ]
6. Manifestation of PTSD in young children. [ ]

Descriptions:

- A. Hypervigilance
- B. Cognitive Processing Therapy
- C. Persistent feelings of guilt
- D. Play reenactment of the trauma
- E. Recurrent, distressing dreams
- F. Avoiding places associated with the trauma

Case Study

A 35-year-old woman survived a car accident one year ago. She frequently has distressing memories of the event and avoids driving or being near busy intersections. She struggles with sleep due to recurring nightmares about the accident and feels constantly on edge, becoming startled by loud noises.

1. Which symptom cluster is most prominently represented in her case?
   - A. Negative alterations in cognition and mood
   - B. Intrusion symptoms
   - C. Arousal and reactivity symptoms
   - D. Avoidance symptoms
2. What would be the most appropriate therapeutic approach for her?
   - A. Cognitive Processing Therapy or Prolonged Exposure Therapy
   - B. Psychoanalysis focusing on unconscious trauma
   - C. Long-term medication with sedatives
   - D. Group therapy without trauma processing
3. Which factor is a likely contributor to her persistent PTSD symptoms?
   - A. Genetic predisposition to anxiety disorders
   - B. Lack of social support after the trauma
   - C. Exposure to secondary trauma unrelated to the accident
   - D. Overexposure to trauma-related stimuli

Answers

Multiple Choice Questions:

1. B
2. D
3. B
4. C
5. C
6. B
7. B

True/False Questions:

1. False
2. True
3. True
4. False
5. True
6. True
7. True
8. False
9. False
10. True

Matching Exercise:

1. E
2. F
3. C
4. A
5. B
6. D

Case Study Answers and Explanations:

1. B Explanation: Distressing memories and nightmares are hallmark intrusion symptoms of PTSD.
2. A Explanation: Evidence-based therapies like Cognitive Processing Therapy or Prolonged Exposure Therapy are effective treatments for PTSD.
3. B Explanation: Lack of social support is a well-documented risk factor for the persistence of PTSD symptoms.

Acute Stress Disorder, ASD

Multiple Choice Questions

1. What is the primary distinction between Acute Stress Disorder (ASD) and PTSD?
   - A. ASD lasts no longer than one month, while PTSD persists beyond one month
   - B. ASD is caused by minor stressors, while PTSD is caused by major trauma
   - C. PTSD is diagnosed in children only, while ASD occurs in adults
   - D. PTSD includes dissociative symptoms, while ASD does not
2. Which of the following is a required diagnostic criterion for ASD?
   - A. Symptoms lasting at least three months
   - B. Symptoms appearing within three days of a traumatic event
   - C. Persistent depressed mood
   - D. Positive symptoms of psychosis
3. Which symptom cluster is included in the diagnostic criteria for ASD?
   - A. Dissociative symptoms
   - B. Persistent compulsions
   - C. Chronic physical pain
   - D. Long-term memory impairment
4. Which of the following is an example of an avoidance symptom in ASD?
   - A. Avoiding places associated with the trauma
   - B. Flashbacks of the traumatic event
   - C. Hypervigilance to potential dangers
   - D. Persistent sadness unrelated to the event
5. How many symptoms must be present across different symptom clusters to meet the diagnostic criteria for ASD?
   - A. At least 5
   - B. At least 9
   - C. At least 12
   - D. At least 15
6. Which of the following best describes the purpose of early intervention for ASD?
   - A. To prevent progression to PTSD
   - B. To eliminate all symptoms of distress within 48 hours
   - C. To provide long-term psychoanalytic therapy
   - D. To focus exclusively on medication management
7. Which therapeutic approach is most effective in managing ASD?
   - A. Supportive therapy and psychoeducation
   - B. Avoidance of discussing the trauma
   - C. Long-term pharmacotherapy
   - D. Hypnosis

True/False

		T	F
1	Acute Stress Disorder requires symptoms to begin within three days of trauma exposure to meet diagnostic criteria.		
2	The DSM-5 states that ASD symptoms may include dissociative manifestations, such as depersonalization or dissociative amnesia.		
3	Unlike PTSD, ASD does not require intrusive symptoms such as flashbacks or recurring dreams related to the trauma.		
4	ASD can only be diagnosed if the traumatic event was directly experienced by the individual and not simply witnessed.		
5	Somatic symptoms, such as excessive sweating or increased heart rate, are not included in the diagnostic criteria for ASD.		
6	The DSM-5 specifies that ASD must last between 3 days and 1 month, without exceptions.		
7	ASD may manifest with avoidance behaviors that limit social interaction or exposure to specific places.		
8	Cognitive-behavioral therapy (CBT) is considered the first-line treatment for ASD, while the use of medication is generally discouraged.		
9	ASD represents a temporary diagnosis that must be reevaluated if symptoms persist beyond one month.		
10	ASD and PTSD share exactly the same diagnostic criteria but differ in symptom duration.		

Matching Exercise

1. Intrusion symptom in ASD. [ ]
2. Dissociative feature of ASD. [ ]
3. Avoidance behavior in ASD. [ ]
4. Onset timeline for ASD symptoms. [ ]
5. Maximum duration of ASD. [ ]
6. Early intervention goal for ASD. [ ]

Descriptions:

- A. Avoiding reminders of the trauma
- B. To prevent progression to PTSD
- C. Recurrent, distressing memories of the event
- D. Depersonalization
- E. Symptoms appearing within three days of the trauma
- F. 30 days

Case Study

A 28-year-old man witnessed a violent robbery four days ago. Since then, he has experienced recurrent distressing memories of the event, avoids walking near the location where it happened, and feels emotionally numb. He reports being easily startled and having difficulty concentrating at work.

1. Which symptom supports a diagnosis of ASD?
   - A. Persistent sadness unrelated to the event
   - B. Recurrent, distressing memories of the event
   - C. Difficulty concentrating due to a pre-existing condition
   - D. Lack of appetite
2. What is the most appropriate initial intervention?
   - A. Psychoeducation and supportive therapy
   - B. Long-term use of sedative medications
   - C. Avoidance of discussing the traumatic event
   - D. Intensive group therapy focused on trauma processing
3. How does the timeline of this individual's symptoms align with the diagnosis of ASD?
   - A. Symptoms appeared too late for ASD diagnosis
   - B. Symptoms appeared within the appropriate window for ASD diagnosis
   - C. Symptoms must persist for at least one month before diagnosis
   - D. Timeline is irrelevant for ASD diagnosis

Answers

Multiple Choice Questions:

1. A
2. B
3. A
4. A
5. B
6. A
7. A

True/False Questions:

1. False
2. True
3. False
4. True
5. True
6. True
7. True
8. False
9. True
10. True

Matching Exercise:

1. C
2. D
3. A
4. E
5. F
6. B

Case Study Answers and Explanations:

1. B - Explanation: Recurrent, distressing memories are an intrusion symptom and a hallmark feature of ASD.
2. A - Explanation: Supportive therapy and psychoeducation are critical components of early intervention for ASD.
3. B - Explanation: Symptoms appearing within three days of the traumatic event meet the timeline criteria for ASD diagnosis.

Adjustment Disorders

Multiple Choice Questions

1. What is the primary feature of adjustment disorders?
    - A. Symptoms that develop in response to an identifiable stressor within three months
    - B. Persistent symptoms unrelated to external stressors
    - C. Symptoms associated with a specific genetic predisposition
    - D. Chronic symptoms lasting more than six months
2. Which of the following symptoms is commonly associated with adjustment disorders?
    - A. Hallucinations and delusions
    - B. Emotional or behavioral symptoms disproportionate to the stressor
    - C. Severe psychomotor retardation
    - D. Persistent memory loss
3. How long do symptoms typically last in adjustment disorders after the stressor or its consequences have resolved?
    - A. Less than one week
    - B. No longer than six months
    - C. One year or longer
    - D. Symptoms persist indefinitely
4. Which of the following is a subcategory of adjustment disorders?
    - A. Adjustment disorder with psychotic features
    - B. Adjustment disorder with anxiety
    - C. Adjustment disorder with dissociation
    - D. Adjustment disorder with mania
5. What distinguishes adjustment disorders from PTSD?
    - A. Adjustment disorders are caused by trauma, while PTSD is not
    - B. Adjustment disorders involve stress reactions that are less severe and shorter in duration than PTSD
    - C. Adjustment disorders are not influenced by external stressors, unlike PTSD
    - D. PTSD occurs only in children, while adjustment disorders affect adults
6. In which population are adjustment disorders most commonly diagnosed?
    - A. Infants and toddlers
    - B. Adolescents and young adults
    - C. Middle-aged adults
    - D. Older adults
7. What is the primary treatment for adjustment disorders?
    - A. Long-term pharmacotherapy
    - B. Cognitive-behavioral therapy and supportive counseling
    - C. Hospitalization for all cases
    - D. Avoidance of discussing the stressor

True/False

		T	F
1	Adjustment Disorders require symptoms to develop within three months of exposure to an identifiable stressor.		
2	According to the DSM-5, symptoms of Adjustment Disorders include both emotional and behavioral manifestations.		
3	Adjustment Disorders cannot be diagnosed if symptoms fully meet the criteria for another mental disorder, such as Major Depressive Disorder.		
4	Symptoms of Adjustment Disorders must resolve within six months after the stressor or its consequences have ended.		
5	Adjustment Disorders include physical symptoms, such as chronic pain, as mandatory diagnostic criteria.		
6	Adjustment Disorders may manifest with anxiety, depression, disruptive behaviors, or a combination of these symptoms.		
7	A diagnosis of Adjustment Disorder requires that the level of emotional or behavioral distress is disproportionate to the severity of the stressor.		
8	Adjustment Disorders can only be diagnosed in the presence of severe or catastrophic stressors, such as the loss of a loved one.		
9	Treatment for Adjustment Disorders often includes psychotherapy, such as cognitive-behavioral therapy, to improve stress management skills.		
10	Adjustment Disorders are considered chronic conditions that often persist for years without significant improvement.		

Matching Exercise

1. Typical duration of symptoms after stressor resolution. [ ]
2. A possible symptom in adjustment disorders. [ ]
3. Stressors that can lead to adjustment disorders. [ ]
4. Age group most commonly affected. [ ]
5. Treatment for adjustment disorders. [ ]
6. Distinction between adjustment disorders and PTSD. [ ]

Descriptions:

- A. No longer than six months
- B. Adolescents and young adults
- C. Emotional or behavioral symptoms disproportionate to the stressor
- D. Divorce or job loss
- E. Cognitive-behavioral therapy
- F. Less severe and shorter reactions than PTSD

Case Study

A 19-year-old college student was recently placed on academic probation after failing several exams. Over the past two months, he has experienced persistent anxiety and frequent crying spells, avoided social activities, and struggled to concentrate. These symptoms began shortly after being informed of the probation. There is no evidence of pre-existing conditions or other psychiatric disorders.

1. Which symptom best illustrates the emotional response characteristic of adjustment disorders?
   - A. Difficulty concentrating due to pre-existing learning disabilities
   - B. Persistent sadness unrelated to external stressors
   - C. Anxiety and tearfulness following an identifiable stressor
   - D. Avoidance of all social contact
2. What would be the most effective treatment approach in this case?
   - A. Psychoeducation and short-term supportive therapy
   - B. Referral for inpatient psychiatric care
   - C. Long-term pharmacological intervention
   - D. Ignoring the symptoms and encouraging academic focus
3. Which feature distinguishes this condition from Generalized Anxiety Disorder?
   - A. The presence of avoidance behaviors
   - B. The temporal connection to an identifiable stressor
   - C. The absence of physical symptoms like restlessness
   - D. The chronic nature of the symptoms

Answers

Multiple Choice Questions:

1. A
2. B
3. B
4. B
5. B
6. B
7. B

True/False Questions:

1. False
2. True
3. False
4. True
5. False
6. True
7. True
8. False
9. True
10. False

Matching Exercise:

1. A
2. C
3. D
4. B
5. E
6. F

Case Study Answers and Explanations:

1. C - Explanation: Anxiety and tearfulness triggered by an identifiable stressor are hallmarks of adjustment disorders.
2. A - Explanation: Psychoeducation and supportive therapy are considered first-line interventions for adjustment disorders.
3. A - Explanation: Adjustment disorders require an identifiable stressor that precedes the onset of symptoms.

Other Trauma- and Stressor-Related Disorders

Multiple Choice Questions

1. Which of the following best describes the purpose of the "Other Specified Trauma- and Stressor-Related Disorder" category?
    - A. To identify symptoms caused by general medical conditions
    - B. To describe cases where full criteria for a specific disorder are not met but the reason is specified
    - C. To diagnose severe psychiatric conditions unrelated to trauma
    - D. To categorize all stress-related disorders as unspecified
2. An example of a presentation that may be categorized under "Other Specified Trauma- and Stressor-Related Disorder" includes:
    - A. Persistent flashbacks with no identifiable stressor
    - B. Subthreshold symptoms of PTSD that do not meet full criteria
    - C. Hallucinations unrelated to traumatic events
    - D. Generalized anxiety with no identifiable trigger
3. When is the "Unspecified Trauma- and Stressor-Related Disorder" diagnosis most appropriately used?
    - A. When detailed clinical information is not available
    - B. When the patient explicitly requests it
    - C. When the symptoms are unrelated to trauma
    - D. When the symptoms meet criteria for multiple disorders
4. Which of the following is **not** included under "Other Specified Trauma- and Stressor-Related Disorder"?
    - A. Adjustment-like disorders with delayed onset
    - B. Persistent complex bereavement disorder
    - C. Dissociative symptoms following minor stressors
    - D. Symptoms that meet full criteria for PTSD
5. What is a key difference between "Other Specified" and "Unspecified" categories in trauma- and stressor-related disorders?
    - A. "Unspecified" requires detailed symptom specification, while "Other Specified" does not
    - B. "Other Specified" identifies specific reasons criteria are not met, while "Unspecified" does not provide further detail
    - C. Both categories are used interchangeably without significant distinction
    - D. "Unspecified" applies only to children under 12
6. What is the primary focus of treatment for these categories of disorders?
    - A. Identifying and managing the stressor causing the symptoms
    - B. Long-term pharmacological treatment
    - C. Ignoring the symptoms to prevent reinforcement of stress
    - D. Emergency hospitalization for all cases
7. Which of the following is an example of a stressor that could lead to symptoms classified under these categories?
    - A. Loss of a job
    - B. Winning a major competition
    - C. Eating a large meal
    - D. Chronic exposure to loud noise

True/False

		T	F
1	The "Unspecified Trauma- and Stressor-Related Disorder" category can only be used in emergency contexts where diagnostic data are limited.		
2	Specified Trauma- and Stressor-Related Disorders include manifestations that partially meet the criteria for PTSD or Acute Stress Disorder but with atypical predominant symptoms.		
3	A diagnosis of Unspecified Trauma- and Stressor-Related Disorder requires the patient to exhibit emotional or behavioral symptoms within one month of the stressor.		
4	Dissociative symptoms, such as amnesia or derealization, cannot be considered in the diagnosis of a Specified Trauma- and Stressor-Related Disorder.		
5	The Specified category requires symptoms to be exclusively explained by a single documented traumatic event.		
6	Trauma- and Stressor-Related Disorders (Specified and Unspecified) can be diagnosed in patients with psychiatric comorbidities, provided the symptoms are not attributable to these conditions.		
7	The minimum duration of symptoms to diagnose an Unspecified Trauma- and Stressor-Related Disorder is at least three months, according to the DSM-5.		
8	The Specified category allows clinicians to describe manifestations that do not meet full diagnostic criteria but cause clinically significant distress.		
9	The Specified and Unspecified categories cannot be used in pediatric patients, as they require a full understanding of emotional impact.		
10	Diagnoses of Specified and Unspecified do not require strict temporal criteria but must always be documented with detailed clinical justification.		

Matching Exercise

1. Subthreshold PTSD symptoms. [ ]
2. Persistent complex bereavement disorder. [ ]
3. Primary focus of treatment. [ ]
4. Reason for using "Unspecified" category. [ ]
5. Stressors commonly associated with these disorders. [ ]
6. Diagnostic requirement for "Other Specified." [ ]

Descriptions:

- A. Subthreshold symptoms of trauma-related disorders
- B. Addressing and managing the identified stressor
- C. Loss of a loved one or major life transition
- D. Lack of detailed clinical information
- E. Job loss or financial stress
- F. Specification of why criteria for a specific disorder are unmet

Case Study

A 45-year-old woman reports persistent sadness, withdrawal from social activities, and difficulty sleeping following the unexpected death of her sibling three months ago. Her symptoms significantly impair her daily functioning. She experiences intrusive memories of her sibling and intense feelings of longing. She does not meet the full criteria for PTSD or Major Depressive Disorder.

1. Which symptom indicates the emotional impact of the stressor in this case?
   - A. Persistent physical pain unrelated to the loss
   - B. Difficulty sleeping and intrusive memories about her sibling
   - C. A sense of relief following the death
   - D. Hyperactivity in daily activities
2. Which therapeutic approach would be most beneficial in addressing her symptoms?
   - A. Cognitive-behavioral therapy focused on grief processing
   - B. Avoiding discussions about the loss
   - C. Long-term pharmacological treatment as the sole intervention
   - D. Referral for inpatient psychiatric care
3. What distinguishes her symptoms as part of an "Other Specified" disorder rather than a fully diagnosed PTSD?
   - A. Symptoms are linked to an identifiable stressor but do not meet full criteria for PTSD
   - B. Lack of distress or impairment in her daily functioning
   - C. Absence of intrusive memories or emotional impact from the event
   - D. Symptoms are primarily physical rather than psychological

Answers

Multiple Choice Questions:

1. B
2. B
3. A
4. D
5. B
6. A
7. A

True/False Questions:

1. True
2. False
3. True
4. False
5. True
6. True
7. True
8. False
9. True
10. False

Matching Exercise:

1. A
2. C
3. B
4. D
5. E
6. F

Case Study Answers and Explanations:

1. B - Explanation: Difficulty sleeping and intrusive memories are hallmark emotional responses to a stressor, reflecting the individual's grief and distress.
2. A - Explanation: Cognitive-behavioral therapy focusing on grief processing is an effective treatment approach to help the individual adapt to their loss.
3. A - Explanation: The "Other Specified" category is used when symptoms are linked to a stressor but do not fully meet criteria for a specific disorder like PTSD.

Dissociative Disorders

Dissociative Disorders involve a disruption or fragmentation of psychological processes that are normally integrated, such as memory, identity, or one's perception of self and the external environment. This category in the DSM-5-TR highlights conditions where these elements no longer work together as they typically would, though the specific symptoms may vary. In practice, clinicians often look for noticeable signs that reveal a break in a person's usual sense of experience—for instance, unexplained memory gaps or feeling as though one is observing oneself from the outside.

Familiar examples include episodes of depersonalization or derealization, as well as situations in which distinct identities surface within the same individual. Beyond formal labels, the common thread is a sense of "being somewhere else" in relation to one's body or surroundings, or a phenomenon where different parts of the self operate without the main consciousness being aware. These occurrences can lead to distress, difficulties in relationships, and challenges in work or academic settings, especially when they appear suddenly or persist for extended periods.

Clinically, evaluating Dissociative Disorders calls for careful collection of personal history, complemented, if possible, by external information (for example, from relatives or medical records). Professionals recognize that these conditions may be tied to trauma, abuse, or severe stress, though a clear trigger is not always identified. In the exercises that follow, you will learn how to differentiate various dissociative experiences, while noting how symptoms might overlap with anxiety, depression, or even psychotic presentations.

The goal of these exercises is to develop the skill to identify key markers such as selective amnesia or the emergence of alternate identities, as well as to rule out any medical or neurological explanations. Cultural factors and context are also important; certain beliefs or rituals might appear dissociative yet be entirely normal within a given community. Additionally, a proper assessment should account for substance use, medication effects, or sleep deprivation, all of which can create altered states of consciousness resembling those seen in these disorders.

In the upcoming multiple-choice and true/false questions, along with case studies, you will encounter examples illustrating how dissociation might present in everyday clinical work. You'll need to consider both the intensity and frequency of symptoms, as well as the coping strategies the individual employs—often without realizing it. By doing so, you can refine your ability to form accurate diagnostic hypotheses and guide intervention appropriately, whether through psychotherapeutic methods or, in some cases, adjunctive medication. This focus on dissociative phenomenology helps distinguish these experiences from psychosis, recognizing them instead as a breakdown in the integration of consciousness and identity.

Dissociative Identity Disorder (DID)

Multiple Choice Questions

1. Which of the following symptoms is characteristic of Dissociative Identity Disorder?
    - A. Memory loss for everyday events
    - B. Obsessive compulsions
    - C. Fear of specific objects
    - D. Repetitive involuntary movements
2. What is the typical age of onset for Dissociative Identity Disorder?
    - A. Childhood or adolescence
    - B. Early childhood (0-3 years)
    - C. Late adulthood
    - D. After the age of 50
3. Which of the following situations is most commonly associated with Dissociative Identity Disorder?
    - A. Childhood physical or emotional abuse
    - B. Substance dependency
    - C. Long-term unemployment
    - D. Loss of a family member in adulthood
4. In Dissociative Identity Disorder, the different identities (or personality states) typically manifest as:
    - A. Different names, characteristics, and experiences
    - B. Minor mood variations
    - C. Intense fear of a single stimulus
    - D. Persistent aggressive tendencies
5. Which of the following diagnostic tools is most commonly used to assess Dissociative Identity Disorder?
    - A. Structured Clinical Interview for DSM-5 (SCID-5)
    - B. IQ test
    - C. Functional Magnetic Resonance Imaging (fMRI)
    - D. Beck Depression Inventory
6. Which of the following best describes the comorbidities often seen with Dissociative Identity Disorder?
    - A. Anxiety and depression
    - B. Anorexia nervosa
    - C. Specific phobias
    - D. Sleep disorders
7. What is one of the primary goals of treatment for Dissociative Identity Disorder?
    - A. Promoting the integration of identity states
    - B. Eliminating all identity states completely
    - C. Ignoring symptoms to focus on other clinical issues
    - D. Reducing treatment duration through anxiolytic medications

True/False Questions

		T	F
1	Dissociative Identity Disorder (DID) is characterized by the presence of two or more distinct personality states that alternately control the individual's behavior.		
2	According to the DSM-5, DID can be diagnosed exclusively if the individual experiences total amnesia regarding the trauma they endured.		
3	Changes in behaviors, memories, or cognitive abilities between personality states in DID can be observed by others or reported by the individual.		
4	A diagnosis of DID requires symptoms to be associated with a single, identifiable traumatic event in the patient's clinical history.		
5	Individuals with DID may exhibit somatic symptoms such as recurrent headaches or chronic pain without an identifiable medical cause.		
6	Dissociative symptoms in DID may include both depersonalization and derealization, but these are not mandatory criteria for diagnosis.		
7	DID can only be diagnosed in adults, as symptoms in children are considered part of normal development.		
8	The use of hypnosis techniques is contraindicated in the treatment of DID, as it may exacerbate identity fragmentation.		
9	A diagnosis of DID excludes the possibility that symptoms are better explained by the effects of a substance or a general medical condition.		
10	Treatment for DID requires an integrated approach aimed at promoting the fusion of separate identities into a cohesive self.		

Matching Exercise

1. A disorder characterized by the presence of two or more distinct identity states. [ ]
2. Memory loss that cannot be explained by medical conditions. [ ]
3. The most commonly used therapy in the treatment of DID. [ ]
4. The typical age when trauma associated with DID occurs. [ ]
5. One of the main therapeutic goals for DID treatment. [ ]
6. A common comorbidity in individuals with DID. [ ]

Descriptions:

- A. Childhood or adolescence
- B. Cognitive-behavioral therapy
- C. Anxiety and depression
- D. Integration of identity states
- E. Dissociative Identity Disorder
- F. Dissociative amnesia

Case Study

A 35-year-old man presents to the clinic with a history of unusual behavior and intermittent memory loss. His wife reports that he sometimes speaks and acts like a completely different person, using a different name and showing distinct behaviors. The man describes a significant history of psychological abuse during childhood and reports frequent episodes of anxiety and depression.

1. Which reported symptom is most significant for diagnosing Dissociative Identity Disorder?
    - A. Intermittent memory loss
    - B. Episodes of anxiety
    - C. History of psychological abuse
    - D. Behavioral changes in response to stress
2. What therapeutic approach would be most appropriate for this patient?
    - A. Medication alone
    - B. Psychodynamic or cognitive-behavioral therapy
    - C. No treatment necessary
    - D. Non-specific group therapy
3. Which symptom should be further investigated to confirm the diagnosis?
    - A. The patient's awareness of their identity states
    - B. Presence of obsessive-compulsive symptoms
    - C. Specific dissociative amnesia
    - D. Substance dependency

Answers

Multiple Choice Questions:

1. A
2. A
3. A
4. A
5. A
6. A
7. A

True/False Questions:

1. True
2. False
3. True
4. False
5. True
6. True
7. False
8. False
9. False
10. True

Matching Exercise:

1. E
2. F
3. B
4. A
5. D
6. C

Case Study Answers and Explanations:

1. A - Explanation: Intermittent memory loss is a hallmark feature of DID.
2. B - Explanation: Psychodynamic or cognitive-behavioral therapy is the recommended treatment.
3. C - Explanation: Dissociative amnesia is a key symptom for confirming the diagnosis.

Dissociative Amnesia

Multiple Choice Questions

1. Which type of memory loss is most commonly observed in Dissociative Amnesia?
    - A. Retrograde amnesia affecting personal information
    - B. Anterograde amnesia affecting the ability to form new memories
    - C. Procedural memory loss affecting learned motor skills
    - D. Sensory memory loss affecting perception
2. What is the primary distinguishing feature of Dissociative Amnesia compared to organic amnesia?
    - A. It primarily affects short-term memory
    - B. It is reversible and often associated with trauma
    - C. It includes significant visual hallucinations
    - D. It progresses with neurodegeneration
3. Which of the following subtypes is NOT part of Dissociative Amnesia?
    - A. Localized amnesia
    - B. Selective amnesia
    - C. Continuous amnesia
    - D. Systemic amnesia
4. Dissociative Amnesia is often associated with:
    - A. Traumatic or stressful events
    - B. Chronic substance abuse
    - C. Genetic predisposition to memory disorders
    - D. Aging and cognitive decline
5. In treating Dissociative Amnesia, what is typically the first step in therapy?
    - A. Immediate pharmacological intervention
    - B. Helping the patient recover their missing memories
    - C. Stabilizing the patient's current emotional state
    - D. Conducting neuroimaging to confirm the diagnosis
6. Which diagnostic tool is most appropriate to assess Dissociative Amnesia?
    - A. Clinical interview with a focus on trauma history
    - B. Standard IQ testing
    - C. Continuous performance task assessments
    - D. Electroencephalogram (EEG)
7. What distinguishes Dissociative Fugue from other forms of Dissociative Amnesia?
    - A. The patient's inability to form new memories
    - B. The presence of unplanned travel or wandering
    - C. Co-occurrence with hallucinations and delusions
    - D. Permanent memory loss affecting all life stages

True/False Questions

		T	F
1	Dissociative amnesia can manifest as an inability to recall autobiographical information relevant to traumatic events.		
2	Symptoms of dissociative amnesia must last at least six months to meet diagnostic criteria.		
3	Dissociative fugue, a subtype of dissociative amnesia, may involve sudden travel without memory of the reason.		
4	A diagnosis of dissociative amnesia requires that symptoms are not explained by substance abuse or documented brain injuries.		
5	Most patients with dissociative amnesia develop intrusive symptoms, such as trauma-related flashbacks.		
6	Dissociative amnesia can include periods of partially recovered memory, alternating with episodes of complete amnesia.		
7	Multiple traumatic events are considered an essential requirement for a diagnosis of dissociative amnesia.		
8	Dissociative amnesia can present with somatic symptoms, such as headaches or nausea, without an apparent medical cause.		
9	Treatment for dissociative amnesia focuses on psychotherapeutic approaches aimed at integrating fragmented memories.		
10	Individuals with dissociative amnesia are aware of missing information but unable to recall it.		

Matching Exercise

1. Memory loss for a specific period of time. [ ]
2. The inability to recall traumatic events despite normal functioning in other areas. [ ]
3. A treatment often used to help recover repressed memories. [ ]
4. Memory loss associated with unplanned travel or wandering. [ ]
5. Emotional state often accompanying Dissociative Amnesia. [ ]
6. A subtype of amnesia characterized by inability to recall categories of information. [ ]

Descriptions:

- A. Hypnosis
- B. Localized amnesia
- C. Selective amnesia
- D. Dissociative Fugue
- E. Anxiety or fear
- F. Systematized amnesia

Case Study

A 29-year-old woman arrives at the clinic accompanied by her partner. She appears visibly anxious and states she cannot remember significant events from the past three months, including her move to a new city and starting a new job. Her partner adds that she has no difficulty performing her daily tasks or recognizing people she interacts with regularly. Upon further questioning, the patient mentions experiencing a traumatic car accident shortly before her memory loss began. She reports no physical injuries but describes feeling "completely detached" since the incident.

1. What type of memory loss does this case most likely represent?
   - A. Generalized amnesia
   - B. Localized amnesia
   - C. Continuous amnesia
   - D. Dissociative Fugue
2. Which therapeutic approach is most appropriate as an initial step?
   - A. Hypnosis to recover lost memories
   - B. Trauma-focused psychotherapy
   - C. Medication to improve memory recall
   - D. Neuroimaging to exclude brain injuries
3. What comorbid condition should be closely monitored in this patient?
   - A. Post-traumatic stress disorder (PTSD)
   - B. Bipolar disorder
   - C. Substance use disorder
   - D. Obsessive-compulsive disorder

Answers

Multiple Choice Questions:

1. A
2. B
3. D
4. A
5. C
6. A
7. B

True/False Questions:

1. True
2. False
3. True
4. False
5. True
6. False
7. True
8. False
9. True
10. False

Matching Exercise:

1. B
2. C
3. A
4. D
5. E
6. F

Case Study Answers and Explanations:

1. B - Explanation: Localized amnesia involves the inability to recall events from a specific period, consistent with the patient's symptoms.
2. B - Explanation: Trauma-focused psychotherapy helps the patient process the triggering event and stabilize emotionally.
3. A - Explanation: PTSD is a common comorbidity in individuals experiencing memory loss after trauma.

Depersonalization/Derealization Disorder (DPDR)

Multiple Choice Questions

1. What is the hallmark feature of Depersonalization/Derealization Disorder?
    - A. Persistent feelings of detachment from oneself or the environment
    - B. Intense fear of specific situations or objects
    - C. Uncontrollable intrusive thoughts and compulsions
    - D. Chronic inability to remember personal details
2. Which of the following is a key characteristic of depersonalization?
    - A. Feeling like a stranger to oneself
    - B. Experiencing frequent auditory hallucinations
    - C. Believing one is being persecuted
    - D. Exhibiting sudden changes in personality states
3. What distinguishes derealization from depersonalization?
    - A. Derealization involves the perception that the external world feels unreal or distorted
    - B. Derealization involves memory impairment rather than perceptual distortion
    - C. Depersonalization is linked to the feeling of external detachment from the environment
    - D. Derealization is caused by substance abuse in all cases
4. Which of the following disorders is most commonly comorbid with Depersonalization/Derealization Disorder?
    - A. Generalized Anxiety Disorder (GAD)
    - B. Schizophrenia
    - C. Anorexia Nervosa
    - D. Autism Spectrum Disorder
5. Which is an essential component of diagnosing Depersonalization/Derealization Disorder?
    - A. Symptoms occur independently of substance use or medical conditions
    - B. Persistent visual hallucinations
    - C. Episodes lasting less than a minute each
    - D. Onset only in individuals over the age of 50
6. Which therapeutic approach is often used to manage Depersonalization/Derealization Disorder?
    - A. Cognitive-behavioral therapy (CBT) with a focus on grounding techniques
    - B. Pharmacological treatment as the sole intervention
    - C. Psychoanalysis focusing solely on childhood experiences
    - D. Behavioral aversion therapy
7. What distinguishes Depersonalization/Derealization Disorder from psychotic disorders?
    - A. Insight into the unreality of the experiences is preserved
    - B. Hallucinations are more prominent in DPDR
    - C. DPDR always includes memory impairment
    - D. Psychotic disorders rarely involve detachment from reality

True/False Questions

		T	F
1	In Depersonalization/Derealization Disorder, an individual may experience recurring episodes of depersonalization, derealization, or both.		
2	A diagnosis of DPDR requires the individual to retain an intact perception of reality despite the experience of detachment.		
3	Symptoms of DPDR must cause clinically significant distress or impairment in social, occupational, or other areas of life.		
4	A diagnosis of DPDR requires symptoms to be associated with a documented traumatic event in the patient's clinical history.		
5	Depersonalization may include feeling as though one is observing oneself from outside the body, as if being an external observer.		
6	DPDR is incompatible with other dissociative disorders and cannot be diagnosed in the presence of comorbidities.		
7	Symptoms of derealization are exclusively limited to distorted perceptions of time, without involving space or surrounding people.		
8	Treatment for DPDR may include cognitive approaches to reduce rumination and improve emotional regulation.		
9	A diagnosis of DPDR is based on strict temporal criteria, excluding episodes of short duration.		
10	Patients with DPDR often report a reduced emotional response to positive or negative events, contributing to the sense of detachment.		

Matching Exercise

1. Persistent detachment from one's own thoughts, feelings, or body. [ ]
2. The perception that the environment feels distorted, foggy, or unreal. [ ]
3. A common grounding technique used in therapy for DPDR. [ ]
4. The most frequently comorbid disorder with DPDR. [ ]
5. A therapeutic approach focusing on identifying and modifying thought patterns. [ ]
6. The key difference between DPDR and psychotic disorders. [ ]

Descriptions:

- A. Derealization
- B. Depersonalization
- C. Five senses grounding technique
- D. Cognitive-behavioral therapy
- E. Insight into the unreality of experiences
- F. Generalized Anxiety Disorder

Case Study

A 24-year-old college student reports feeling "disconnected" from herself for the past six months. She describes episodes where her body feels "unreal" and her surroundings seem like a movie set. She states that these sensations began during a period of extreme stress before her exams. Despite these experiences, she recognizes that her perceptions are not real and is distressed by the inability to control them. The patient denies substance use and has no history of neurological conditions. She reports difficulty focusing on daily tasks due to constant rumination about her symptoms.

1. Which symptom in this case strongly supports a diagnosis of Depersonalization/Derealization Disorder?
   - A. Feeling disconnected from her body
   - B. Difficulty concentrating on tasks
   - C. A history of stressful events
   - D. Awareness that her perceptions are not real
2. What is the first-line therapeutic approach for this patient?
   - A. Long-term psychoanalysis
   - B. Cognitive-behavioral therapy with grounding techniques
   - C. Antipsychotic medication
   - D. Hypnosis to alter her perception
3. Which factor rules out an alternative diagnosis?
   - A. Awareness of the unreality of her experiences
   - B. Stressful events triggering the symptoms
   - C. Absence of substance use or neurological conditions
   - D. Persistent difficulty focusing

Answers

Multiple Choice Questions:

1. A
2. A
3. A
4. A
5. A
6. A
7. A

True/False Questions:

1. True
2. True
3. True
4. False
5. True
6. False
7. False
8. True
9. False
10. True

Matching Exercise:

1. B
2. A
3. C
4. F
5. D
6. E

Case Study Answers and Explanations:

1. A - Explanation: Feeling disconnected from one's body is a hallmark of depersonalization.
2. B - Explanation: Cognitive-behavioral therapy with grounding techniques helps address the patient's detachment and rumination.
3. C - Explanation: The absence of substance use or medical conditions is necessary to confirm a primary diagnosis of DPDR.

Other Specified and Unspecified Dissociative Disorders

Multiple Choice Questions

1. Which of the following features most commonly defines Other Specified Dissociative Disorders (OSDD)?
    - A. Dissociative symptoms that do not fully meet the criteria for any specific dissociative disorder
    - B. Symptoms limited to episodes of generalized amnesia
    - C. Persistent detachment without associated distress
    - D. Dissociative symptoms caused by substance use
2. What differentiates Other Specified Dissociative Disorder from Unspecified Dissociative Disorder?
    - A. OSDD includes a clear specification of the clinical presentation
    - B. OSDD requires comorbid anxiety or depression
    - C. Unspecified Dissociative Disorder is diagnosed in cases of malingering
    - D. There is no difference between the two diagnoses
3. Which of the following examples may be categorized under Other Specified Dissociative Disorder?
    - A. Identity disturbance due to prolonged and intense coercion
    - B. Hallucinations without insight into their unreality
    - C. Chronic and untreated substance-induced dissociation
    - D. Memory loss associated with neurodegenerative conditions
4. Unspecified Dissociative Disorder is typically used in which of the following situations?
    - A. When the clinician lacks sufficient information for a more specific diagnosis
    - B. When symptoms align with multiple dissociative disorders equally
    - C. For cases limited to acute dissociative episodes
    - D. When the patient reports substance use as a primary factor
5. Which clinical scenario would likely be categorized as Other Specified Dissociative Disorder?
    - A. Dissociative trance where the patient appears unresponsive but retains awareness
    - B. Generalized amnesia after a neurological event
    - C. A single, brief episode of derealization
    - D. Chronic stress resulting in sleep disturbance
6. What is the primary purpose of the Unspecified Dissociative Disorder category?
    - A. To provide a flexible diagnostic option when full criteria are not met
    - B. To diagnose conditions with clear biological markers
    - C. To identify dissociative symptoms caused solely by trauma
    - D. To categorize dissociative symptoms exclusively in children
7. Which of the following interventions is often prioritized in managing Other Specified and Unspecified Dissociative Disorders?
    - A. Stabilizing the patient's immediate emotional and physical state
    - B. Prescribing high-dose antipsychotics
    - C. Conducting neuroimaging as a diagnostic prerequisite
    - D. Avoiding therapy until symptoms resolve on their own

True/False Questions

		T	F
1	Other Specified Dissociative Disorders include clinical presentations that do not fully meet the diagnostic criteria for a specific dissociative disorder in the DSM-5.		
2	Symptoms of Other Specified Dissociative Disorders may include episodes of dissociative trance that are not culturally accepted.		
3	The Unspecified category is used in situations where the clinician lacks sufficient information for a more detailed diagnosis.		
4	A diagnosis of Unspecified Dissociative Disorder requires symptoms to be exclusively linked to documented traumatic events.		
5	Dissociative fugue is a condition exclusive to Dissociative Identity Disorder and cannot be part of Other Specified Dissociative Disorders.		
6	Other Specified and Unspecified Dissociative Disorders may include symptoms such as amnesia, depersonalization, and derealization.		
7	A diagnosis of Unspecified Dissociative Disorder requires a minimum symptom duration of at least six months.		
8	Other Specified Dissociative Disorders allow clinicians to describe atypical manifestations causing significant distress or functional impairment.		
9	The Unspecified category is frequently used in emergency settings where complete documentation of clinical history is unavailable.		
10	Both categories are limited to symptoms that can exclusively be explained by other medical conditions or substance use.		

Matching Exercise

1. Symptoms that do not fully meet the criteria for a specific dissociative disorder. [ ]
2. A temporary diagnostic category used when detailed evaluation is incomplete. [ ]
3. A culturally specific dissociative episode. [ ]
4. An example of OSDD involving identity disturbance under coercion. [ ]
5. The first therapeutic focus in managing these disorders. [ ]
6. A dissociative condition requiring significant clinician judgment to categorize. [ ]

Descriptions:

- A. Other Specified Dissociative Disorder
- B. Unspecified Dissociative Disorder
- C. Dissociative trance
- D. Identity disturbance
- E. Immediate stabilization
- F. Flexible diagnostic approach

Case Study

A 38-year-old man reports episodes of identity confusion, during which he feels disconnected from his preferences and decisions, stating he feels as though he is "not himself." He has a history of prolonged emotional coercion in a past relationship. His symptoms have caused significant impairment in his daily functioning. He also describes cultural beliefs about spirit possession, which influence his understanding of his dissociative experiences.

1. Which aspect of the patient's presentation requires further exploration to confirm a diagnosis?
   - A. The duration and consistency of identity confusion episodes
   - B. The presence of a medical condition causing his symptoms
   - C. The role of cultural beliefs in shaping his perception of symptoms
   - D. His awareness of the unreality of his experiences
2. What is the primary clinical feature that distinguishes this case from Dissociative Identity Disorder?
   - A. Lack of distinct identity states with separate characteristics
   - B. Presence of cultural influences in symptom expression
   - C. The patient's reluctance to disclose traumatic experiences
   - D. The absence of memory gaps for daily events
3. What therapeutic goal should be prioritized in this case?
   - A. Helping the patient integrate his dissociative experiences into a coherent sense of self
   - B. Reducing his belief in cultural explanations of his symptoms
   - C. Encouraging the patient to avoid emotionally triggering situations
   - D. Using pharmacological intervention to alleviate distress

Answers

Multiple Choice Questions:

1. A
2. A
3. A
4. A
5. A
6. A
7. A

True/False Questions:

1. True
2. True
3. True
4. False
5. False
6. True
7. False
8. True
9. True
10. False

Matching Exercise:

1. A
2. B
3. C
4. D
5. E
6. F

Case Study Answers and Explanations:

1. A - Explanation: Understanding the duration and consistency of symptoms helps to differentiate between dissociative disorders.
2. A - Explanation: Dissociative Identity Disorder involves distinct identity states, which are not present in this case.
3. A - Explanation: Integration of dissociative experiences into the patient's self-concept is a key therapeutic goal.

Somatic Symptom and Related Disorders

This category encompasses various forms of discomfort in which individuals experience persistent or intense physical symptoms, often without sufficient clinical evidence to explain their severity. This does not imply that the disorders are "imagined": the pain, distress, or worry are real and have a substantial effect on daily life, leading to frequent medical visits, requests for tests, and a notable impact on personal activities and relationships.

A key characteristic of these disorders involves pronounced anxiety about one's body, which can affect any bodily system or function—ranging from the fear of having a serious illness, as seen in Illness Anxiety Disorder (formerly Hypochondriasis), to functional neurological symptoms not explained by any identified neurological condition (Conversion Disorder). It is important to determine whether the somatic discomfort is sustained by unresolved emotional issues or conflicts, as well as to check for other co-occurring psychological conditions (such as anxiety or depression) that could heighten the perception of pain or physical discomfort.

From a diagnostic standpoint, the challenge lies in distinguishing these disorders from actual medical conditions that may not yet be identified, while avoiding both excessive clinical examinations and the possibility of overlooking a genuine organic problem. It is crucial to analyze how the person interprets and reacts to their symptoms: catastrophic beliefs, a continual search for reassurance, or lifestyle changes aimed at "preventing escalation" are clues that excessive body focus may be restricting normal daily life.

In clinical practice, the ability to spot warning signs of Somatic Symptom Disorder or related conditions is crucial for guiding individuals toward an integrated approach that includes both psychological support and appropriate medical evaluation. In many cases, pairing relaxation methods or cognitive techniques can help reduce catastrophic perceptions of symptoms and improve anxiety management. It is also important to establish a collaborative relationship among the patient, clinician, and other professionals involved, minimizing unnecessary tests and avoiding the oversimplification of labeling the discomfort as "just psychological."

A thorough understanding of Somatic Symptom and Related Disorders therefore requires special attention to emotional factors, the contexts in which pain or symptoms arise, and how these symptoms fit into the person's life history. A careful assessment allows for targeted interventions, helping lower the burden of health-related stress and restoring better balance between physical health and psychological well-being.

Somatic Symptom Disorder

Multiple Choice Questions

1. What is a key feature of Somatic Symptom Disorder?
    - A. A single physical symptom without associated emotional distress
    - B. Excessive thoughts, feelings, or behaviors related to physical symptoms
    - C. Delusions of physical disease despite normal diagnostic results
    - D. Symptoms intentionally fabricated for external gain
2. How does Somatic Symptom Disorder differ from Illness Anxiety Disorder?
    - A. Somatic Symptom Disorder involves physical symptoms that are distressing, while Illness Anxiety Disorder involves minimal or no symptoms
    - B. Illness Anxiety Disorder always includes panic attacks
    - C. Somatic Symptom Disorder is exclusively linked to medical conditions
    - D. Illness Anxiety Disorder is more common in men
3. Which of the following is an appropriate first-line treatment for Somatic Symptom Disorder?
    - A. Antipsychotic medication
    - B. Cognitive-behavioral therapy (CBT)
    - C. Long-term psychoanalysis
    - D. Hospitalization to address functional impairment
4. A patient with Somatic Symptom Disorder is most likely to:
    - A. Avoid discussing their symptoms for fear of embarrassment
    - B. Frequently seek medical care and reassurance
    - C. Exhibit complete unawareness of their physical complaints
    - D. Present symptoms only in response to specific triggers
5. What distinguishes Somatic Symptom Disorder from malingering?
    - A. The absence of external incentives for symptom presentation
    - B. The presence of multiple physical symptoms
    - C. Symptoms that are intentionally produced or feigned
    - D. The lack of emotional distress related to physical symptoms
6. Which of the following statements is true about Somatic Symptom Disorder?
    - A. It is most commonly associated with severe delusions
    - B. Symptoms are intentionally fabricated to obtain medication
    - C. It involves genuine physical symptoms with excessive psychological distress
    - D. It is diagnosed only when no medical explanation exists
7. Which of these strategies is central to managing Somatic Symptom Disorder?
    - A. Focusing exclusively on finding a medical explanation for symptoms
    - B. Addressing the patient's emotional response to their symptoms
    - C. Avoiding discussions about the psychological components of their distress
    - D. Reinforcing the patient's belief in a specific medical cause

True/False Questions

		T	F
1	A distinctive feature of Somatic Symptom Disorder is that somatic symptoms must necessarily be accompanied by documented physical damage through clinical tests.		
2	The diagnostic criteria for Somatic Symptom Disorder include the idea that somatic symptoms are deliberately created or exaggerated by the patient.		
3	The presence of high levels of health-related anxiety is considered a central criterion for the diagnosis of Somatic Symptom Disorder.		
4	The diagnosis of Somatic Symptom Disorder cannot be made if the somatic symptoms can be explained by a documented medical condition.		
5	The diagnosis can be made even in the absence of physical symptoms if the patient exhibits excessive worry about their health.		
6	The minimum duration to consider symptoms relevant for Somatic Symptom Disorder is three consecutive months.		
7	A patient with Somatic Symptom Disorder may have symptoms that vary over time, including symptoms that shift from one bodily system to another.		
8	An important factor in the diagnosis is the impact of somatic symptoms on the patient's daily life, rather than the objective severity of the symptoms themselves.		
9	The diagnosis requires a detailed analysis of maladaptive behaviors associated with somatic symptoms.		
10	Patients with Somatic Symptom Disorder can never have a comorbid diagnosis of Major Depressive Disorder.		

Matching Exercise

1. Persistent preoccupation with physical symptoms despite medical reassurance. [ ]
2. Excessive worry about the severity of symptoms. [ ]
3. Treatment focusing on altering maladaptive thoughts about symptoms. [ ]
4. A common comorbid condition with Somatic Symptom Disorder. [ ]
5. A behavior often seen in patients seeking validation for their symptoms. [ ]
6. The primary goal of therapy for Somatic Symptom Disorder. [ ]

Descriptions:

- A. Catastrophic thinking
- B. Anxiety
- C. Reassurance seeking
- D. Cognitive-behavioral therapy
- E. Emotional and functional stabilization
- F. Somatic preoccupation

Case Study

A 35-year-old woman reports chronic headaches and fatigue that have persisted for over a year. Despite undergoing multiple medical evaluations, no clear cause has been identified. The patient expresses excessive concern about her symptoms, fearing they indicate a severe neurological disorder. She frequently visits her physician and insists on additional diagnostic tests. Her symptoms have significantly disrupted her work and family life. She becomes visibly distressed when reassured that her test results are normal.

1. Which clinical feature is most characteristic of Somatic Symptom Disorder in this case?
    - A. The persistence of unexplained physical symptoms
    - B. Her emotional distress and preoccupation with symptoms
    - C. Her request for additional diagnostic tests
    - D. The chronic nature of her symptoms
2. What would be the most appropriate initial treatment approach for this patient?
    - A. Prescribing high-dose painkillers to alleviate her headaches
    - B. Initiating cognitive-behavioral therapy to address her health-related anxiety
    - C. Repeating diagnostic tests to provide further reassurance
    - D. Referring her to a neurologist for specialized evaluation
3. How might the clinician address the patient's reassurance-seeking behavior?
    - A. Encourage frequent visits to reduce her anxiety
    - B. Focus on the psychological impact of her symptoms while validating her concerns
    - C. Avoid discussing the psychological aspects to prevent further distress
    - D. Suggest the symptoms are entirely psychological in nature

Answers

Multiple Choice Questions:
1. B
2. A
3. B
4. B
5. A
6. C
7. B

True/False Questions:
1. True
2. False
3. True
4. False
5. True
6. False
7. True
8. True
9. True
10. False

Matching Exercise:
1. F
2. A
3. D
4. B
5. C
6. E

Case Study Answers and Explanations:
1. B - Explanation: The patient's excessive distress and preoccupation with symptoms are hallmark features of Somatic Symptom Disorder.
2. B - Explanation: Cognitive-behavioral therapy is an evidence-based treatment to address health-related anxiety and maladaptive thinking patterns.
3. B - Explanation: Addressing the emotional impact while validating the patient's concerns can help reduce reassurance-seeking behaviors.

Illness Anxiety Disorder

Multiple Choice Questions

1. Which of the following is the most distinguishing feature of Illness Anxiety Disorder?
    - A. Minimal or no somatic symptoms with intense preoccupation about having a serious illness
    - B. Multiple unexplained physical symptoms with significant emotional distress
    - C. Persistent belief in a diagnosis despite contradictory medical evidence
    - D. Symptoms that are intentionally fabricated for external rewards
2. What differentiates Illness Anxiety Disorder from Somatic Symptom Disorder?
    - A. Illness Anxiety Disorder involves a heightened focus on possible illness with minimal symptoms
    - B. Illness Anxiety Disorder requires the presence of comorbid anxiety disorders
    - C. Illness Anxiety Disorder is diagnosed only in patients with chronic medical conditions
    - D. Illness Anxiety Disorder involves physical symptoms with functional impairment
3. A clinician is evaluating a 50-year-old man with persistent health concerns despite normal medical findings. He is preoccupied with the idea of having cancer and frequently monitors his body for signs. Which cognitive feature supports a diagnosis of Illness Anxiety Disorder?
    - A. Catastrophic misinterpretation of normal bodily sensations
    - B. Complete denial of medical reassurance
    - C. Persistent avoidance of medical consultations
    - D. Hallucinations related to illness
4. Which therapeutic approach is most appropriate for Illness Anxiety Disorder?
    - A. Psychoeducation combined with cognitive-behavioral therapy (CBT)
    - B. Long-term antipsychotic therapy to reduce intrusive thoughts
    - C. Frequent reassurance from multiple medical providers
    - D. Diagnostic testing at regular intervals to reduce patient anxiety
5. Which of the following criteria from the DSM-5 excludes a diagnosis of Illness Anxiety Disorder?
    - A. Symptoms that occur exclusively during acute panic attacks
    - B. Health anxiety lasting less than one month
    - C. Beliefs about illness that are fixed and delusional in nature
    - D. Functional impairment due to comorbid conditions
6. Which scenario is most consistent with Illness Anxiety Disorder?
    - A. A patient with chronic back pain seeking multiple pain medications
    - B. A patient frequently checking their pulse and avoiding exercise out of fear of heart disease despite normal tests
    - C. A patient insisting on surgery for unexplained abdominal pain despite a lack of evidence
    - D. A patient experiencing severe fatigue after a traumatic life event
7. Which cognitive bias is commonly observed in patients with Illness Anxiety Disorder?
    - A. Selective attention to bodily sensations
    - B. Overgeneralization based on past traumatic experiences
    - C. Cognitive dissonance regarding health beliefs
    - D. Denial of the need for medical intervention

True/False Questions

		T	F
1	Physical symptoms in Illness Anxiety Disorder are often multiple and variable, resembling Somatic Symptom Disorder.		
2	Health-related worries persist in Illness Anxiety Disorder only if reassurance comes from specialists.		
3	Illness Anxiety Disorder includes avoidance behaviors related to healthcare settings.		
4	The diagnosis is excluded if physical symptoms, even mild ones, are present.		
5	Beliefs about serious illness can exist without reaching delusional intensity.		
6	Illness Anxiety Disorder focuses exclusively on current physical symptoms.		
7	The six-month duration applies to the overall cycle of health-related anxiety and behaviors.		
8	Health-related rituals can make Illness Anxiety Disorder resemble Obsessive-Compulsive Disorder.		
9	Differential evaluation with Generalized Anxiety Disorder is unnecessary.		
10	Psychological therapy is effective only when combined with pharmacological treatments.		

Matching Exercise

1. Excessive preoccupation with having or acquiring a serious illness. [ ]
2. A psychological intervention targeting maladaptive health-related thoughts. [ ]
3. A common cognitive pattern in Illness Anxiety Disorder involving misinterpretation of bodily sensations. [ ]
4. Behavior often seen in Illness Anxiety Disorder, such as avoiding exercise or seeking reassurance. [ ]
5. A criterion that excludes a diagnosis of Illness Anxiety Disorder. [ ]
6. A common comorbid condition. [ ]

Descriptions:

- A. Selective attention
- B. Avoidance or reassurance seeking
- C. Delusional health beliefs
- D. Anxiety or depression
- E. Illness preoccupation
- F. Cognitive-behavioral therapy

Case Study

A 28-year-old man reports persistent fears of having a serious heart condition. He frequently checks his pulse and avoids physical activity, stating, "What if I push myself too hard and trigger a heart attack?" He has undergone multiple evaluations, including a cardiac stress test, which showed no abnormalities. Despite reassurances from his cardiologist, he remains convinced something is wrong. His symptoms began six months ago after witnessing his father suffer a heart attack. He reports trouble focusing at work due to constant worry and frequently seeks reassurance from his partner.

1. What aspect of this patient's presentation is most consistent with Illness Anxiety Disorder?
   - A. His fear of triggering a heart attack through physical activity
   - B. His history of witnessing his father's medical emergency
   - C. His avoidance of physical activity and reliance on reassurance
   - D. His trouble focusing at work
2. What therapeutic approach would be most effective for this patient?
   - A. Frequent medical tests to rule out all possible conditions
   - B. Psychoeducation and cognitive-behavioral therapy focusing on catastrophic thinking
   - C. Prescribing anxiolytic medication to reduce his worry
   - D. Encouraging him to avoid seeking medical reassurance
3. Which criterion from the DSM-5 confirms the diagnosis of Illness Anxiety Disorder in this case?
   - A. Symptoms persisting for at least six months
   - B. Lack of insight into the unreality of his fears
   - C. Significant functional impairment due to health-related anxiety
   - D. Excessive focus on a past traumatic event

Answers

Multiple Choice Questions:
1. A
2. A
3. A
4. A
5. C
6. B
7. A

True/False Questions:
1. True
2. False
3. True
4. False
5. True
6. False
7. True
8. True
9. False
10. True

Matching Exercise:
1. E
2. F
3. A
4. B
5. C
6. D

Case Study Answers and Explanations:
1. C - Explanation: Avoidance and reassurance seeking are hallmark behaviors in Illness Anxiety Disorder.
2. B - Explanation: CBT is the evidence-based treatment for reducing catastrophic thinking and health-related anxiety.
3. A - Explanation: DSM-5 requires symptoms to persist for at least six months for a diagnosis of Illness Anxiety Disorder.

Conversion Disorder

Multiple Choice Questions

1. Which of the following is a defining feature of Conversion Disorder?
    - A. Neurological symptoms that are incompatible with recognized medical or neurological conditions
    - B. Symptoms intentionally produced to gain external rewards
    - C. Persistent cognitive impairments without physical symptoms
    - D. Symptoms exclusively related to substance use
2. What clinical presentation would most strongly suggest Conversion Disorder?
    - A. Weakness or paralysis that fluctuates depending on the patient's attention
    - B. Chronic pain with no apparent cause
    - C. Fear of specific neurological conditions despite normal test results
    - D. Episodes of memory loss unrelated to trauma
3. Which finding is most commonly associated with Conversion Disorder during clinical evaluation?
    - A. The Hoover sign, indicating inconsistency in weakness
    - B. Diffuse atrophy on imaging studies
    - C. Worsening symptoms with cognitive-behavioral therapy
    - D. Fixed delusional beliefs about a specific condition
4. What is a key factor differentiating Conversion Disorder from malingering?
    - A. The absence of external incentives in Conversion Disorder
    - B. The intentional exaggeration of symptoms in Conversion Disorder
    - C. The presence of clear medical findings in malingering
    - D. The rapid resolution of symptoms with reassurance
5. Which of the following therapeutic interventions is most appropriate for managing Conversion Disorder?
    - A. Encouraging a focus on symptom minimization during therapy
    - B. Collaborative treatment involving physical therapy and psychotherapy
    - C. Immediate pharmacological intervention to address symptoms
    - D. Repeated diagnostic testing to reassure the patient
6. Which symptom is most indicative of a motor subtype of Conversion Disorder?
    - A. Sudden blindness with normal eye examination results
    - B. Seizure-like episodes without electrical abnormalities on EEG
    - C. Inability to move a limb despite normal muscle strength on testing
    - D. Persistent dizziness with normal neurological findings
7. Which psychological factor is most commonly associated with Conversion Disorder?
    - A. Recent exposure to significant emotional stress
    - B. A history of specific phobias
    - C. Cognitive impairments following a neurological injury
    - D. Substance-induced alterations in perception

True/False Questions

		T	F
1	Diagnosis of Conversion Disorder requires the presence of a documented neurological deficit.		
2	Symptoms of Conversion Disorder can include paralysis, but without an evident physiological basis.		
3	Conversion Disorder is distinct from Factitious Disorder because the symptoms are not intentionally produced.		
4	Diagnosis of Conversion Disorder is excluded if the patient has a documented neurological condition.		
5	Diagnosis requires clear incompatibility between symptoms and recognized medical conditions.		
6	Psychogenic seizures can be included in the diagnostic criteria for Conversion Disorder.		
7	Onset of Conversion Disorder symptoms is never associated with stressful or traumatic events.		
8	The duration of Conversion Disorder symptoms can be brief but must be clinically significant.		
9	For Conversion Disorder diagnosis, all possible underlying medical conditions must be completely ruled out.		
10	Patients with Conversion Disorder may exhibit sensory symptoms like blindness or hearing loss without organic causes.		

Matching Exercise

1. A motor symptom often observed in Conversion Disorder. [ ]
2. A psychological intervention commonly used in treatment. [ ]
3. A clinical finding that supports the diagnosis of Conversion Disorder. [ ]
4. A factor commonly associated with the onset of Conversion Disorder. [ ]
5. A subtype of Conversion Disorder involving sensory impairments. [ ]
6. A key characteristic distinguishing Conversion Disorder from malingering. [ ]

Descriptions:

- A. Stress or trauma
- B. Hoover sign
- C. Collaborative care with CBT
- D. Paralysis or weakness
- E. Sensory loss (e.g., blindness)
- F. Lack of external incentives

Case Study

A 30-year-old woman presents with sudden weakness in her right leg, which began three days after a heated argument with her partner. She describes being unable to move her leg and is using a wheelchair. A neurological examination reveals inconsistencies, including normal reflexes and strength in the supine position but an inability to bear weight. She has no history of neurological conditions, and imaging studies, including an MRI, are unremarkable. The patient reports significant stress in her personal life, describing feelings of being "trapped." She denies intentional symptom exaggeration and appears distressed by her condition.

1. Which clinical finding most strongly supports a diagnosis of Conversion Disorder in this case?
   - A. Normal imaging studies
   - B. Inconsistencies between reported symptoms and physical examination findings
   - C. The presence of recent stressors
   - D. The use of a wheelchair to manage symptoms
2. What is the most appropriate initial intervention for this patient?
   - A. Referring her for comprehensive diagnostic testing to exclude rare neurological conditions
   - B. Initiating cognitive-behavioral therapy to address underlying stress and maladaptive thought patterns
   - C. Providing reassurance and advising rest until symptoms improve
   - D. Prescribing anxiolytic medications to address her distress
3. Which factor in the patient's history complicates the diagnostic process?
   - A. The presence of stressors in her personal life
   - B. The lack of prior neurological symptoms
   - C. Her visible distress about her condition
   - D. Her reliance on a wheelchair

Answers

Multiple Choice Questions:

1. A
2. A
3. A
4. A
5. B
6. C
7. A

True/False Questions:

1. False
2. True
3. True
4. False
5. True
6. True
7. False
8. True
9. False
10. True

Matching Exercise:

1. D
2. C
3. B
4. A
5. E
6. F

Case Study Answers and Explanations:

1. B - Explanation: The inconsistencies between symptoms and examination findings are characteristic of Conversion Disorder.
2. B - Explanation: CBT is an effective first-line intervention to address stress and maladaptive responses contributing to symptoms.
3. A - Explanation: The presence of stressors could suggest psychological contributions but may also lead to diagnostic overshadowing if not carefully evaluated.

Psychological Factors Affecting Other Medical Conditions

Multiple Choice Questions

1. Which of the following best defines Psychological Factors Affecting Other Medical Conditions?
   - A. A mental disorder caused by a chronic medical condition
   - B. The presence of psychological or behavioral factors that adversely affect a medical condition
   - C. Physical symptoms caused entirely by psychological distress
   - D. Intentional exaggeration of symptoms for secondary gain
2. Which example best illustrates Psychological Factors Affecting Other Medical Conditions?
   - A. Anxiety exacerbating symptoms of asthma
   - B. Chronic pain due to a somatic disorder
   - C. Psychogenic seizures without any neurological findings
   - D. Persistent fatigue attributed to unresolved grief
3. Which of the following psychological factors would most likely worsen a medical condition?
   - A. Denial of the need for medical treatment
   - B. Excessive focus on emotional well-being
   - C. Over-reliance on prescribed medication
   - D. Development of supportive coping strategies
4. What distinguishes Psychological Factors Affecting Other Medical Conditions from Somatic Symptom Disorder?
   - A. The presence of a diagnosed medical condition in Psychological Factors Affecting Other Medical Conditions
   - B. The absence of psychological distress in Somatic Symptom Disorder
   - C. Intentional exaggeration of symptoms in Psychological Factors Affecting Other Medical Conditions
   - D. The exclusive focus on mental health in Psychological Factors Affecting Other Medical Conditions
5. Which intervention is most appropriate for managing Psychological Factors Affecting Other Medical Conditions?
   - A. Focusing on the medical condition without addressing psychological factors
   - B. Integrated care combining medical and psychological treatments
   - C. Prescribing medications for the medical condition only
   - D. Avoiding psychological discussions to reduce patient distress
6. Which of the following scenarios most accurately reflects Psychological Factors Affecting Other Medical Conditions?
   - A. A patient with diabetes whose blood sugar levels are poorly controlled due to stress and inconsistent medication use
   - B. A patient reporting chronic fatigue with no identifiable medical cause
   - C. A patient with multiple physical complaints but normal diagnostic findings
   - D. A patient avoiding exercise due to fear of physical injury
7. Which psychological factor is commonly associated with worsening of medical conditions?
   - A. Catastrophic thinking about symptoms
   - B. Increased adherence to medical recommendations
   - C. Improved emotional regulation
   - D. Reduced focus on physical symptoms

True/False Questions

		T	F
1	Diagnosis of Psychological Factors Affecting Other Medical Conditions requires that a psychological factor worsens an existing medical condition.		
2	Psychological factors affecting a medical condition must necessarily be intentional and conscious.		
3	Poor or absent adherence to medical recommendations can be among the psychological factors worsening a medical condition.		
4	Psychological factors must cause a measurable worsening of the medical condition to be diagnosed.		
5	Anxiety can contribute to the onset or worsening of cardiovascular diseases and be considered in this diagnosis.		
6	The disorder is distinct from somatoform disorders as it requires the presence of a documented medical condition.		
7	Maladaptive behaviors, such as ignoring significant symptoms, can worsen the prognosis of an existing medical condition.		
8	Diagnosis of Psychological Factors Affecting Other Medical Conditions excludes the presence of unconscious psychological factors.		
9	To make the diagnosis, the relationship between the psychological factor and the medical condition must be proven with clinical tests.		
10	Psychological factors affecting a medical condition can never include cultural or environmental aspects.		

Matching Exercise

1. A psychological factor that can delay recovery from a medical condition. [ ]
2. An intervention commonly used to address psychological factors affecting medical conditions. [ ]
3. A medical condition commonly worsened by psychological stress. [ ]
4. A behavior that negatively impacts adherence to medical treatment. [ ]
5. The primary goal of treatment in this condition. [ ]
6. A distinguishing feature of this condition compared to Somatic Symptom Disorder. [ ]

Descriptions:

- A. Stress management therapy
- B. Anxiety exacerbating asthma
- C. Improving physical and emotional outcomes
- D. Denial of illness severity
- E. The presence of a diagnosed medical condition
- F. Catastrophic thinking

Case Study

A 52-year-old man with a history of hypertension presents with worsening blood pressure despite being prescribed appropriate medication. His physician notes that he is inconsistent in taking his medication and frequently skips follow-up appointments. When questioned, the patient reports that he "doesn't believe the medication is necessary" because he "feels fine." He acknowledges recent stress at work but insists that it is "not a big deal." He denies depressive symptoms but mentions occasional difficulty sleeping.

1. Which psychological factor is most likely affecting this patient's medical condition?
    - A. Catastrophic thinking about his blood pressure
    - B. Denial of the severity of his condition
    - C. Maladaptive coping mechanisms
    - D. Anxiety about his treatment plan
2. What would be the most effective initial intervention for this patient?
    - A. Prescribing additional antihypertensive medications
    - B. Addressing his denial and educating him about the risks of untreated hypertension
    - C. Referring him to a psychiatrist for a mood disorder evaluation
    - D. Reducing workplace stress through immediate lifestyle changes
3. Which outcome measure would indicate successful management of this condition?
    - A. Improved adherence to his medication regimen
    - B. Reduction in workplace stress
    - C. Stabilization of his blood pressure through medication changes
    - D. Decreased frequency of follow-up visits

Answers

Multiple Choice Questions:
1. B
2. A
3. A
4. A
5. B
6. A
7. A

True/False Questions:
1. True
2. False
3. True
4. False
5. True
6. True
7. True
8. False
9. False
10. False

Matching Exercise:
1. F
2. A
3. B
4. D
5. C
6. E

Case Study Answers and Explanations:
1. B - Explanation: Denial of the severity of his condition is interfering with his adherence to treatment.
2. B - Explanation: Educating the patient and addressing his denial are critical for improving adherence and outcomes.
3. A - Explanation: Improved adherence to his medication regimen directly impacts the management of his hypertension.

Factitious Disorder

Multiple Choice Questions

1. Which characteristic distinguishes Factitious Disorder from other similar conditions?
   - A. Intentionally produced symptoms without evident external gain
   - B. Non-intentional symptoms associated with psychological stress
   - C. Symptoms fully explained by an underlying medical condition
   - D. Behaviors aimed at avoiding anxiety-provoking situations
2. A patient presents with unusual symptoms and repeated hospitalizations at different facilities. Which factor would suggest Factitious Disorder?
   - A. Resistance to providing a complete medical history
   - B. Immediate acceptance of diagnosis and treatment
   - C. Symptoms that consistently improve with treatment
   - D. Absence of psychological comorbidities
3. Which of the following is a subtype of Factitious Disorder?
   - A. Factitious Disorder imposed on another
   - B. Somatic Symptom Disorder with related anxiety
   - C. Malingering Disorder
   - D. Conversion Disorder
4. What is a risk associated with patients who have Factitious Disorder imposed on another?
   - A. Physical or emotional harm to the person under their care
   - B. Memory loss for traumatic events
   - C. Persistent social isolation without family involvement
   - D. Physical symptoms inconsistent with clinical findings
5. Which therapeutic intervention is most suitable for Factitious Disorder?
   - A. Confronting the patient directly about falsified symptoms
   - B. A multidisciplinary approach focusing on psychological support
   - C. Avoiding any therapeutic intervention to prevent symptom reinforcement
   - D. Leaving the management solely to a primary care physician
6. Which of the following is a common feature in patients with Factitious Disorder?
   - A. An inconsistent and contradictory medical history
   - B. Total avoidance of contact with medical personnel
   - C. Symptoms that spontaneously resolve without treatment
   - D. Complete acceptance of provided diagnoses
7. What is the best method to differentiate Factitious Disorder from malingering?
   - A. The absence of evident external motives in Factitious Disorder
   - B. The use of advanced diagnostic tests to confirm symptoms
   - C. The presence of psychotic symptoms in malingering
   - D. Differential diagnosis is not possible

True/False Questions

		T	F
1	Factitious Disorder is characterized by the intentional production of symptoms without an obvious external gain.		
2	Symptoms in Factitious Disorder must necessarily be physical, not psychological.		
3	Patients with Factitious Disorder may tamper with medical tests to simulate illness.		
4	Factitious Disorder is always diagnosed exclusively in hospital settings.		
5	The primary motivation in Factitious Disorder is the desire to assume the sick role.		
6	In Factitious Disorder imposed on another, the victim is usually a minor or a vulnerable person.		
7	Factitious Disorder is distinct from somatic disorders because symptoms are produced consciously.		
8	Diagnosis requires direct evidence, such as a confession, to confirm the intentional production of symptoms.		
9	Patients with Factitious Disorder may undergo unnecessary medical procedures as a result of their behaviors.		
10	Behaviors associated with Factitious Disorder can pose significant health risks to the patient.		

Matching Exercise

1. Intentional production of symptoms without evident external gain. [ ]
2. A form of Factitious Disorder where symptoms are imposed on another person. [ ]
3. A key intervention in managing Factitious Disorder. [ ]
4. A factor distinguishing Factitious Disorder from malingering. [ ]
5. A possible risk associated with Factitious Disorder imposed on another. [ ]
6. The main characteristic of symptoms in Factitious Disorder. [ ]

Descriptions:

- A. Physical harm to the person under care
- B. Psychological support and multidisciplinary approach
- C. Absence of external motives
- D. Factitious Disorder imposed on another
- E. Intentional production of symptoms
- F. Symptoms unexplained by medical conditions

Case Study

A 40-year-old man presents to the hospital complaining of severe abdominal pain. Despite numerous diagnostic tests, no organic cause is identified. The patient repeatedly requests painkillers but refuses to provide a complete medical history. During hospitalization, staff observe that he administers non-prescribed medications to himself. Further investigation reveals frequent hospitalizations at other facilities, always with different symptoms and no definitive diagnoses.

1. Which clinical feature suggests Factitious Disorder in this case?
    - A. Frequent hospitalizations at other facilities
    - B. Abdominal pain with no identifiable cause
    - C. Self-administration of non-prescribed medications
    - D. Requests for painkillers
2. What would be the most appropriate therapeutic approach in this case?
    - A. Confronting the patient directly about falsified symptoms
    - B. Integrating a multidisciplinary team to manage the case
    - C. Administering painkillers to reduce the patient's suffering
    - D. Avoiding further investigation to prevent symptom worsening
3. Which of the following factors should be carefully monitored to prevent complications?
    - A. Presence of psychiatric comorbidities
    - B. The patient's response to administered medications
    - C. Risk of self-inflicted harm
    - D. Potential diagnostic errors

Answers

Multiple Choice Questions:
1. A
2. A
3. A
4. A
5. B
6. A
7. A

True/False Questions:
1. True
2. False
3. True
4. False
5. True
6. True
7. True
8. False
9. True
10. True

Matching Exercise:
1. E
2. D
3. B
4. C
5. A
6. F

Case Study Answers and Explanations:
1. C - Explanation: Self-administration of non-prescribed medications is indicative of intentionally produced symptoms.
2. B - Explanation: A multidisciplinary team is essential to manage the complexities of Factitious Disorder.
3. C - Explanation: Self-inflicted harm is a significant risk that requires close monitoring.

Other Somatic Symptom and Related Disorder

Multiple Choice Questions

1. What defines "Specified Somatic Symptom and Related Disorders"?
    - A. Somatic symptoms that do not fully meet criteria for a specific disorder but have detailed clinical explanations
    - B. Somatic symptoms entirely attributable to a medical condition
    - C. Absence of physical symptoms with significant health-related worry
    - D. Symptoms meeting criteria for Factitious Disorder
2. An example of "Specified Somatic Symptom and Related Disorder" could include:
    - A. A presentation that does not fully meet criteria for Conversion Disorder
    - B. A differential diagnosis between Malingering and Factitious Disorder
    - C. Psychosomatic symptoms in the presence of a severe medical condition
    - D. Chronic pain symptoms entirely explained by radiologic findings
3. When is the "Unspecified Somatic Symptom and Related Disorder" category appropriate?
    - A. When insufficient clinical information is available for a more precise diagnosis
    - B. When somatic symptoms resolve spontaneously
    - C. When symptoms meet criteria for Factitious Disorder
    - D. When a patient refuses diagnostic testing
4. Which of the following is a common risk for patients with Unspecified Somatic Symptom and Related Disorders?
    - A. Over-medicalization and unnecessary invasive treatments
    - B. Absence of physical symptoms associated with psychological distress
    - C. High satisfaction with medical treatment received
    - D. Easy diagnostic clarity
5. What is the most appropriate treatment strategy for managing a patient with Unspecified Somatic Symptom and Related Disorders?
    - A. Integration of medical and psychological interventions
    - B. Avoiding any treatment to prevent reinforcing the symptoms
    - C. Repeating diagnostic tests until all organic causes are ruled out
    - D. Prescribing medication to immediately reduce physical discomfort
6. What is the primary goal of treating Specified Somatic Symptom and Related Disorders?
    - A. Improving the patient's quality of life, even in the absence of a specific diagnosis
    - B. Completely eliminating physical symptoms
    - C. Confronting the patient about their mistaken health beliefs
    - D. Referring the patient to a single medical specialist
7. In what context is the Unspecified category most frequently used?
    - A. Emergency situations or short-term hospitalizations
    - B. Chronic diagnoses with predictable progression
    - C. Neurological illnesses with prominent somatic symptoms
    - D. Only in pediatric psychiatric contexts

True/False Questions

		T	F
1	The diagnosis can be made even if the patient shows no somatic symptoms at the time of evaluation.		
2	Excessive health-related behaviors must persist continuously for at least six months.		
3	This diagnosis may include patients with a partial medical explanation for their symptoms.		
4	Somatic symptoms must be proportional to the perceived effect on the patient's life.		
5	It cannot be diagnosed if somatic symptoms are attributable to a cultural or religious belief.		
6	The diagnosis applies when the intensity of concern exceeds the severity of documented somatic symptoms.		
7	The diagnosis requires an evident temporal relationship between somatic symptoms and psychological stressors.		
8	Patients with this diagnosis cannot have comorbidities with other somatic disorders.		
9	This diagnosis applies exclusively to patients seeking medical care for their symptoms.		
10	Patients may present somatic symptoms that change over time without a coherent medical explanation.		

Matching Exercise

1. A temporary diagnosis when insufficient information is available. [ ]
2. A somatic symptom that does not fully meet criteria for a specific disorder. [ ]
3. A common therapeutic approach for these disorders. [ ]
4. A characteristic shared by both categories. [ ]
5. A common risk in patients with an Unspecified diagnosis. [ ]
6. The primary goal of treatment. [ ]

Descriptions:

- A. Improving quality of life
- B. Excessive health-related worry
- C. Use of the Unspecified category
- D. Integrated medical-psychological approach
- E. Symptoms partially compatible with Conversion Disorder
- F. Over-medicalization

Case Study

A 50-year-old woman presents to the emergency room with diffuse muscle pain and fatigue lasting six months. She reports slight improvement after initial treatments, but symptoms persist. The patient expresses concern that the cause remains unidentified, yet refuses to consult a psychologist. Diagnostic tests, including an MRI, are normal. Her physician notes that she frequently seeks multiple medical evaluations but rarely completes recommended treatments.

1. Which feature of this case suggests Specified Somatic Symptom and Related Disorder?
   - A. Persistence of symptoms without a precise diagnosis
   - B. Initial improvement with medical treatments
   - C. Refusal of psychological consultation
   - D. Normal diagnostic results
2. What would be the most appropriate therapeutic approach in this case?
   - A. Proposing an integrated medical and psychological approach
   - B. Prescribing painkillers until symptoms resolve
   - C. Repeating diagnostic tests to rule out other pathologies
   - D. Avoiding any treatment to prevent patient worry
3. Which patient behavior should be closely monitored to optimize treatment?
   - A. Continuous requests for new diagnostic tests
   - B. Slight improvement with initial treatments
   - C. Tendency to frequently change physicians
   - D. Refusal of psychological consultation

Answers

Multiple Choice Questions:
1. A
2. A
3. A
4. A
5. A
6. A
7. A

True/False Questions:
1. True
2. False
3. True
4. True
5. False
6. True
7. False
8. True
9. True
10. False

Matching Exercise:
1. C
2. E
3. D
4. B
5. F
6. A

Case Study Answers and Explanations:
1. A - Explanation: Persistence of symptoms without a clear diagnosis is characteristic of Specified Somatic Symptom and Related Disorder.
2. A - Explanation: An integrated approach helps address both physical symptoms and psychological distress.
3. A - Explanation: Continuous requests for new tests can complicate treatment and lead to over-medicalization.

Feeding and Eating Disorders

This diagnostic category includes conditions where eating behavior, or the individual's self-perception regarding food and body weight, is significantly disrupted. In addition to the unique features of each disorder, these conditions share a major impact on physical health, psychological well-being, and family or social dynamics. In severe cases, they can lead to immediate medical concerns, due to possible nutritional imbalances or physical complications.

Among the more widely recognized disorders, Anorexia Nervosa and Bulimia Nervosa differ in some respects yet share certain traits, such as an excessive focus on weight or body shape and a powerful influence of these factors on self-esteem. In Anorexia Nervosa, people severely limit their food intake, resulting in pronounced weight loss, along with an intense fear of gaining weight and a distorted body image. Bulimia Nervosa, by contrast, involves episodes of binge eating followed by compensatory behaviors (such as self-induced vomiting or the misuse of laxatives) aimed at countering the calorie intake.

Another relevant condition is Binge-Eating Disorder, where periods of overeating are not followed by purging but often bring on guilt and shame. This can lead to weight-related concerns, including obesity, and related physical or emotional issues. In addition to these well-known disorders, the DSM-5-TR includes other, less common or more specific conditions, like Pica (consuming items that are not typically considered food) or Rumination Disorder, which entails regurgitating and partly rechewing food.

From a diagnostic standpoint, it is key to look at both behavioral patterns (binging, restrictive eating, use of diuretics or laxatives) and psychological aspects (distorted thoughts, excessive worries about weight or body shape). Clinicians also need to rule out any medical problems that could either mimic or worsen the condition, as well as explore environmental or interpersonal factors that affect eating habits (such as family expectations, cultural standards favoring thinness, or traumatic experiences).

In clinical practice, managing these disorders often demands a collaborative effort: nutritionists, psychotherapists, psychiatrists, and other health professionals work together to restore more balanced eating habits and address the emotional factors that drive the disorder. In some situations—especially when body weight becomes dangerously low or serious physical complications arise—hospitalization may be required. Recognizing how these issues affect self-image and relationships is a central concern: feelings of shame, the need for control, and fear of judgment can delay help-seeking and complicate the recovery process. Tackling the motivational and emotional aspects tied to eating behaviors is thus an important step in effectively addressing these conditions.

Pica

Multiple Choice Questions

1. What defines Pica according to the DSM-5?
    - A. Persistent consumption of non-nutritive, non-food substances for at least one month
    - B. Voluntary restriction of caloric intake to lose weight
    - C. Episodes of binge eating followed by compensatory behaviors
    - D. Loss of appetite associated with psychological stress
2. Which of the following behaviors could be considered an example of Pica?
    - A. Occasional consumption of chalk during a stressful period
    - B. Persistent chewing of ice without medical reasons
    - C. Regularly eating sand for over a month without nutritional benefits
    - D. Avoiding certain food groups for dietary reasons
3. Which underlying condition is often associated with Pica in adults?
    - A. Iron metabolism disorders or iron deficiency anemia
    - B. Cluster B personality disorders
    - C. Psychotic disorders with delusional eating habits
    - D. Substance abuse causing gastrointestinal disorders
4. In which population is Pica most commonly diagnosed?
    - A. Pregnant women and young children
    - B. Adolescents with anxiety disorders
    - C. Adults with substance dependence
    - D. Elderly individuals with chronic illnesses
5. Which DSM-5 criterion excludes a diagnosis of Pica?
    - A. The consumption of non-food substances is culturally accepted
    - B. Symptoms occur in the context of pregnancy
    - C. The behavior occurs only in the presence of a primary eating disorder
    - D. Symptoms have been present for less than one month
6. What is the primary clinical risk associated with Pica?
    - A. Intoxication or intestinal obstruction caused by ingested materials
    - B. Psychological dependence on the ingested substances
    - C. Severe weight loss due to the consumption of non-food substances
    - D. Episodes of binge eating without compensatory behaviors
7. Which treatment is often recommended for patients with Pica?
    - A. Cognitive-behavioral therapy (CBT) to identify triggers
    - B. Administration of anxiolytics to reduce compulsive behaviors
    - C. Surgery to remove ingested substances from the stomach
    - D. High-calorie diet to compensate for nutritional deficiencies

True/False Questions

		T	F
1	Diagnosis of PICA requires that the behavior of ingesting non-nutritive substances persists for at least one month.		
2	Eating behavior associated with PICA is always limited to a specific age group.		
3	PICA can be diagnosed in patients with developmental disorders, provided the behavior is inappropriate for the developmental level.		
4	PICA can be diagnosed independently of other medical or psychiatric conditions.		
5	Patients with PICA may ingest substances like chalk, paper, or hair.		
6	Diagnosis of PICA cannot be attributed to culturally accepted practices.		
7	PICA is diagnosed exclusively in children under six years old.		
8	The behavior of ingesting non-nutritive substances may be associated with specific nutritional deficiencies.		
9	Diagnosis requires thorough evaluation to rule out other conditions that may explain the behavior.		
10	PICA can never cause medical complications such as intestinal obstructions or poisonings.		

Matching Exercise

1. Persistent ingestion of non-food substances such as dirt or paper. [ ]
2. A medical factor often associated with Pica in adults. [ ]
3. A population in which Pica is commonly diagnosed. [ ]
4. A common treatment for patients with Pica. [ ]
5. A clinical risk associated with Pica. [ ]
6. A criterion that excludes a diagnosis of Pica. [ ]

Descriptions:

- A. Intoxication or intestinal obstruction
- B. Iron deficiency anemia
- C. Cognitive-behavioral therapy
- D. Pregnant women and young children
- E. Culturally accepted consumption of non-food substances
- F. Persistent consumption of non-nutritive substances

Case Study

A 7-year-old girl is brought to the clinic by her parents, who are concerned about her regular consumption of paper and sand for the past three months. The family reports that the behavior started gradually but has become more frequent in recent weeks. Despite this, the girl has no apparent gastrointestinal symptoms. Blood tests reveal iron deficiency anemia. The mother mentions that she had a similar habit of eating ice during pregnancy.

1. Which element of this case supports a diagnosis of Pica?
   - A. The persistence of the behavior for more than one month
   - B. The absence of gastrointestinal symptoms
   - C. The maternal history of unusual eating habits
   - D. The gradual onset of the behavior
2. What therapeutic intervention would be most appropriate in this case?
   - A. Treating the iron deficiency anemia with iron supplementation
   - B. Monitoring the behavior without further intervention
   - C. Intensive psychological intervention for both the mother and child
   - D. A high-protein diet
3. Which clinical risk should be carefully monitored for this child?
   - A. Risk of intestinal obstruction or toxicity
   - B. Worsening untreated anemia
   - C. Secondary food refusal
   - D. Psychological dependence on the behavior

Answers

Multiple Choice Questions:
1. A
2. C
3. A
4. A
5. A
6. A
7. A

True/False Questions:
1. True
2. False
3. True
4. True
5. True
6. True
7. False
8. True
9. True
10. False

Matching Exercise:
1. F
2. B
3. D
4. C
5. A
6. E

Case Study Answers and Explanations:
1. A - Explanation: The persistence of the behavior for more than one month meets a DSM-5 criterion for Pica.
2. A - Explanation: Treating the iron deficiency is crucial to reducing the behavior associated with Pica.
3. A - Explanation: Ingesting non-food substances can lead to serious gastrointestinal complications.

Rumination Disorder

Multiple Choice Questions

1. What distinguishes Rumination Disorder from other feeding and eating disorders?
    - A. Repeated regurgitation of food not attributed to a medical condition
    - B. Persistent restriction of caloric intake leading to significant weight loss
    - C. Frequent binge eating episodes followed by compensatory behaviors
    - D. Avoidance of certain food textures or types due to sensory sensitivity
2. In which population is Rumination Disorder most commonly diagnosed?
    - A. Infants and young children
    - B. Adolescents with anxiety disorders
    - C. Adults with gastrointestinal conditions
    - D. Elderly individuals with dementia
3. Which clinical feature is most indicative of Rumination Disorder?
    - A. Regurgitation of food followed by re-chewing, re-swallowing, or spitting out
    - B. Avoidance of eating in social settings due to fear of embarrassment
    - C. Persistent lack of interest in eating or food
    - D. Consuming non-nutritive substances for at least one month
4. Which of the following must be ruled out to diagnose Rumination Disorder?
    - A. Gastroesophageal reflux disease (GERD) or pyloric stenosis
    - B. Anemia or iron deficiency
    - C. A history of physical or emotional trauma
    - D. Sensory sensitivity to specific food textures
5. What psychological factor is commonly associated with Rumination Disorder in adults?
    - A. Maladaptive coping mechanisms for managing stress or anxiety
    - B. Preoccupation with body weight or shape
    - C. Fear of contamination from specific foods
    - D. Uncontrollable cravings for high-calorie foods
6. Which therapeutic approach is most appropriate for Rumination Disorder in children?
    - A. Behavioral therapy focusing on diaphragmatic breathing and distraction techniques
    - B. Pharmacological intervention with antiemetics or antacids
    - C. Long-term hospitalization to monitor nutritional intake
    - D. Avoidance of structured meals to reduce regurgitation episodes
7. Which complication is most likely associated with untreated Rumination Disorder?
    - A. Malnutrition and failure to thrive
    - B. Psychological dependence on specific eating patterns
    - C. Obstruction of the gastrointestinal tract
    - D. Development of substance abuse disorders

True/False Questions

		T	F
1	Rumination Disorder is characterized by repeated regurgitation of food that may be re-chewed, re-swallowed, or spit out.		
2	Diagnosis of Rumination Disorder requires that the behavior is associated with nausea or spontaneous vomiting.		
3	Regurgitation behavior in Rumination Disorder is always associated with underlying medical conditions.		
4	Diagnosis of Rumination Disorder requires that the behavior persists for at least one month.		
5	Rumination Disorder cannot be diagnosed if an eating disorder such as anorexia nervosa is present.		
6	This disorder can be observed in both children and adults.		
7	Rumination Disorder is not attributable to cultural or religious practices related to food.		
8	The behavior is not better explained by a gastrointestinal condition, such as gastroesophageal reflux disease.		
9	Diagnosis of Rumination Disorder excludes cases where the behavior occurs solely during acute stress episodes.		
10	Treatment of Rumination Disorder may include specific behavioral interventions, such as biofeedback.		

Matching Exercise

1. Persistent regurgitation of food not caused by a medical condition. [ ]
2. A key psychological factor often associated with Rumination Disorder. [ ]
3. A therapeutic intervention commonly used for treating Rumination Disorder. [ ]
4. A medical condition that must be ruled out before diagnosis. [ ]
5. A common complication of untreated Rumination Disorder. [ ]
6. A population in which Rumination Disorder is frequently observed. [ ]

Descriptions:

- A. Diaphragmatic breathing and distraction techniques
- B. Gastroesophageal reflux disease (GERD)
- C. Malnutrition or failure to thrive
- D. Maladaptive stress coping mechanisms
- E. Infants and young children
- F. Regurgitation of food

Case Study

A 9-year-old boy is brought to a pediatric clinic by his parents, who are concerned about his repeated regurgitation of food after meals over the past two months. The parents report that the boy re-chews and occasionally re-swallows the food but does not appear distressed by the behavior. Physical examination and diagnostic tests, including an upper gastrointestinal series, are normal. The boy has a history of mild intellectual disability. He denies any nausea or abdominal pain. His school reports that he often avoids eating with peers and prefers to eat alone.

1. Which aspect of this case supports a diagnosis of Rumination Disorder?
   - A. The absence of underlying medical causes
   - B. The child's history of intellectual disability
   - C. Avoidance of eating in social settings
   - D. The duration of symptoms
2. What therapeutic intervention would be most appropriate for this patient?
   - A. Behavioral therapy focusing on diaphragmatic breathing and structured meals
   - B. Pharmacological intervention with anti-reflux medications
   - C. Referral for long-term inpatient treatment
   - D. Psychoeducation for the parents without additional interventions
3. Which complication should be closely monitored in this case?
   - A. Malnutrition or failure to thrive
   - B. Development of a primary eating disorder
   - C. Gastrointestinal obstruction
   - D. Psychological dependence on regurgitation

Answers

Multiple Choice Questions:
1. A
2. A
3. A
4. A
5. A
6. A
7. A

True/False Questions:
1. True
2. False
3. False
4. True
5. False
6. True
7. True
8. True
9. False
10. True

Matching Exercise:
1. F
2. D
3. A
4. B
5. C
6. E

Case Study Answers and Explanations:
1. A - Explanation: The absence of medical causes, combined with persistent regurgitation and lack of distress, aligns with Rumination Disorder.
2. A - Explanation: Behavioral therapy is effective in addressing maladaptive eating behaviors in children.
3. A - Explanation: Malnutrition is a common complication of untreated Rumination Disorder and must be carefully monitored.

Avoidant/Restrictive Food Intake Disorder (ARFID)

Multiple Choice Questions

1. Which of the following is a defining characteristic of ARFID?
   - A. Persistent failure to meet appropriate nutritional and energy needs without concern for body weight or shape
   - B. Restrictive eating patterns specifically aimed at weight loss
   - C. Episodes of binge eating followed by purging behaviors
   - D. Preoccupation with perceived flaws in physical appearance
2. Which clinical feature would most strongly differentiate ARFID from Anorexia Nervosa?
   - A. Lack of interest in eating or food without body image concerns
   - B. Significant weight loss over a short period of time
   - C. Fear of gaining weight or becoming fat
   - D. Nutritional deficiencies due to limited food intake
3. A 10-year-old child is evaluated for ARFID. Which of the following parental reports would most strongly support this diagnosis?
   - A. The child refuses to eat certain foods due to their texture and avoids meals with peers
   - B. The child occasionally skips meals during stressful times but compensates later
   - C. The child reports a desire to lose weight to "fit in" at school
   - D. The child overeats during celebrations and feels guilty afterward
4. What psychological factor is commonly associated with ARFID?
   - A. Avoidance behaviors linked to sensory sensitivities or fear of choking
   - B. Cognitive distortions about body image and weight
   - C. Compulsive behaviors to neutralize caloric intake
   - D. Obsessive focus on specific macronutrients in the diet
5. Which medical complication is most likely in patients with untreated ARFID?
   - A. Growth delays and developmental impairments
   - B. Gastrointestinal obstruction
   - C. Cardiac arrhythmias due to purging behaviors
   - D. Severe electrolyte imbalances
6. What is the primary goal of therapy in treating ARFID?
   - A. Restoring appropriate nutritional intake and addressing food-related anxieties
   - B. Eliminating all food-related sensitivities or fears
   - C. Encouraging self-monitoring of caloric intake and body weight
   - D. Prescribing medications to reduce appetite suppression
7. Which of the following treatments is commonly used in managing ARFID?
   - A. Exposure-based therapy targeting food avoidance
   - B. High-dose antipsychotics to reduce obsessive behaviors
   - C. Long-term hospitalization for nutritional deficiencies
   - D. Frequent use of appetite stimulants

True/False Questions

		T	F
1	ARFID is characterized by a clear restriction in food intake not related to concerns about weight or body shape.		
2	Diagnosis of ARFID requires nausea or vomiting as primary symptoms.		
3	ARFID can lead to significant nutritional deficiencies and reliance on nutritional supplements.		
4	Diagnosis of ARFID is excluded if eating behavior is attributable to a medical condition.		
5	ARFID can manifest in childhood but persist into adulthood.		
6	Patients with ARFID always show fear of weight gain or concern about body weight.		
7	ARFID cannot be diagnosed alongside other eating disorders.		
8	Patients with ARFID may avoid specific foods due to their texture or color.		
9	Significant weight loss can be a consequence of ARFID.		
10	Restrictive eating behavior in ARFID is always associated with previous eating-related trauma.		

Matching Exercise

1. Persistent avoidance of food due to fear of choking or vomiting. [ ]
2. A medical complication commonly observed in untreated ARFID. [ ]
3. A psychological intervention used in ARFID treatment. [ ]
4. A distinguishing feature of ARFID compared to other eating disorders. [ ]
5. A population where ARFID is more frequently diagnosed. [ ]
6. A goal of exposure-based therapy for ARFID. [ ]

Descriptions:

- A. Addressing sensory sensitivities or fear of eating
- B. Children or individuals with autism spectrum disorder
- C. Growth and developmental delays
- D. Lack of body image concerns
- E. Exposure therapy
- F. Avoidance due to fear of adverse consequences

Case Study

A 7-year-old boy is referred for evaluation due to significant weight loss and nutritional deficiencies over the past six months. His parents report that he avoids eating foods with certain textures, such as mashed potatoes and yogurt, and gags at the sight of some foods. He expresses fear of choking after witnessing a family member experience a choking episode. Despite their efforts, his parents struggle to get him to try new foods. His pediatrician notes slowed growth and developmental delays consistent with malnutrition.

1. Which feature most strongly supports a diagnosis of ARFID in this case?
   - A. The child's persistent avoidance of certain textures and foods
   - B. Weight loss and nutritional deficiencies
   - C. Fear of choking linked to a specific incident
   - D. Parental challenges in introducing new foods
2. What therapeutic approach would be most effective in this case?
   - A. Exposure therapy targeting his fear of choking and sensory sensitivities
   - B. Immediate prescription of appetite stimulants
   - C. Long-term inpatient care for malnutrition management
   - D. Behavioral therapy focusing on caloric intake monitoring
3. Which clinical outcome should be prioritized in treatment?
   - A. Restoration of appropriate weight and growth
   - B. Elimination of all food-related fears and sensitivities
   - C. Complete dietary diversity within three months
   - D. Avoidance of hospitalizations related to malnutrition

Answers

Multiple Choice Questions:

1. A
2. A
3. A
4. A
5. A
6. A
7. A

True/False Questions:

1. True
2. False
3. True
4. False
5. True
6. False
7. False
8. True
9. True
10. False

Matching Exercise:

1. F
2. C
3. E
4. D
5. B
6. A

Case Study Answers and Explanations:

1. C - Explanation: The fear of choking following a specific incident is a key factor in ARFID.
2. A - Explanation: Exposure therapy helps address specific fears and sensory sensitivities that lead to food avoidance.
3. A - Explanation: Restoring appropriate weight and growth is essential for mitigating the health impacts of ARFID.

Anorexia Nervosa

Multiple Choice Questions

1. Which of the following is a diagnostic criterion for Anorexia Nervosa according to the DSM-5?
   - A. Intense fear of gaining weight or becoming fat, even when underweight
   - B. Episodes of binge eating followed by compensatory behaviors
   - C. Persistent avoidance of food due to sensory sensitivities
   - D. Persistent lack of interest in eating or food without weight concerns
2. What is a distinguishing feature of the restrictive type of Anorexia Nervosa?
   - A. Weight loss through excessive dieting and exercise without binge eating or purging
   - B. Alternating periods of binge eating and excessive restriction
   - C. Frequent use of laxatives to compensate for overeating
   - D. Severe food aversion unrelated to body image concerns
3. Which medical complication is most commonly associated with Anorexia Nervosa?
   - A. Bradycardia and hypotension
   - B. Elevated blood pressure
   - C. Insulin resistance
   - D. Hyperlipidemia
4. Which psychological feature is often present in patients with Anorexia Nervosa?
   - A. Distorted body image with overvaluation of thinness
   - B. Frequent binge eating episodes followed by guilt
   - C. Fear of specific food textures or sensory properties
   - D. Obsessive focus on cleanliness in food preparation
5. Which therapeutic intervention is most appropriate for patients with severe Anorexia Nervosa?
   - A. Multidisciplinary treatment combining nutritional rehabilitation and psychotherapy
   - B. Long-term pharmacological therapy to restore appetite
   - C. Avoidance of discussions about body weight to reduce anxiety
   - D. Immediate hospitalization for all patients regardless of severity
6. In the DSM-5, what differentiates Anorexia Nervosa from Avoidant/Restrictive Food Intake Disorder (ARFID)?
   - A. Anorexia Nervosa involves body image disturbance, while ARFID does not
   - B. ARFID is associated with significant weight loss, while Anorexia Nervosa is not
   - C. Anorexia Nervosa is diagnosed only in females, while ARFID occurs in both genders
   - D. ARFID primarily affects adults, while Anorexia Nervosa is limited to adolescents
7. Which clinical sign would indicate the need for immediate medical intervention in a patient with Anorexia Nervosa?
   - A. Heart rate below 40 beats per minute
   - B. Weight loss of 5% over one month
   - C. Persistent refusal to attend therapy sessions
   - D. Increased preoccupation with food

True/False Questions

		T	F
1	Amenorrhea is an indispensable diagnostic criterion for anorexia nervosa according to the DSM-5.		
2	In patients with anorexia nervosa, body weight must be below 85% of the expected weight to make the diagnosis.		
3	People with anorexia nervosa may experience binge episodes followed by compensatory behaviors, but this does not exclude the diagnosis of anorexia.		
4	The "restrictive" subtype of anorexia nervosa excludes any use of compensatory behaviors such as self-induced vomiting.		
5	A patient with anorexia nervosa may have a normal body mass index (BMI) if the diagnosis is based on intense fear of weight gain and dietary restriction.		
6	The severity of anorexia nervosa in the DSM-5 is based solely on body mass index (BMI).		
7	Anorexia nervosa may present with psychotic-like symptoms such as an extremely rigid distorted body image, but this does not imply the presence of a separate psychotic disorder.		
8	Physical symptoms such as bradycardia and hypothermia are common in patients with anorexia nervosa and indicate the severity of the disorder.		
9	To be diagnosed with anorexia nervosa, there must be documented episodes of self-harm or suicide attempts.		
10	Anorexia nervosa is more common in men than in women, according to the DSM-5 epidemiological statistics.		

Matching Exercise

1. Persistent fear of gaining weight despite being underweight. [ ]
2. A medical complication frequently observed in Anorexia Nervosa. [ ]
3. A distinguishing psychological feature of Anorexia Nervosa. [ ]
4. A key component of treatment for Anorexia Nervosa. [ ]
5. A type of Anorexia Nervosa involving episodes of purging behaviors. [ ]
6. A sign requiring immediate hospitalization in severe cases. [ ]

Descriptions:

- A. Body image disturbance
- B. Bradycardia
- C. Binge-eating/purging type
- D. Nutritional rehabilitation
- E. Electrolyte imbalance
- F. Heart rate below 40 beats per minute

Case Study

A 16-year-old girl is referred to a clinic for significant weight loss over the past six months. Her parents report that she has become increasingly restrictive with her food intake, avoids meals with family, and exercises excessively. The girl expresses intense fear of gaining weight and believes she looks "overweight" despite being underweight. Her BMI is 16. Physical examination reveals bradycardia, cold extremities, and lanugo. Lab results indicate mild hypokalemia. The girl denies any episodes of binge eating or purging behaviors.

1. What aspect of this case supports a diagnosis of restrictive-type Anorexia Nervosa?
    - A. Avoidance of meals and excessive exercise
    - B. BMI of 16 and mild hypokalemia
    - C. Parental concerns about weight loss
    - D. Presence of lanugo and cold extremities
2. What is the most appropriate first-line treatment approach for this patient?
    - A. Multidisciplinary treatment focusing on nutritional rehabilitation and psychotherapy
    - B. Long-term use of appetite stimulants to encourage weight gain
    - C. Behavioral therapy aimed at reducing exercise frequency
    - D. Hospitalization for electrolyte imbalance correction only
3. Which clinical outcome should be prioritized during the initial treatment phase?
    - A. Restoration of vital signs and nutritional stabilization
    - B. Immediate resolution of distorted body image
    - C. Elimination of excessive exercise within the first week
    - D. Rapid achievement of a normal BMI

Answers

Multiple Choice Questions:
1. A
2. A
3. A
4. A
5. A
6. A
7. A

True/False Questions:
1. True
2. False
3. True
4. False
5. True
6. False
7. True
8. True
9. False
10. False

Matching Exercise:
1. A
2. B
3. A
4. D
5. C
6. F

Case Study Answers and Explanations:
1. A - Explanation: Restrictive behaviors, such as avoiding meals and excessive exercise, are hallmarks of restrictive-type Anorexia Nervosa.
2. A - Explanation: Multidisciplinary treatment is essential to address both the physical and psychological components of Anorexia Nervosa.
3. A - Explanation: Initial treatment focuses on restoring vital signs and nutritional health to prevent medical complications.

Bulimia Nervosa

Multiple Choice Questions

1. A patient with Bulimia Nervosa reports recurrent episodes of binge eating. Which of the following criteria is required to define a binge eating episode?
   - A. Eating an abnormally large amount of food in a discrete period of time accompanied by a sense of lack of control
   - B. Avoiding meals with family due to embarrassment about eating habits
   - C. Consuming only specific food groups during meals
   - D. Eating until physical discomfort occurs, without compensatory behaviors
2. A 20-year-old female reports frequent binge-purge episodes but maintains a normal BMI. Which aspect of her presentation would differentiate Bulimia Nervosa from Anorexia Nervosa?
   - A. Presence of compensatory behaviors like vomiting or laxative use
   - B. Persistent weight below the minimally normal range
   - C. Lack of body image concerns
   - D. Frequent avoidance of social situations involving food
3. Which behavior is NOT typical of Bulimia Nervosa?
   - A. Self-induced vomiting following binge eating episodes
   - B. Excessive exercise as a compensatory behavior
   - C. Severe food restriction without episodes of binge eating
   - D. Use of diuretics or laxatives to compensate for overeating
4. A patient with Bulimia Nervosa is at risk for which of the following medical complications?
   - A. Hypokalemia leading to cardiac arrhythmias
   - B. Gastrointestinal bleeding due to stress ulcers
   - C. Severe weight loss below 85% of expected body weight
   - D. Persistent hypoglycemia due to poor dietary intake
5. Which psychosocial factor is most likely to perpetuate Bulimia Nervosa in an affected individual?
   - A. A cycle of guilt and shame following binge-purge episodes
   - B. Preoccupation with food safety and contamination
   - C. Anxiety triggered by specific textures of food
   - D. Over-reliance on a rigid meal schedule
6. Which scenario best illustrates the clinical presentation of Bulimia Nervosa?
   - A. A 19-year-old athlete who consumes large meals and compensates with hours of exercise but denies distress
   - B. A 25-year-old woman who binge eats when stressed but does not use compensatory behaviors
   - C. A 21-year-old college student who eats excessively in private, followed by vomiting and a sense of relief
   - D. A 30-year-old man who avoids meals entirely to lose weight
7. What is the primary goal during the initial phase of treatment for Bulimia Nervosa?
   - A. Reducing the frequency of binge-purge episodes and normalizing eating patterns
   - B. Eliminating distorted body image within the first month
   - C. Achieving significant weight loss through structured meal plans
   - D. Minimizing exercise-related injuries

True/False Questions

		T	F
1	The minimum duration for a diagnosis of bulimia nervosa is three months, with recurrent episodes of binge eating and inappropriate compensatory behaviors.		
2	Patients with bulimia nervosa may maintain a normal or even above-average weight, according to DSM-5 criteria.		
3	Episodes of binge eating in bulimia nervosa are characterized by a sense of loss of control over food intake.		
4	Inappropriate compensatory behaviors, such as self-induced vomiting, laxative use, or excessive exercise, are central elements in the diagnosis of bulimia nervosa.		
5	To diagnose bulimia nervosa, the patient must exhibit an intense fear of gaining weight, regardless of the presence of binge eating or compensatory behaviors.		
6	Bulimia nervosa can be diagnosed even if the patient does not present severe physical symptoms such as bradycardia or hypothermia.		
7	Patients with bulimia nervosa often report significant concern about body shape and weight.		
8	According to the DSM-5, the exclusive use of compensatory behaviors without recurrent binge eating episodes excludes a diagnosis of bulimia nervosa.		
9	Bulimia nervosa is more commonly observed in men than in women, according to DSM-5 epidemiological statistics.		
10	The severity of bulimia nervosa is determined solely by the number of weekly binge eating episodes reported.		

Matching Exercise

1. A psychological feature that perpetuates the binge-purge cycle. [ ]
2. A common medical complication in Bulimia Nervosa. [ ]
3. A compensatory behavior other than vomiting. [ ]
4. A diagnostic criterion differentiating Bulimia Nervosa from Anorexia Nervosa. [ ]
5. The first-line therapy for Bulimia Nervosa. [ ]
6. A population in which Bulimia Nervosa is most prevalent. [ ]

Descriptions:

- A. Hypokalemia
- B. Excessive exercise
- C. Cognitive-behavioral therapy (CBT)
- D. Normal or above-normal weight
- E. Guilt and shame after binge eating
- F. Adolescent and young adult females

Case Study

A 24-year-old woman presents to a clinic reporting recurrent episodes of uncontrollable eating where she consumes large amounts of food in a short time. She describes feeling guilty afterward and uses laxatives and self-induced vomiting to "make up for it." Despite these behaviors, she maintains a normal weight. Lab tests reveal mild hypokalemia and elevated amylase levels. She reports significant distress and preoccupation with her body image but denies a desire to lose significant weight.

1. Which clinical feature most strongly supports a diagnosis of Bulimia Nervosa in this case?
   - A. Use of laxatives and self-induced vomiting after binge eating
   - B. Normal body weight with mild hypokalemia
   - C. Elevated amylase levels due to vomiting behaviors
   - D. Preoccupation with body image without significant weight loss
2. What is the most appropriate therapeutic approach for this patient?
   - A. Cognitive-behavioral therapy targeting binge-purge behaviors and body image concerns
   - B. Pharmacological treatment with antidepressants to reduce binge episodes
   - C. Long-term hospitalization to monitor medical complications
   - D. Nutritional counseling as the sole intervention
3. Which complication should be closely monitored in this patient?
   - A. Electrolyte imbalances leading to arrhythmias
   - B. Persistent hypoglycemia due to reduced caloric intake
   - C. Gastrointestinal obstruction caused by binge eating
   - D. Weight loss below the normal BMI range

Answers

Multiple Choice Questions:
1. A
2. A
3. C
4. A
5. A
6. C
7. A

True/False Questions:
1. False
2. True
3. True
4. True
5. False
6. True
7. True
8. False
9. False
10. False

Matching Exercise:
1. E
2. A
3. B
4. D
5. C
6. F

Case Study Answers and Explanations:
1. A - Explanation: The use of laxatives and self-induced vomiting after binge eating is a hallmark feature of Bulimia Nervosa.
2. A - Explanation: CBT is the most effective first-line treatment for addressing binge-purge behaviors and cognitive distortions.
3. A - Explanation: Electrolyte imbalances, such as hypokalemia, can cause serious medical complications and must be closely monitored.

Binge-Eating Disorder (BED)

Multiple Choice Questions

1. What distinguishes Binge-Eating Disorder from Bulimia Nervosa?
   - A. Absence of inappropriate compensatory behaviors following binge episodes
   - B. Higher frequency of binge episodes in Binge-Eating Disorder
   - C. Significant weight loss in patients with Binge-Eating Disorder
   - D. Preoccupation with body image in Binge-Eating Disorder
2. Which of the following is NOT a diagnostic feature of Binge-Eating Disorder?
   - A. Recurrent episodes of eating an unusually large amount of food in a discrete period
   - B. Feeling a lack of control during binge episodes
   - C. Persistent use of purging behaviors to prevent weight gain
   - D. Marked distress regarding binge eating
3. A 30-year-old patient with Binge-Eating Disorder reports binge episodes followed by feelings of shame. Which aspect of this presentation would differentiate BED from emotional overeating?
   - A. Episodes occur at least once a week for three months
   - B. The patient eats when experiencing negative emotions
   - C. The patient consumes food until feeling uncomfortably full
   - D. There is no significant weight gain over time
4. Which psychological factor is most commonly associated with Binge-Eating Disorder?
   - A. Low self-esteem and emotional dysregulation
   - B. Obsessive preoccupation with food safety
   - C. Anxiety related to food textures or choking
   - D. Rigid adherence to specific dietary restrictions
5. What is the most appropriate first-line treatment for Binge-Eating Disorder?
   - A. Cognitive-behavioral therapy (CBT) targeting eating patterns and emotional regulation
   - B. Pharmacological treatment with antipsychotic medications
   - C. Hospitalization to monitor nutritional intake
   - D. Long-term use of appetite suppressants
6. Which medical complication is most likely in patients with untreated Binge-Eating Disorder?
   - A. Obesity and related comorbidities
   - B. Malnutrition and failure to thrive
   - C. Severe electrolyte imbalances
   - D. Gastrointestinal bleeding
7. Which patient behavior would most strongly suggest a diagnosis of Binge-Eating Disorder?
   - A. Eating large quantities of food in secret without subsequent compensatory behaviors
   - B. Consuming non-nutritive substances for at least one month
   - C. Restricting caloric intake to avoid weight gain after overeating
   - D. Avoiding meals entirely due to fear of gaining weight

True/False Questions

		T	F
1	Binge-eating disorder (BED) is characterized by recurrent episodes of binge eating without the use of inappropriate compensatory behaviors.		
2	To diagnose BED, binge eating episodes must necessarily occur in the presence of other medical or psychiatric conditions.		
3	Individuals with BED often report significant distress associated with binge eating episodes.		
4	In BED, binge eating episodes may involve consuming an amount of food larger than what is normal within a limited time period.		
5	Patients with BED must have a body mass index (BMI) over 30 to meet DSM-5 diagnostic criteria.		
6	BED differs from bulimia nervosa due to the absence of inappropriate compensatory behaviors, such as self-induced vomiting.		
7	The severity of BED is determined solely by the patient's body weight.		
8	Binge-eating disorder is more common than other forms of eating disorders according to DSM-5 epidemiological statistics.		
9	To diagnose BED, binge eating episodes must occur at least five times per week for a minimum of three months.		
10	Individuals with BED never report psychological symptoms such as shame or guilt associated with binge eating episodes.		

Matching Exercise

1. A key emotional trigger for binge episodes. [ ]
2. A psychological treatment commonly used for BED. [ ]
3. A medical complication frequently associated with BED. [ ]
4. A feature that distinguishes BED from Bulimia Nervosa. [ ]
5. A behavior commonly reported by patients with BED. [ ]
6. A diagnostic criterion for Binge-Eating Disorder. [ ]

Descriptions:

- A. Cognitive-behavioral therapy (CBT)
- B. Absence of compensatory behaviors
- C. Obesity or metabolic syndrome
- D. Eating alone due to embarrassment
- E. Eating until feeling uncomfortably full
- F. Emotional dysregulation

Case Study

A 35-year-old man presents to his primary care physician with concerns about his eating habits and recent weight gain. He describes episodes of eating large amounts of food, often at night, during which he feels "out of control." These episodes occur at least twice a week and are followed by feelings of guilt and shame. The patient does not use vomiting, laxatives, or excessive exercise to compensate for overeating. He reports eating alone because he feels embarrassed about the quantity of food he consumes. His BMI is 32, and he has been diagnosed with hypertension.

1. Which aspect of this patient's presentation most strongly supports a diagnosis of Binge-Eating Disorder?
    - A. Recurrent episodes of eating large amounts of food with a sense of loss of control
    - B. BMI of 32 and hypertension
    - C. Eating alone due to embarrassment about food consumption
    - D. Guilt and shame following overeating
2. What therapeutic intervention would be most appropriate for this patient?
    - A. Cognitive-behavioral therapy focusing on eating patterns and emotional triggers
    - B. Immediate prescription of appetite suppressants to reduce binge episodes
    - C. Referral for bariatric surgery to address weight concerns
    - D. Hospitalization for hypertension management
3. Which clinical outcome should be prioritized during the initial phase of treatment?
    - A. Reduction in binge eating episodes and improved emotional regulation
    - B. Immediate weight loss through structured meal plans
    - C. Elimination of feelings of guilt and shame
    - D. Achieving normal blood pressure without medications

Answers

Multiple Choice Questions:
1. A
2. C
3. A
4. A
5. A
6. A
7. A

True/False Questions:
1. True
2. False
3. True
4. True
5. False
6. True
7. False
8. True
9. False
10. False

Matching Exercise:
1. F
2. A
3. C
4. B
5. D
6. E

Case Study Answers and Explanations:
1. A - Explanation: Recurrent episodes of eating large amounts of food with a sense of loss of control are the hallmark of BED.
2. A - Explanation: CBT is an evidence-based treatment that targets the emotional and behavioral aspects of BED.
3. A - Explanation: Reducing binge eating episodes is essential to improving the patient's overall health and emotional well-being.

Other Feeding or Eating Disorders

Multiple Choice Questions

1. What defines an "Other Specified Feeding or Eating Disorder"?
   - A. A condition that does not fully meet the criteria for a specific eating disorder but has a clearly identified clinical presentation
   - B. Episodes of binge eating without compensatory behaviors
   - C. A condition exclusively associated with primary psychiatric disorders
   - D. An eating disorder diagnosed only in children
2. Which scenario represents an example of an "Other Specified Feeding or Eating Disorder"?
   - A. An atypical presentation of Anorexia Nervosa with normal weight
   - B. Binge eating episodes with frequent compensatory behaviors
   - C. Avoidance of certain foods for cultural or religious reasons
   - D. Loss of appetite associated with a chronic medical condition
3. When is the "Unspecified Feeding or Eating Disorder" category used?
   - A. When available information is insufficient for a more precise diagnosis
   - B. When the patient's symptoms fully meet the criteria for a specific disorder
   - C. When symptoms are associated with a recent psychological trauma
   - D. Only in pediatric contexts
4. Which of the following conditions justifies using the Unspecified category?
   - A. A patient in an emergency setting who refuses to provide detailed information about eating behaviors
   - B. A chronic case of Bulimia Nervosa diagnosed years ago
   - C. A diagnosed ARFID case with clearly identified symptoms
   - D. A patient with a history of caloric restriction for aesthetic purposes
5. What is the most common clinical risk for patients with an Unspecified Feeding or Eating Disorder?
   - A. Malnutrition and metabolic complications
   - B. Psychological dependence on specific foods
   - C. Progression to less severe eating disorders
   - D. Spontaneous resolution without intervention
6. Which treatment approach is most suitable for patients with Other Specified Feeding or Eating Disorders?
   - A. A multidisciplinary approach including medical and psychological support
   - B. Pharmacological therapy alone to reduce physical symptoms
   - C. Long-term monitoring without active intervention
   - D. Restrictive diets to minimize symptoms
7. What is the primary treatment goal for Unspecified Feeding or Eating Disorders?
   - A. Establishing a stable eating routine and reducing emotional distress associated with food
   - B. Achieving rapid weight gain
   - C. Eliminating all behavioral symptoms immediately
   - D. Reducing interaction with environmental triggers

True/False Questions

		T	F
1	Other specified feeding or eating disorders (OSFED) include conditions that do not fully meet the criteria for anorexia nervosa, bulimia nervosa, or binge-eating disorder.		
2	The diagnosis of OSFED requires the patient to have a BMI below 18.5.		
3	OSFED does not include specific diagnostic subtypes in the DSM-5, as it is considered a single generalized category.		
4	Night Eating Syndrome is classified as a specific disorder within OSFED.		
5	Rumination disorder is a subcategory of avoidant/restrictive food intake disorder according to the DSM-5.		
6	Individuals with OSFED may exhibit intense concern about body weight or shape.		
7	OSFED can include diagnoses such as atypical anorexia, where all features of anorexia are present except significant weight loss.		
8	To receive a diagnosis of OSFED, symptoms must be present for at least six months.		
9	OSFED can cause significant impairment in social or occupational functioning, despite not meeting criteria for another specific disorder.		
10	Individuals with OSFED cannot experience binge eating, as this would automatically classify them as having bulimia nervosa or binge-eating disorder.		

Matching Exercise

1. A temporary diagnosis due to insufficient clinical information. [ ]
2. A common treatment for Other Specified Feeding or Eating Disorders. [ ]
3. A medical complication associated with both categories. [ ]
4. A feature of an Other Specified Feeding or Eating Disorder. [ ]
5. A population frequently diagnosed with Unspecified Disorders. [ ]
6. The primary treatment goal for both categories. [ ]

Descriptions:

- A. Establishing a stable eating routine
- B. Adolescents and young adults
- C. Multidisciplinary approach
- D. Malnutrition
- E. Atypical presentations of Anorexia Nervosa
- F. Unspecified category

Case Study

A 25-year-old woman is admitted to the hospital for malnutrition and fatigue. She reports episodes of intense caloric restriction followed by brief periods of normal eating but denies binge eating or compensatory behaviors. The patient expresses significant anxiety about consuming certain foods but denies concerns about weight or body image. Medical evaluations rule out diagnoses of Anorexia Nervosa or Bulimia Nervosa, but her symptoms persist.

1. Which aspect of this case supports a diagnosis of an Other Specified Feeding or Eating Disorder?
   - A. Intermittent caloric restriction without weight concerns
   - B. Malnutrition and fatigue
   - C. Absence of compensatory behaviors
   - D. Periods of normal eating between restrictions
2. What therapeutic intervention would be most appropriate for this patient?
   - A. Cognitive-behavioral therapy focusing on food-related anxiety
   - B. Pharmacological treatment with anxiolytics to reduce food-related concerns
   - C. Non-interventionist approach with passive monitoring
   - D. Exclusive consultation with a dietitian
3. Which clinical complication should be closely monitored in this case?
   - A. Worsening malnutrition
   - B. Psychological dependence on restricted foods
   - C. Progression to Bulimia Nervosa
   - D. Onset of acute hypoglycemia

Answers

Multiple Choice Questions:
1. A
2. A
3. A
4. A
5. A
6. A
7. A

True/False Questions:
1. True
2. False
3. False
4. True
5. False
6. True
7. True
8. False
9. True
10. False

Matching Exercise:
1. F
2. C
3. D
4. E
5. B
6. A

Case Study Answers and Explanations:
1. A - Explanation: Intermittent caloric restriction without weight concerns is characteristic of a Specified Disorder.
2. A - Explanation: Cognitive-behavioral therapy is effective in addressing food-related anxiety and improving eating behaviors.
3. A - Explanation: Malnutrition can worsen without appropriate intervention and requires close monitoring.

Elimination Disorders

Elimination Disorders involve voluntary or involuntary passage of urine or feces at an age and under circumstances where these functions are generally expected to be well controlled. Although sometimes overlooked, they can have a substantial impact on daily life, as well as on family dynamics, school performance, and social interactions.

Enuresis is characterized by inappropriate urination—commonly at night but sometimes during the day—without any underlying medical explanation (for example, a urinary tract infection). It typically occurs in children older than the usual age by which bladder control has been established. Encopresis, on the other hand, involves inappropriate defecation (such as soiling clothing or floors) without a medical cause. This diagnosis applies only when the child has reached an age at which bowel control is normally expected.

When evaluating these conditions, it is important to distinguish potential physiological contributors from psychological or environmental factors. Some children may have developmental delays or reduced sensation of the urge to eliminate, while others may be influenced by emotional aspects or relational problems (such as stress, family conflicts, or anxiety). Certain medical issues—like chronic constipation or endocrine and neurological problems—can also play a role, so careful assessment is necessary before a diagnosis is made.

Treatment frequently combines behavioral strategies (for instance, setting specific toilet times, using positive reinforcement, or employing nighttime alarms for enuresis) with psychological support if emotional or interpersonal difficulties are present. Parents and caregivers have a key role: a supportive attitude that focuses on collaboration and encourages the child tends to be more helpful than punishments or scolding, which may exacerbate the issue and heighten anxiety.

With proper understanding and management, most children can overcome Elimination Disorders, reducing the negative effects on their emotional and social development. It is also important to identify and address any underlying factors to prevent enuresis or encopresis from becoming a source of frustration, shame, or social withdrawal. Ongoing monitoring and personalized interventions can guide both the child and the family toward effective control and improved well-being.

Enuresis

Multiple Choice Questions

1. Which of the following is a diagnostic criterion for Enuresis according to the DSM-5?
   - A. Repeated voiding of urine into bed or clothes, occurring at least twice a week for three months
   - B. Persistent difficulty initiating or maintaining sleep due to fear of incontinence
   - C. Repeated episodes of urinary retention despite a desire to void
   - D. Involuntary defecation occurring during the night
2. A 6-year-old child has episodes of nighttime bedwetting three times a week. Which factor would suggest primary enuresis?
   - A. The child has never achieved consistent nighttime dryness
   - B. The child previously achieved dryness for six months but relapsed
   - C. The bedwetting occurs exclusively after consuming caffeinated beverages
   - D. The bedwetting is accompanied by daytime urinary accidents
3. What is the primary psychological impact of untreated Enuresis in school-aged children?
   - A. Social embarrassment and reduced self-esteem
   - B. Persistent behavioral issues unrelated to enuresis
   - C. Increased risk of developing a comorbid eating disorder
   - D. Difficulty in academic performance due to daytime fatigue
4. Which of the following conditions must be ruled out to diagnose Enuresis?
   - A. Urinary tract infections or diabetes mellitus
   - B. Obsessive-compulsive disorder
   - C. Generalized Anxiety Disorder
   - D. Sleep-related breathing disorders
5. A parent reports that their 8-year-old has begun wetting the bed after their recent divorce. What type of enuresis is most likely?
   - A. Secondary enuresis triggered by a psychosocial stressor
   - B. Primary enuresis due to delayed bladder control development
   - C. Diurnal enuresis with comorbid anxiety
   - D. Enuresis caused by an undiagnosed neurological condition
6. Which therapeutic approach is considered most effective for managing nocturnal enuresis in children?
   - A. Enuresis alarms combined with positive reinforcement techniques
   - B. Restriction of fluid intake before bedtime without further intervention
   - C. Long-term use of anticholinergic medications
   - D. Immediate referral to a urologist for invasive diagnostic testing
7. Which outcome measure is most appropriate for evaluating treatment progress in a child with enuresis?
   - A. Decrease in the frequency of bedwetting episodes over time
   - B. Improvement in overall academic performance
   - C. Reduction in nighttime awakenings unrelated to voiding
   - D. Increased fluid intake during the day

True/False Questions

		T	F
1	The diagnosis of enuresis in the DSM-5 requires the child to be at least 4 years old.		
2	To be diagnosed, enuresis must occur at least twice a week for a minimum of three consecutive months or cause clinically significant distress.		
3	Enuresis can be classified as "nocturnal," "diurnal," or "mixed" depending on when the involuntary urination occurs.		
4	Enuresis is always considered a primary psychological disorder and cannot be caused by underlying medical conditions.		
5	In cases of secondary enuresis, the child has had a period of at least six months of bladder control before the onset of the disorder.		
6	According to the DSM-5, pharmacological therapy is the recommended first-line treatment for primary nocturnal enuresis.		
7	Nocturnal enuresis is more common in males, while diurnal enuresis tends to be more frequent in females.		
8	For the diagnosis of enuresis, the behavior must be considered abnormal relative to the child's developmental level.		
9	Diurnal enuresis is always associated with a structural problem in the lower urinary tract.		
10	In children with enuresis, it is essential to assess the impact of the disorder on social functioning and emotional well-being.		

Matching Exercise

1. Episodes of bedwetting in a child who has never achieved nighttime dryness. [ ]
2. A medical condition that must be ruled out before diagnosing enuresis. [ ]
3. A behavioral intervention commonly used to manage enuresis. [ ]
4. A common psychological impact of untreated enuresis. [ ]
5. Enuresis that begins following a significant life stressor. [ ]
6. A pharmacological option sometimes used for enuresis. [ ]

Descriptions:

- A. Secondary enuresis
- B. Desmopressin
- C. Urinary tract infection
- D. Social embarrassment
- E. Enuresis alarms
- F. Primary enuresis

Case Study

A 7-year-old boy is referred to a pediatric clinic for nighttime bedwetting occurring 4–5 times per week. The child has never achieved consistent nighttime dryness. His parents note that he often sleeps deeply and does not wake up after wetting the bed. The boy appears otherwise healthy, with no history of urinary tract infections or diabetes. The family recently moved to a new home, which the parents believe has been stressful for him.

1. Which aspect of this case supports a diagnosis of primary enuresis?
   - A. The child has never achieved consistent nighttime dryness
   - B. The bedwetting occurs 4–5 times per week
   - C. The family recently experienced a stressful move
   - D. The child sleeps deeply and does not wake up
2. What is the most appropriate first-line treatment for this child?
   - A. Enuresis alarms combined with behavioral reinforcement strategies
   - B. Immediate use of pharmacological agents like desmopressin
   - C. Fluid restriction for several hours before bedtime
   - D. Referral to a sleep specialist to evaluate deep sleep patterns
3. What complication should be monitored during treatment?
   - A. Potential psychological effects of bedwetting, such as low self-esteem
   - B. Risk of developing a urinary tract infection due to behavioral therapy
   - C. Dehydration caused by fluid restriction
   - D. Increased frequency of diurnal enuresis

Answers

Multiple Choice Questions:
1. A
2. A
3. A
4. A
5. A
6. A
7. A

True/False Questions:
1. False
2. True
3. True
4. False
5. True
6. False
7. True
8. True
9. False
10. True

Matching Exercise:
1. F
2. C
3. E
4. D
5. A
6. B

Case Study Answers and Explanations:
1. A - Explanation: The child has never achieved nighttime dryness, indicating primary enuresis.
2. A - Explanation: Enuresis alarms and behavioral strategies are first-line treatments for primary nocturnal enuresis.
3. A - Explanation: Untreated enuresis can affect a child's self-esteem and social interactions, requiring close monitoring.

Encopresis

Multiple Choice Questions

1. Which of the following scenarios is most consistent with a diagnosis of Encopresis?
    - A. A 6-year-old child has repeated episodes of involuntary fecal soiling in inappropriate places despite no evidence of a medical condition.
    - B. A 4-year-old child has occasional bowel movements outside the toilet while toilet training.
    - C. A 10-year-old child refuses to eat solid foods due to fear of constipation.
    - D. A 7-year-old child has diarrhea due to a chronic gastrointestinal illness.
2. A 9-year-old boy has been experiencing fecal incontinence for the past six months, mostly during the day, and often avoids using the toilet at school. What factor would differentiate retentive from non-retentive encopresis?
    - A. The presence of underlying constipation or hard stools
    - B. The absence of soiling at night
    - C. Avoidance of using public restrooms
    - D. Persistent fear of abdominal pain
3. Which of the following interventions is most appropriate as a first step in managing retentive encopresis?
    - A. Addressing constipation through laxatives and dietary changes
    - B. Behavioral therapy focusing on anxiety management
    - C. Immediate referral to a pediatric gastroenterologist for invasive testing
    - D. Long-term use of antidiarrheal medications
4. Which psychosocial factor is commonly associated with Encopresis in school-aged children?
    - A. Social embarrassment leading to avoidance of peer interactions
    - B. Cognitive deficits impairing recognition of the need to defecate
    - C. Intense fear of gaining weight linked to food restriction
    - D. Obsessive cleaning rituals after bowel movements
5. A child with Encopresis is frequently reprimanded by caregivers for soiling. What impact might this response have on the child's condition?
    - A. Increased anxiety and worsening of the soiling behavior
    - B. Immediate improvement in toilet training adherence
    - C. Resolution of symptoms through behavior suppression
    - D. Development of comorbid eating disorders
6. What is the primary goal of treatment in Encopresis?
    - A. Establishing regular bowel habits and reducing fecal incontinence episodes
    - B. Minimizing fluid intake to reduce the frequency of bowel movements
    - C. Rapid elimination of all behavioral symptoms within one week
    - D. Preventing the use of public restrooms
7. Which medical condition must be ruled out before diagnosing Encopresis?
    - A. Hirschsprung's disease or other structural abnormalities
    - B. Attention-deficit/hyperactivity disorder (ADHD)
    - C. Obsessive-compulsive disorder (OCD)
    - D. Generalized anxiety disorder (GAD)

True/False Questions

		T	F
1	The diagnosis of encopresis requires that the child's chronological age be at least 4 years or equivalent in terms of development.		
2	Encopresis can be either voluntary or involuntary, according to DSM-5 criteria.		
3	To diagnose encopresis, the behavior must occur exclusively during stressful events, such as family or school changes.		
4	Encopresis can be classified as "with constipation and overflow incontinence" or "without constipation and overflow incontinence."		
5	In children with encopresis, a history of chronic constipation or painful defecation is commonly found.		
6	The diagnosis of encopresis requires that the behavior be present for at least 12 consecutive months.		
7	Encopresis can cause clinically significant distress or impairment in social, school, or other important areas of functioning.		
8	Behavioral interventions, such as biofeedback therapy, are often used to treat encopresis associated with constipation.		
9	Untreated encopresis is expected to resolve spontaneously without medical or psychological intervention.		
10	In cases of encopresis, it is important to rule out organic causes, such as anatomical abnormalities or gastrointestinal disorders.		

Matching Exercise

1. Fecal incontinence in the absence of constipation. [ ]
2. A behavioral intervention commonly used to treat Encopresis. [ ]
3. A medical condition that must be ruled out before diagnosis. [ ]
4. A psychological impact commonly seen in children with Encopresis. [ ]
5. A key goal in managing retentive Encopresis. [ ]
6. A population in which Encopresis is more prevalent. [ ]

Descriptions:

- A. Hirschsprung's disease
- B. Toilet training with positive reinforcement
- C. Social embarrassment and low self-esteem
- D. Establishing regular bowel habits
- E. Non-retentive Encopresis
- F. School-aged boys

Case Study

A 7-year-old boy is referred for frequent episodes of fecal soiling during the day over the past five months. His parents report that he avoids using the toilet, stating that it "hurts" to poop. On examination, the child has a distended abdomen and reduced bowel sounds. His stool is hard and pellet-like. The family has tried encouraging him to use the toilet, but he becomes anxious and resists. There is no history of developmental delay or significant medical conditions.

1. Which clinical feature most strongly supports a diagnosis of retentive Encopresis?
   - A. Distended abdomen with hard, pellet-like stools
   - B. Avoidance of toilet use due to anxiety
   - C. Five-month history of daytime soiling
   - D. No history of developmental delay
2. What is the most appropriate initial intervention for this patient?
   - A. Use of stool softeners and dietary modifications to address constipation
   - B. Behavioral therapy targeting toilet anxiety
   - C. Referral for psychological counseling before medical treatment
   - D. Immediate imaging studies to rule out structural abnormalities
3. What complication should be monitored in this child during treatment?
   - A. Recurrence of stool withholding behaviors
   - B. Increased risk of urinary tract infections
   - C. Progression to nocturnal enuresis
   - D. Development of anxiety-related eating behaviors

Answers

Multiple Choice Questions:
1. A
2. A
3. A
4. A
5. A
6. A
7. A

True/False Questions:
1. True
2. True
3. False
4. True
5. True
6. False
7. True
8. True
9. False
10. True

Matching Exercise:
1. E
2. B
3. A
4. C
5. D
6. F

Case Study Answers and Explanations:
1. A - Explanation: Distended abdomen and hard stools suggest underlying constipation, characteristic of retentive Encopresis.
2. A - Explanation: Stool softeners and dietary modifications address the root cause of stool withholding.
3. A - Explanation: Stool withholding behaviors may recur if constipation is not managed effectively.

Other Specified and Unspecified Elimination Disorders

Multiple Choice Questions

1. When is the "Specified Elimination Disorder" category used?
    - A. When an elimination disorder does not fully meet criteria for Enuresis or Encopresis but has defined clinical characteristics
    - B. When the patient meets all criteria for Encopresis but also has episodes of enuresis
    - C. When the elimination disorder is caused by a known medical condition
    - D. When enuresis symptoms occur exclusively during the day
2. Which scenario represents an example of a "Specified Elimination Disorder"?
    - A. A 7-year-old child with occasional fecal incontinence episodes that do not meet the duration criteria for Encopresis
    - B. An adolescent with frequent urinary incontinence secondary to a urinary tract infection
    - C. A child with nocturnal enuresis occurring at least three times per week
    - D. An adult with difficulty voiding due to primary psychological factors
3. What is the primary goal of treatment for Specified Elimination Disorders?
    - A. Improving bowel and/or bladder function through personalized interventions
    - B. Preventing excessive bathroom use during school hours
    - C. Minimizing the impact of the disorder without active treatment
    - D. Administering medication to address anxiety related to symptoms
4. When is the "Unspecified Elimination Disorder" category used?
    - A. When insufficient information is available to make a complete diagnosis
    - B. When symptoms meet the criteria for both Encopresis and Enuresis
    - C. When a patient has occasional symptoms of incontinence
    - D. When the disorder is exclusively associated with a chronic medical condition
5. What is a common clinical risk for patients with an Unspecified Elimination Disorder?
    - A. Progression to more defined disorders such as Encopresis or Enuresis
    - B. Malnutrition due to excessive stool retention
    - C. Reduced quality of life due to social stigma
    - D. Recurrent episodes of gastrointestinal infections
6. Which therapeutic intervention is most appropriate for Specified Elimination Disorders?
    - A. A combined approach of behavioral therapy and medical management
    - B. Pharmacological treatment to reduce the frequency of episodes
    - C. Passive monitoring with minimal interventions
    - D. Dietary changes without additional treatment
7. Which complication is common in patients with Unspecified Elimination Disorders?
    - A. Development of generalized anxiety
    - B. Prolonged dependence on aids such as diapers or catheters
    - C. Behavioral problems related to frustration
    - D. Need for surgical intervention to correct intestinal complications

True/False Questions

		T	F
1	Other specified and unspecified elimination disorders include conditions that do not fully meet the criteria for enuresis or encopresis.		
2	To diagnose an unspecified elimination disorder, all psychological or environmental factors contributing to the symptom must be excluded.		
3	Other specified elimination disorder requires the presence of a structural abnormality for diagnosis.		
4	An example of "Other Specified Elimination Disorder" includes episodes of urinary incontinence occurring exclusively during the day without identifiable medical causes.		
5	In other specified and unspecified elimination disorders, symptoms can cause clinically significant distress or impairment in social or school functioning.		
6	The DSM-5 requires that other specified elimination disorder always be diagnosed alongside an underlying medical condition.		
7	Unspecified elimination disorders can include atypical symptoms of incontinence that do not fall into primary categories.		
8	The diagnosis of an other specified elimination disorder may be used when sufficient information is available to provide a detailed description of the condition.		
9	In elimination disorders, cultural and family factors influencing the behavior are essential considerations.		
10	Other specified and unspecified elimination disorders can manifest at any age, including beyond childhood, if the symptoms meet diagnostic criteria.		

Matching Exercise

1. A temporary diagnosis due to insufficient clinical information. [ ]
2. A common goal in treating Specified Elimination Disorders. [ ]
3. A psychological complication associated with Elimination Disorders. [ ]
4. A population in which Elimination Disorders are frequently diagnosed. [ ]
5. A condition that must be ruled out before diagnosing an Elimination Disorder. [ ]
6. An intervention commonly used for managing Specified Disorders. [ ]

Descriptions:

- A. Education for patients and families
- B. School-aged children
- C. Intestinal or urological abnormalities
- D. Reducing emotional and social impact
- E. Unspecified category
- F. Reduced quality of life

Case Study

An 8-year-old child is brought to the clinic for occasional episodes of daytime fecal incontinence. There are no signs of constipation or abdominal pain. The mother reports that the symptoms occur mainly at school and have worsened after a recent class change. Initial medical evaluations reveal no physical abnormalities.

1. Which aspect of this case supports a diagnosis of a Specified Elimination Disorder?
   - A. Episodes of incontinence without evidence of constipation
   - B. Worsening symptoms after a class change
   - C. Absence of physical abnormalities on medical exams
   - D. Symptoms that occur primarily at school
2. What therapeutic intervention would be most appropriate for this patient?
   - A. Behavioral therapy to reduce school-related anxiety
   - B. Use of laxatives to prevent constipation
   - C. Immediate referral to a specialist for further diagnostic evaluation
   - D. Passive monitoring until symptoms worsen
3. What complication should be monitored during treatment?
   - A. Development of social anxiety related to incontinence
   - B. Progression to episodes of nocturnal enuresis
   - C. Dependence on laxatives
   - D. Onset of gastrointestinal infections

Answers

Multiple Choice Questions:
1. A
2. A
3. A
4. A
5. C
6. A
7. C

True/False Questions:
1. True
2. False
3. False
4. True
5. True
6. False
7. True
8. True
9. True
10. True

Matching Exercise:
1. E
2. D
3. F
4. B
5. C
6. A

Case Study Answers and Explanations:
1. A - Explanation: Episodes of incontinence without constipation support the Specified category.
2. A - Explanation: Behavioral therapy can address emotional factors linked to the school environment.
3. A - Explanation: Social anxiety is a common complication in patients with elimination disorders and should be closely monitored.

Sleep-Wake Disorders

This category includes a range of conditions in which the quality, quantity, or timing of sleep is disturbed, affecting daytime functioning and overall well-being. Sleep is not merely "rest," but a biological process that supports physical and mental recovery. Ongoing difficulty with falling asleep, staying asleep, or regulating sleep-wake rhythms can significantly interfere with everyday life.

Among the more common disorders is **Insomnia**, marked by trouble initiating sleep, staying asleep, or waking too early, often accompanied by a sense of non-restorative rest. Worrying about poor sleep can worsen the situation, setting up a cycle that impacts mood, concentration, and energy. At the opposite extreme are **Hypersomnolence Disorders**, involving excessive daytime sleepiness or prolonged sleep that still doesn't feel refreshing. A well-known example is **Narcolepsy**, characterized by sudden onset of sleep during waking hours, sometimes combined with brief episodes of muscle weakness or vivid experiences upon falling asleep or waking up.

Breathing-related sleep issues, such as obstructive sleep apnea, involve repeated pauses in breathing, leading to frequent awakenings and undermining overall sleep quality. In **Circadian Rhythm Sleep-Wake Disorders**, the primary challenge is a mismatch between an individual's internal sleep-wake cycle and social or environmental demands (for example, work schedules or daylight exposure), causing insomnia or excessive sleepiness at inappropriate times. **Parasomnias** encompass behaviors like sleepwalking, night terrors, and frequent nightmares—experiences that disrupt rest and, in some cases, pose risks if the person engages in complicated actions while asleep.

When evaluating Sleep-Wake Disorders, clinicians consider personal history, daily habits (light exposure, work routines, exercise), any medical or psychiatric conditions, and the use of medications or other substances. Chronic pain, depression, or acid reflux can all interfere with proper rest, as can rotating shift work or persistent jet lag.

Treatment can range from basic "sleep hygiene" recommendations—maintaining consistent bedtimes, minimizing noise and light, limiting screen use before bedtime—to more specialized therapies. In cases like insomnia or narcolepsy, medication may be used alongside cognitive-behavioral approaches aimed at unhelpful beliefs about sleep. With obstructive sleep apnea, positive airway pressure (CPAP) devices may be needed during the night, whereas circadian rhythm disorders often call for planned light exposure or gradually shifting sleep schedules.

Understanding the interplay of factors that affect sleep and wakefulness is essential for choosing an effective strategy, tailored to each person's circumstances and any coexisting conditions. By addressing these concerns early on and in a focused manner, individuals can often experience a notable improvement in sleep quality, energy levels, emotional balance, and overall daily functioning.

Insomnia Disorder

Multiple Choice Questions

1. A patient reports difficulty falling asleep, staying asleep, and waking up too early for the past two months. Which feature differentiates insomnia disorder from occasional sleep disturbances?
    - A. Significant distress or impairment in daily functioning due to sleep issues
    - B. Trouble sleeping only on specific days of the week
    - C. Sleep disturbances resolving without intervention
    - D. Symptoms occurring exclusively during periods of high stress
2. Which of the following conditions must be ruled out before diagnosing Insomnia Disorder?
    - A. Obstructive sleep apnea or restless legs syndrome
    - B. Major Depressive Disorder without sleep disturbances
    - C. Chronic fatigue syndrome with no associated sleep issues
    - D. Diabetes mellitus affecting nighttime activity
3. A 40-year-old patient reports difficulty falling asleep despite a consistent bedtime routine. Which factor would most strongly support a diagnosis of Insomnia Disorder?
    - A. The patient spends more than 30 minutes trying to fall asleep at least three nights per week
    - B. The patient consumes caffeinated beverages during the day
    - C. The patient works long hours and feels fatigued after work
    - D. The patient occasionally naps for short durations during the day
4. Which therapeutic intervention is considered first-line for treating chronic insomnia?
    - A. Cognitive-behavioral therapy for insomnia (CBT-I)
    - B. Long-term use of benzodiazepines
    - C. Hypnotic medications as a standalone treatment
    - D. Referral for sleep studies in all cases
5. What is a key psychological factor commonly associated with Insomnia Disorder?
    - A. Anxiety or preoccupation with sleep difficulties
    - B. Hallucinations during the early morning hours
    - C. Paranoia about being unable to wake up
    - D. Obsessive focus on body weight and appearance
6. Which of the following lifestyle changes would most benefit a patient with Insomnia Disorder?
    - A. Establishing a consistent sleep schedule and avoiding screen time before bed
    - B. Exercising vigorously late in the evening to promote fatigue
    - C. Consuming small amounts of alcohol to aid relaxation
    - D. Increasing daytime napping to compensate for nighttime sleep loss
7. What distinguishes Insomnia Disorder from other sleep-wake disorders?
    - A. Persistent difficulty initiating or maintaining sleep despite adequate opportunity
    - B. Symptoms occurring exclusively in the context of substance use
    - C. Recurrent episodes of excessive sleepiness during the day
    - D. Difficulty sleeping due to irregular work shifts

True/False Questions

		T	F
1	The diagnosis of insomnia disorder requires difficulty initiating or maintaining sleep, or early awakening accompanied by an inability to return to sleep.		
2	Insomnia disorder can only be diagnosed if the symptoms cause clinically significant distress or impairment in social, occupational, or other important areas of functioning.		
3	According to the DSM-5, to diagnose insomnia disorder, the patient must exhibit noticeable daytime symptoms such as chronic fatigue or irritability.		
4	Insomnia disorder must occur at least three times per week for a minimum of three months to meet DSM-5 diagnostic criteria.		
5	Insomnia can only be considered a primary disorder if the presence of an underlying mental or physical condition is excluded.		
6	Patients with insomnia disorder may report a subjective perception of sleep quality significantly worse than indicated by objective monitoring data.		
7	Situational insomnia, which occurs exclusively during periods of acute stress and resolves quickly, meets the diagnostic criteria for insomnia disorder.		
8	In patients with insomnia disorder, the sleep problems are not better explained by the effects of substances such as caffeine or medications.		
9	Treatment for insomnia disorder can include both behavioral interventions, such as cognitive behavioral therapy for insomnia (CBT-I), and pharmacological approaches.		
10	Insomnia disorder occurs exclusively in adults and is not considered a clinical issue in children or adolescents.		

Matching Exercise

1. Persistent difficulty falling or staying asleep despite adequate opportunity. [ ]
2. A first-line psychological treatment for Insomnia Disorder. [ ]
3. A condition that must be ruled out before diagnosing Insomnia Disorder. [ ]
4. A behavioral recommendation to improve sleep quality. [ ]
5. A common daytime consequence of untreated Insomnia Disorder. [ ]
6. A population where Insomnia Disorder is more prevalent. [ ]

Descriptions:

- A. Cognitive-behavioral therapy for insomnia (CBT-I)
- B. Fatigue or impaired functioning
- C. Obstructive sleep apnea
- D. Older adults
- E. Consistent sleep schedule
- F. Insomnia Disorder

Case Study

A 35-year-old man presents to his physician with complaints of difficulty falling asleep and frequent nighttime awakenings for the past four months. He reports spending hours in bed trying to sleep, but often feels frustrated and anxious about his inability to do so. Despite feeling tired during the day, he avoids napping. He works a standard schedule and denies irregular shifts or recent travel. His partner reports loud snoring and occasional gasping sounds during sleep.

1. Which feature of this case suggests a diagnosis other than Insomnia Disorder?
   - A. Frequent nighttime awakenings with feelings of frustration
   - B. Loud snoring and gasping sounds during sleep
   - C. Persistent sleep difficulties for four months
   - D. Avoidance of daytime napping
2. What is the most appropriate next step in managing this patient?
   - A. Referral for a sleep study to evaluate for sleep apnea
   - B. Initiation of hypnotic medications to address sleep difficulties
   - C. Cognitive-behavioral therapy for insomnia (CBT-I)
   - D. Recommending over-the-counter sleep aids
3. Which lifestyle change would most benefit this patient?
   - A. Establishing a consistent bedtime and wake time, including weekends
   - B. Reducing fluid intake before bedtime to avoid interruptions
   - C. Avoiding exercise in the late afternoon
   - D. Consuming herbal supplements to promote relaxation

Answers

Multiple Choice Questions:

1. A
2. A
3. A
4. A
5. A
6. A
7. A

True/False Questions:

1. True
2. True
3. False
4. True
5. False
6. True
7. False
8. True
9. True
10. False

Matching Exercise:

1. F
2. A
3. C
4. E
5. B
6. D

Case Study Answers and Explanations:

1. B - Explanation: Loud snoring and gasping sounds suggest the possibility of obstructive sleep apnea rather than primary insomnia.
2. A - Explanation: A sleep study is indicated to rule out sleep apnea, given the reported symptoms.
3. A - Explanation: A consistent sleep schedule helps regulate circadian rhythms and improve sleep quality.

Hypersomnolence Disorder

Multiple Choice Questions

1. A patient reports excessive daytime sleepiness despite sleeping 9–10 hours per night. Which feature would most strongly support a diagnosis of Hypersomnolence Disorder?
   - A. Difficulty waking up in the morning accompanied by sleep inertia
   - B. Recurrent naps during the day after inadequate nighttime sleep
   - C. Sleep disturbances related to environmental factors
   - D. Trouble initiating sleep due to anxiety
2. Which of the following medical conditions must be ruled out before diagnosing Hypersomnolence Disorder?
   - A. Obstructive sleep apnea or narcolepsy
   - B. Generalized anxiety disorder
   - C. Chronic insomnia
   - D. Post-traumatic stress disorder
3. Which characteristic distinguishes Hypersomnolence Disorder from Narcolepsy?
   - A. Lack of cataplexy or other REM sleep-related symptoms
   - B. Episodes of sudden sleep onset during physical activity
   - C. Hallucinations occurring at sleep onset or upon awakening
   - D. Sleep paralysis episodes during nocturnal awakenings
4. A 28-year-old patient complains of excessive daytime sleepiness that has persisted for over three months. Which behavioral factor would suggest Hypersomnolence Disorder rather than a lifestyle-related sleep problem?
   - A. Consistently feeling unrested despite adequate sleep duration
   - B. Irregular work hours affecting the sleep-wake cycle
   - C. Occasional nighttime awakenings due to noise disturbances
   - D. Reduced caffeine consumption leading to fatigue
5. Which therapeutic intervention is most appropriate for managing Hypersomnolence Disorder?
   - A. Stimulant medications to promote wakefulness during the day
   - B. Benzodiazepines to improve nighttime sleep quality
   - C. Cognitive-behavioral therapy for insomnia (CBT-I)
   - D. Bright light therapy to regulate the sleep-wake cycle
6. What psychological impact is commonly associated with untreated Hypersomnolence Disorder?
   - A. Impaired social or occupational functioning due to persistent fatigue
   - B. Excessive preoccupation with body weight and caloric intake
   - C. Obsessive focus on sleep hygiene practices
   - D. Panic attacks triggered by episodes of sleep inertia
7. Which lifestyle modification is most likely to benefit a patient with Hypersomnolence Disorder?
   - A. Maintaining a consistent sleep schedule and avoiding extended naps
   - B. Limiting fluid intake before bed to prevent nighttime awakenings
   - C. Increasing evening physical activity to promote sleep depth
   - D. Using over-the-counter sleep aids to improve nighttime rest

True/False Questions

		T	F
1	The diagnosis of hypersomnolence disorder requires excessive sleepiness despite a main sleep period of at least seven hours.		
2	Hypersomnolence disorder can only be diagnosed if the patient exhibits episodes of cataplexy or sleep paralysis.		
3	Patients with hypersomnolence disorder may experience significant difficulty waking up, such as sleep inertia or confusion.		
4	Symptoms of hypersomnolence disorder must occur at least three times per week for a minimum of three months to meet DSM-5 criteria.		
5	To diagnose hypersomnolence disorder, the patient must have a concomitant sleep-related breathing disorder.		
6	Hypersomnolence disorder may include unrefreshing naps that do not alleviate feelings of tiredness.		
7	The diagnosis of hypersomnolence disorder requires the exclusion of other causes, such as medication effects or underlying medical conditions.		
8	In patients with hypersomnolence disorder, social, occupational, or other important areas of functioning are frequently impaired due to sleepiness.		
9	Hypersomnolence disorder is more common in women than in men, according to DSM-5 epidemiological statistics.		
10	Treatment for hypersomnolence disorder may include pharmacological interventions, such as stimulants, and behavioral strategies to improve the sleep-wake cycle.		

Matching Exercise

1. Excessive sleepiness despite sleeping 9 or more hours per night. [ ]
2. A first-line pharmacological treatment for Hypersomnolence Disorder. [ ]
3. A symptom distinguishing Hypersomnolence Disorder from Narcolepsy. [ ]
4. A common daytime consequence of untreated Hypersomnolence Disorder. [ ]
5. A lifestyle recommendation for patients with Hypersomnolence Disorder. [ ]
6. A condition that must be ruled out before diagnosing Hypersomnolence Disorder. [ ]

Descriptions:

- A. Stimulants such as modafinil
- B. Lack of cataplexy
- C. Fatigue and impaired functioning
- D. Obstructive sleep apnea
- E. Consistent sleep schedule
- F. Hypersomnolence Disorder

Case Study

A 25-year-old woman reports feeling excessively sleepy during the day despite sleeping 9–10 hours each night. She struggles to wake up in the morning and often feels groggy for an hour after getting up. She denies nighttime awakenings but says her sleep feels unrefreshing. A review of her sleep habits reveals a consistent sleep schedule, and no evidence of snoring or breathing irregularities is found. Symptoms have persisted for the past four months and interfere with her ability to focus at work.

1. Which clinical feature most strongly supports a diagnosis of Hypersomnolence Disorder?
    - A. Difficulty waking up in the morning with persistent sleep inertia
    - B. Nocturnal awakenings or breathing irregularities during sleep
    - C. Unrefreshing sleep despite adequate duration
    - D. A consistent sleep schedule over the past four months
2. What is the most appropriate first step in managing this patient?
    - A. Initiating stimulant medications to address daytime sleepiness
    - B. Referring her for a sleep study to rule out other sleep disorders
    - C. Recommending bright light therapy to improve alertness
    - D. Suggesting over-the-counter sleep aids to improve sleep quality
3. What complication should be monitored in this patient during treatment?
    - A. Impaired occupational functioning due to persistent fatigue
    - B. Development of symptoms consistent with obstructive sleep apnea
    - C. Increased reliance on hypnotic medications for sleep initiation
    - D. Worsening anxiety related to preoccupation with sleep quality

Answers

Multiple Choice Questions:
1. A
2. A
3. A
4. A
5. A
6. A
7. A

True/False Questions:
1. True
2. False
3. True
4. True
5. False
6. True
7. True
8. True
9. False
10. True

Matching Exercise:
1. F
2. A
3. B
4. C
5. E
6. D

Case Study Answers and Explanations:
1. C - Explanation: Unrefreshing sleep despite adequate duration is a hallmark of Hypersomnolence Disorder.
2. B - Explanation: A sleep study helps rule out other conditions such as sleep apnea that may mimic Hypersomnolence Disorder.
3. A - Explanation: Persistent fatigue can interfere with occupational functioning and must be monitored during treatment.

Narcolepsy

Multiple Choice Questions

1. Which of the following is a hallmark symptom of Narcolepsy?
   - A. Recurrent episodes of sudden, uncontrollable sleep during the day
   - B. Difficulty falling asleep despite fatigue
   - C. Persistent early morning awakenings with difficulty returning to sleep
   - D. Episodes of excessive movement during REM sleep
2. A 24-year-old patient reports episodes of sudden muscle weakness triggered by laughter. Which feature of Narcolepsy does this describe?
   - A. Cataplexy
   - B. Sleep paralysis
   - C. Hypnagogic hallucinations
   - D. Sleep attacks
3. What is the primary physiological cause of Narcolepsy with cataplexy (type 1)?
   - A. Loss of hypocretin-producing neurons in the hypothalamus
   - B. Dysfunction of the circadian rhythm
   - C. Overproduction of melatonin during the day
   - D. Excessive stimulation of the autonomic nervous system
4. Which symptom would most strongly suggest Narcolepsy rather than another sleep disorder?
   - A. Hypnagogic or hypnopompic hallucinations
   - B. Difficulty maintaining sleep due to environmental factors
   - C. Daytime sleepiness exclusively after insufficient nighttime sleep
   - D. Episodes of nighttime sleep paralysis without daytime sleepiness
5. Which therapeutic intervention is most appropriate for managing excessive daytime sleepiness in Narcolepsy?
   - A. Stimulants such as modafinil or armodafinil
   - B. Benzodiazepines to improve sleep onset
   - C. Antipsychotic medications to reduce hallucinations
   - D. Long-term use of sedative hypnotics
6. Which lifestyle modification is most beneficial for patients with Narcolepsy?
   - A. Scheduled daytime naps to reduce sleep attacks
   - B. Limiting fluid intake to prevent nighttime awakenings
   - C. Exercising vigorously before bedtime to promote better nighttime sleep
   - D. Avoiding carbohydrates to maintain energy levels
7. What distinguishes Narcolepsy Type 1 (with cataplexy) from Narcolepsy Type 2?
   - A. The presence of cataplexy and lower hypocretin levels in Type 1
   - B. Higher frequency of sleep paralysis in Type 2
   - C. Absence of daytime sleepiness in Type 1
   - D. Occurrence of REM sleep behavior disorder in Type 2

True/False Questions

		T	F
1	Narcolepsy is characterized by recurrent episodes of an irresistible need to sleep or lapsing into sleep, occurring within the same day, at least three times per week over three months.		
2	The presence of cataplexy, a sudden loss of muscle tone in response to strong emotions, is a diagnostic criterion for narcolepsy type 1.		
3	A diagnosis of narcolepsy can be made even in the absence of reduced hypocretin levels in the cerebrospinal fluid.		
4	Narcolepsy is never associated with episodes of sleep paralysis or hypnagogic hallucinations.		
5	In patients with narcolepsy, REM sleep may occur within 15 minutes of sleep onset, a phenomenon known as early-onset REM sleep.		
6	Treatment for narcolepsy often includes the use of stimulants to manage daytime sleepiness and specific medications to control cataplexy.		
7	Narcolepsy is more commonly observed in men than in women, according to DSM-5 epidemiological statistics.		
8	Symptoms of narcolepsy can cause significant impairment in social, school, or occupational functioning.		
9	Narcolepsy is considered a chronic neurological condition without a definitive cure, but with treatments that can improve symptoms.		
10	To diagnose narcolepsy, it is sufficient for the patient to report a history of daytime sleepiness without further diagnostic tests.		

Matching Exercise

1. Sudden loss of muscle tone triggered by strong emotions. [ ]
2. A pharmacological treatment for excessive daytime sleepiness. [ ]
3. A lifestyle intervention beneficial for Narcolepsy. [ ]
4. A distinguishing feature of Narcolepsy Type 1. [ ]
5. Vivid hallucinations that occur at sleep onset. [ ]
6. A condition that must be ruled out before diagnosing Narcolepsy. [ ]

Descriptions:

- A. Cataplexy
- B. Modafinil
- C. Scheduled daytime naps
- D. Low hypocretin levels
- E. Hypnagogic hallucinations
- F. Obstructive sleep apnea

Case Study

A 19-year-old college student reports excessive daytime sleepiness that has persisted for the past six months. He describes falling asleep suddenly during lectures and feeling refreshed after short naps. He also reports episodes of muscle weakness triggered by laughter, vivid dream-like experiences while falling asleep, and occasional inability to move upon waking. His nighttime sleep is otherwise unremarkable, and there is no history of significant medical conditions.

1. Which feature of this case strongly suggests a diagnosis of Narcolepsy Type 1?
    - A. Muscle weakness triggered by laughter
    - B. Feeling refreshed after short naps
    - C. Vivid dream-like experiences while falling asleep
    - D. Persistent daytime sleepiness
2. What is the most appropriate next step in managing this patient?
    - A. Conducting a multiple sleep latency test (MSLT) to confirm the diagnosis
    - B. Prescribing benzodiazepines to improve nighttime sleep quality
    - C. Recommending sleep hygiene practices without further testing
    - D. Initiating antidepressants to manage excessive daytime sleepiness
3. What therapeutic outcome should be prioritized during treatment?
    - A. Reducing the frequency and severity of daytime sleep attacks
    - B. Complete elimination of all sleep-related symptoms within the first month
    - C. Achieving eight hours of uninterrupted nighttime sleep
    - D. Preventing future episodes of sleep paralysis

Answers

Multiple Choice Questions:
1. A
2. A
3. A
4. A
5. A
6. A
7. A

True/False Questions:
1. True
2. True
3. False
4. False
5. True
6. True
7. False
8. True
9. True
10. False

Matching Exercise:
1. A
2. B
3. C
4. D
5. E
6. F

Case Study Answers and Explanations:
1. A - Explanation: Muscle weakness triggered by laughter (cataplexy) is a hallmark feature of Narcolepsy Type 1.
2. A - Explanation: The multiple sleep latency test (MSLT) is used to confirm Narcolepsy and assess REM sleep abnormalities.
3. A - Explanation: Reducing daytime sleep attacks is a primary goal to improve the patient's daily functioning and quality of life.

Sleep-Related Breathing Disorders

Multiple Choice Questions

1. A 45-year-old patient reports loud snoring and excessive daytime sleepiness. His partner describes episodes of breathing cessation during sleep. Which subtype of Sleep-Related Breathing Disorder is most likely?
    - A. Obstructive Sleep Apnea (OSA)
    - B. Central Sleep Apnea (CSA)
    - C. Sleep-Related Hypoventilation
    - D. Cheyne-Stokes Breathing Pattern
2. Which clinical feature distinguishes Obstructive Sleep Apnea (OSA) from Central Sleep Apnea (CSA)?
    - A. Presence of respiratory effort during apneic episodes in OSA
    - B. Episodes of loud snoring in CSA
    - C. Association with obesity in CSA
    - D. Occurrence exclusively in individuals without underlying medical conditions
3. Which diagnostic tool is most commonly used to confirm Sleep-Related Breathing Disorders?
    - A. Polysomnography (sleep study)
    - B. Home blood pressure monitoring
    - C. Electroencephalogram (EEG)
    - D. Spirometry
4. A 60-year-old man with a history of heart failure experiences periodic breathing patterns during sleep with alternating hyperventilation and apnea. Which subtype of Sleep-Related Breathing Disorder is most likely?
    - A. Cheyne-Stokes Breathing
    - B. Obstructive Sleep Apnea
    - C. Complex Sleep Apnea Syndrome
    - D. Primary Hypoventilation Syndrome
5. What is the primary treatment for moderate-to-severe Obstructive Sleep Apnea (OSA)?
    - A. Continuous Positive Airway Pressure (CPAP) therapy
    - B. Weight loss and dietary modifications alone
    - C. Long-term use of hypnotic medications
    - D. Referral for surgical correction in all cases
6. Which complication is most commonly associated with untreated Sleep-Related Breathing Disorders?
    - A. Cardiovascular diseases such as hypertension and arrhythmias
    - B. Progressive vision loss due to increased intraocular pressure
    - C. Severe malnutrition due to disrupted eating patterns
    - D. Cognitive enhancement during the day due to hyperventilation
7. Which lifestyle modification is most effective for reducing symptoms of Obstructive Sleep Apnea?
    - A. Weight loss in overweight or obese patients
    - B. Increasing fluid intake before bedtime
    - C. Consuming small doses of caffeine to reduce sleepiness
    - D. Engaging in high-intensity exercise late at night

True/False Questions

		T	F
1	Sleep-related breathing disorders include conditions such as obstructive sleep apnea, central sleep apnea, and sleep-related hypoventilation syndrome.		
2	Obstructive sleep apnea is characterized by recurrent episodes of partial or complete obstruction of the upper airway during sleep, causing oxygen desaturation.		
3	Sleep-related hypoventilation syndrome can be diagnosed in the absence of apneas or hypopneas, based solely on CO_2 accumulation during sleep.		
4	In sleep-related breathing disorders, excessive daytime sleepiness is a mandatory symptom for diagnosis.		
5	The diagnosis of central sleep apnea can be confirmed via polysomnography, showing recurrent episodes of breathing cessation without airway obstruction.		
6	Sleep-related breathing disorder can cause hypertension, cardiovascular problems, and reduced quality of life if untreated.		
7	Obstructive sleep apnea syndrome occurs exclusively in patients with severe obesity.		
8	Treatment for sleep-related breathing disorders may include the use of continuous positive airway pressure (CPAP) devices or other interventions such as weight loss.		
9	Obesity hypoventilation syndrome is diagnosed only in patients with a body mass index (BMI) over 40.		
10	In sleep-related breathing disorders, it is important to distinguish between central and obstructive causes to choose the most appropriate treatment.		

Matching Exercise

1. Episodes of breathing cessation during sleep with preserved respiratory effort. [ ]
2. A condition often associated with Cheyne-Stokes Breathing. [ ]
3. A non-invasive device used to treat Obstructive Sleep Apnea. [ ]
4. A diagnostic test commonly used for Sleep-Related Breathing Disorders. [ ]
5. A risk factor commonly associated with Obstructive Sleep Apnea. [ ]
6. A subtype of SRBD characterized by lack of respiratory effort. [ ]

Descriptions:

- A. Polysomnography
- B. CPAP therapy
- C. Obesity
- D. Central Sleep Apnea
- E. Obstructive Sleep Apnea
- F. Heart failure

Case Study

A 50-year-old woman presents with complaints of excessive daytime sleepiness and fatigue. Her partner reports loud snoring and observed episodes of gasping and choking during sleep. The patient has a BMI of 32 and a history of poorly controlled hypertension. She denies significant nighttime awakenings but feels unrefreshed in the morning. A polysomnography reveals an Apnea-Hypopnea Index (AHI) of 18, consistent with moderate Obstructive Sleep Apnea.

1. Which clinical feature strongly supports a diagnosis of Obstructive Sleep Apnea in this patient?
    - A. Episodes of gasping and choking during sleep
    - B. BMI of 32 with poorly controlled hypertension
    - C. Unrefreshed sleep despite adequate duration
    - D. Excessive daytime sleepiness and fatigue
2. What is the most appropriate next step in managing this patient?
    - A. Initiating CPAP therapy to reduce apneic episodes
    - B. Recommending hypnotic medications to improve sleep quality
    - C. Advising weight loss as the sole intervention
    - D. Referral for surgical correction of airway obstruction
3. Which complication should be closely monitored in this patient?
    - A. Development of arrhythmias due to untreated OSA
    - B. Onset of hypoglycemia related to disrupted sleep
    - C. Vision impairment secondary to nocturnal hypoxia
    - D. Neurological deficits caused by frequent awakenings

Answers

Multiple Choice Questions:
1. A
2. A
3. A
4. A
5. A
6. A
7. A

True/False Questions:
1. True
2. True
3. True
4. False
5. True
6. True
7. False
8. True
9. False
10. True

Matching Exercise:
1. E
2. F
3. B
4. A
5. C
6. D

Case Study Answers and Explanations:
1. A - Explanation: Gasping and choking episodes during sleep are hallmark symptoms of Obstructive Sleep Apnea.
2. A - Explanation: CPAP therapy is the first-line treatment for moderate-to-severe OSA.
3. A - Explanation: Arrhythmias are a common cardiovascular complication of untreated OSA and must be closely monitored.

Circadian Rhythm Sleep-Wake Disorders

Multiple Choice Questions

1. A patient reports difficulty falling asleep until 3 a.m. and trouble waking up before 10 a.m., despite having sufficient sleep opportunity. Which subtype of Circadian Rhythm Sleep-Wake Disorder does this most likely indicate?
    - A. Delayed Sleep Phase Type
    - B. Advanced Sleep Phase Type
    - C. Non-24-Hour Sleep-Wake Type
    - D. Irregular Sleep-Wake Type
2. Which of the following distinguishes Advanced Sleep Phase Type from Delayed Sleep Phase Type?
    - A. Consistently earlier sleep onset and wake times in Advanced Sleep Phase Type
    - B. Inability to achieve restorative sleep in Advanced Sleep Phase Type
    - C. Disrupted sleep patterns caused by external factors in Delayed Sleep Phase Type
    - D. Complete absence of sleep-wake rhythms in both subtypes
3. A 35-year-old blind man reports difficulty maintaining a regular sleep schedule, with sleep and wake times shifting later each day. Which subtype of Circadian Rhythm Sleep-Wake Disorder does this suggest?
    - A. Non-24-Hour Sleep-Wake Type
    - B. Irregular Sleep-Wake Type
    - C. Shift Work Type
    - D. Delayed Sleep Phase Type
4. What is the primary physiological mechanism underlying Circadian Rhythm Sleep-Wake Disorders?
    - A. Misalignment between the endogenous circadian clock and external environmental cues
    - B. Chronic overproduction of melatonin during the day
    - C. Structural abnormalities in the suprachiasmatic nucleus
    - D. Prolonged periods of sleep deprivation due to environmental factors
5. Which therapeutic intervention is most appropriate for managing Delayed Sleep Phase Type?
    - A. Bright light therapy in the morning and melatonin in the evening
    - B. Long-term use of hypnotic medications to induce sleep
    - C. Avoidance of daytime napping to prevent phase delay
    - D. Restriction of screen time without additional interventions
6. A nurse working rotating night shifts reports excessive daytime sleepiness and trouble falling asleep after night shifts. Which subtype of Circadian Rhythm Sleep-Wake Disorder is most likely?
    - A. Shift Work Type
    - B. Advanced Sleep Phase Type
    - C. Irregular Sleep-Wake Type
    - D. Non-24-Hour Sleep-Wake Type
7. Which complication is most commonly associated with untreated Circadian Rhythm Sleep-Wake Disorders?
    - A. Impaired occupational or social functioning due to sleep-wake misalignment
    - B. Increased risk of seizure activity during nocturnal hours
    - C. Development of obsessive-compulsive behaviors related to sleep hygiene
    - D. Chronic malnutrition due to disrupted eating patterns

True/False Questions

		T	F
1	Circadian rhythm sleep-wake disorders are characterized by a misalignment between a person's endogenous sleep-wake cycle and the demands of their social or professional environment.		
2	Delayed sleep phase syndrome is a type of circadian rhythm disorder where the biological clock is significantly delayed compared to conventional schedules.		
3	Circadian rhythm disorders can cause daytime sleepiness, difficulty concentrating, and impairment in social or occupational functioning.		
4	The diagnosis of circadian rhythm disorders always requires the use of an actigraph or sleep diary for a minimum of six months.		
5	Advanced sleep phase syndrome is more common in older adults than in young adults.		
6	Circadian rhythm disorders can be treated with behavioral interventions such as light therapy and sleep hygiene strategies.		
7	Shift work disorder occurs exclusively in people who work night shifts.		
8	Irregular sleep-wake rhythm disorder is characterized by a fragmented sleep-wake pattern without a consolidated cycle.		
9	Jet lag disorder is considered a temporary circadian rhythm disorder that occurs after transmeridian travel.		
10	Circadian rhythm disorders are always associated with underlying medical conditions, such as neurological or psychiatric disorders.		

Matching Exercise

1. A subtype associated with sleep-wake times shifting later each day. [ ]
2. A therapeutic intervention for Delayed Sleep Phase Type. [ ]
3. A population commonly affected by Delayed Sleep Phase Type. [ ]
4. A subtype commonly linked to occupational demands. [ ]
5. A diagnostic test used to assess circadian rhythm misalignment. [ ]
6. A potential complication of untreated Circadian Rhythm Sleep-Wake Disorders. [ ]

Descriptions:

- A. Non-24-Hour Sleep-Wake Type
- B. Bright light therapy
- C. Adolescents and young adults
- D. Shift Work Type
- E. Actigraphy or sleep diary
- F. Impaired social and occupational functioning

Case Study

A 42-year-old woman presents with complaints of fatigue and difficulty maintaining a regular sleep schedule. She reports going to bed at varying times and frequently waking up multiple times during the night. She works irregular shifts at a hospital and struggles with excessive daytime sleepiness. Sleep history and actigraphy reveal irregular sleep-wake patterns with no consistent 24-hour rhythm.

1. Which subtype of Circadian Rhythm Sleep-Wake Disorder is most likely in this patient?
    - A. Irregular Sleep-Wake Type
    - B. Shift Work Type
    - C. Non-24-Hour Sleep-Wake Type
    - D. Delayed Sleep Phase Type
2. What is the most appropriate initial intervention for this patient?
    - A. Establishing a consistent sleep schedule aligned with her work shifts
    - B. Prescribing sedative-hypnotic medications to regulate sleep
    - C. Initiating bright light therapy during her waking hours
    - D. Recommending dietary changes to reduce fatigue
3. What complication should be closely monitored during treatment?
    - A. Impaired cognitive performance due to ongoing circadian misalignment
    - B. Development of dependency on sleep medications
    - C. Progression to chronic insomnia
    - D. Neurological deficits caused by sleep deprivation

Answers

Multiple Choice Questions:
1. A
2. A
3. A
4. A
5. A
6. A
7. A

True/False Questions:
1. True
2. True
3. True
4. False
5. True
6. True
7. False
8. True
9. True
10. False

Matching Exercise:
1. A
2. B
3. C
4. D
5. E
6. F

Case Study Answers and Explanations:
1. A - Explanation: Irregular Sleep-Wake Type is characterized by inconsistent sleep patterns with no discernible 24-hour rhythm.
2. A - Explanation: Establishing a consistent sleep schedule aligned with work shifts helps manage circadian misalignment.
3. A - Explanation: Cognitive impairment is a common complication of untreated circadian rhythm disorders.

Parasomnias

Multiple Choice Questions

1. A 10-year-old child is brought to the clinic for episodes of sleepwalking. His parents report he gets out of bed and wanders the house with no memory of the events. Which subtype of parasomnia does this describe?
    - A. Non-REM Sleep Arousal Disorder
    - B. Nightmare Disorder
    - C. REM Sleep Behavior Disorder
    - D. Sleep-Related Hypoventilation
2. Which of the following differentiates REM Sleep Behavior Disorder (RBD) from Non-REM Sleep Arousal Disorders?
    - A. RBD involves dream enactment behaviors during REM sleep
    - B. Non-REM Sleep Arousal Disorders occur primarily in adults
    - C. RBD is characterized by loud snoring and apneic episodes
    - D. Non-REM Sleep Arousal Disorders are associated with vivid, recallable dreams
3. Which condition is most strongly associated with REM Sleep Behavior Disorder?
    - A. Neurodegenerative diseases such as Parkinson's disease
    - B. Anxiety disorders in adolescents
    - C. Obstructive Sleep Apnea Syndrome
    - D. Primary Hypersomnia
4. A 35-year-old man reports frequent episodes of waking up in the middle of the night, unable to move, and feeling a "presence" in the room. Which type of parasomnia is most likely?
    - A. Isolated Sleep Paralysis
    - B. Non-REM Sleep Arousal Disorder
    - C. Nightmare Disorder
    - D. REM Sleep Behavior Disorder
5. What is the most appropriate first-line intervention for a patient with REM Sleep Behavior Disorder?
    - A. Clonazepam to reduce dream enactment behaviors
    - B. Antidepressants to address underlying emotional distress
    - C. Bright light therapy to regulate sleep patterns
    - D. Cognitive-behavioral therapy for sleep hygiene
6. Which behavioral recommendation is most appropriate for managing Non-REM Sleep Arousal Disorders?
    - A. Ensuring a safe sleep environment to prevent injury during episodes
    - B. Introducing daytime naps to reduce sleep inertia
    - C. Using sleep trackers to monitor nocturnal awakenings
    - D. Restricting fluid intake to minimize nocturnal arousals
7. Which of the following clinical features is most indicative of Nightmare Disorder?
    - A. Recurrent, vivid dreams that cause distress and lead to awakenings
    - B. Episodes of screaming or thrashing during sleep without recall
    - C. Enactment of violent behaviors during sleep with associated injury
    - D. Persistent difficulty falling asleep due to pre-sleep anxiety

True/False Questions

		T	F
1	Sleepwalking episodes are exclusive to REM sleep and involve full awareness of actions performed during the episode.		
2	NREM parasomnias, such as night terrors, typically occur during the first third of the sleep period.		
3	REM sleep behavior disorder (RBD) can be diagnosed even in the absence of an underlying neurological condition, such as Parkinson's disease.		
4	Night terrors are more common in adults than in children and are associated with vivid dreams.		
5	Sleep paralysis is a parasomnia characterized by the inability to move or speak during sleep-wake transitions, despite full awareness of the surrounding environment.		
6	Nightmares are distinguished from night terrors by the individual's ability to recall specific details of the dream content.		
7	For REM sleep behavior disorder, abnormal behaviors must be documented exclusively through polysomnography.		
8	Parasomnias may include potentially dangerous behaviors, such as eating or driving during sleep, without the individual's awareness upon waking.		
9	The use of alcohol or sedatives can exacerbate NREM parasomnias, such as sleepwalking.		
10	The diagnosis of a parasomnia does not require symptoms to cause distress or significant impairment in daily functioning.		

Matching Exercise

1. Recurrent, vivid dreams that cause distress and frequent awakenings. [ ]
2. Dream enactment behaviors during REM sleep. [ ]
3. Episodes of screaming or thrashing during sleep without memory. [ ]
4. A pharmacological treatment for REM Sleep Behavior Disorder. [ ]
5. A parasomnia commonly associated with neurodegenerative diseases. [ ]
6. A behavioral recommendation for managing sleepwalking. [ ]

Descriptions:

- A. REM Sleep Behavior Disorder
- B. Clonazepam
- C. Night terrors
- D. Nightmare Disorder
- E. Ensuring a safe sleep environment
- F. Parkinson's disease

Case Study

A 60-year-old man is referred to a sleep clinic for violent behaviors during sleep. His wife reports he frequently shouts, kicks, and punches while asleep, nearly injuring her on multiple occasions. The patient recalls vivid dreams of being chased or attacked but denies daytime sleepiness. He has a history of anxiety and was recently diagnosed with Parkinson's disease.

1. Which parasomnia is most likely in this case?
   - A. REM Sleep Behavior Disorder
   - B. Nightmare Disorder
   - C. Non-REM Sleep Arousal Disorder
   - D. Isolated Sleep Paralysis
2. What is the most appropriate intervention for this patient?
   - A. Prescribing clonazepam to reduce dream enactment behaviors
   - B. Initiating cognitive-behavioral therapy to address anxiety
   - C. Recommending antidepressants to improve sleep quality
   - D. Using bright light therapy to stabilize the sleep-wake cycle
3. Which complication should be closely monitored in this patient?
   - A. Progression of neurodegenerative disease symptoms
   - B. Development of obstructive sleep apnea due to medication use
   - C. Increased frequency of nightmares during treatment
   - D. Cognitive impairments caused by excessive daytime sleepiness

Answers

Multiple Choice Questions:
1. A
2. A
3. A
4. A
5. A
6. A
7. A

True/False Questions:
1. False
2. True
3. True
4. False
5. True
6. True
7. False
8. True
9. True
10. False

Matching Exercise:
1. D
2. A
3. C
4. B
5. F
6. E

Case Study Answers and Explanations:
1. A - Explanation: Dream enactment behaviors during REM sleep are characteristic of REM Sleep Behavior Disorder.
2. A - Explanation: Clonazepam is the first-line treatment for reducing violent dream enactment behaviors.
3. A - Explanation: REM Sleep Behavior Disorder is associated with an increased risk of neurodegenerative conditions like Parkinson's disease.

Other Sleep-Wake Disorders

Multiple Choice Questions

1. When is the "Other Specified Insomnia Disorder" category used?
    - A. When the patient presents with insomnia symptoms that do not fully meet the criteria for Insomnia Disorder but cause significant distress
    - B. When the patient's insomnia symptoms are secondary to a diagnosed medical condition
    - C. When symptoms of insomnia occur less than once per week
    - D. When the patient's insomnia resolves spontaneously without intervention
2. Which example best illustrates "Other Specified Hypersomnolence Disorder"?
    - A. Recurrent episodes of excessive daytime sleepiness without a clear underlying cause
    - B. Difficulty falling asleep due to preoccupation with stress
    - C. Sleep-related hallucinations occurring exclusively in REM sleep
    - D. Sleep attacks during physical activity accompanied by muscle weakness
3. A patient presents with disrupted sleep-wake patterns that do not align with any specific circadian rhythm disorder. Which category would be most appropriate?
    - A. Other Specified Sleep-Wake Disorder
    - B. Delayed Sleep Phase Disorder
    - C. Unspecified Hypersomnolence Disorder
    - D. Obstructive Sleep Apnea Syndrome
4. Which scenario justifies the use of the "Unspecified Sleep-Wake Disorder" category?
    - A. A patient in an emergency setting presents with significant sleep disturbances, but insufficient information is available for a precise diagnosis
    - B. A patient with a clear diagnosis of REM Sleep Behavior Disorder refuses treatment
    - C. A patient meets full criteria for Insomnia Disorder but declines therapy
    - D. A patient experiences occasional nightmares without functional impairment
5. What is the primary treatment goal for patients with "Other Specified Insomnia Disorder"?
    - A. Improving sleep quality and reducing associated daytime impairments
    - B. Identifying and treating the underlying medical cause
    - C. Eliminating all symptoms of nighttime awakenings immediately
    - D. Preventing further episodes without lifestyle modifications
6. Which of the following is a key distinguishing feature between "Specified" and "Unspecified" Sleep-Wake Disorders?
    - A. Specified disorders include a clear explanation of why the criteria are not fully met
    - B. Unspecified disorders occur exclusively in pediatric populations
    - C. Specified disorders require a minimum symptom duration of six months
    - D. Unspecified disorders are only diagnosed in the presence of comorbid conditions
7. A patient with significant daytime fatigue reports a pattern of sleep that varies in duration and timing but does not meet criteria for a specific sleep disorder. Which category would be most appropriate?
    - A. Other Specified Hypersomnolence Disorder
    - B. Other Specified Insomnia Disorder
    - C. Unspecified Sleep-Wake Disorder
    - D. Non-24-Hour Sleep-Wake Disorder

True/False Questions

		T	F
1	Other sleep-wake disorders include conditions that do not fully meet the criteria for disorders such as insomnia or hypersomnolence but cause clinically significant distress.		
2	The diagnosis of "Other Specified Sleep-Wake Disorder" requires the exclusion of environmental factors, such as excessive noise, as a primary cause of the disorder.		
3	Insufficient sleep syndrome is an example of a specified sleep-wake disorder, characterized by a chronically inadequate sleep duration relative to individual needs.		
4	Unspecified sleep-wake disorders are always transient and do not require specific therapeutic interventions.		
5	The DSM-5 allows for the diagnosis of specified sleep-wake disorders based on a combination of subjective symptoms and objective data, such as actigraphy results.		
6	A patient with mixed symptoms of insomnia and hypersomnolence that do not meet criteria for any specific diagnosis may be classified as having an unspecified sleep-wake disorder.		
7	In unspecified sleep-wake disorders, treatment often focuses on identifying and managing underlying factors, such as chronic stress or undiagnosed medical conditions.		
8	Specified sleep-wake disorders may include rare conditions like time-zone change syndrome in individuals who frequently travel.		
9	The diagnosis of an unspecified sleep-wake disorder always requires polysomnographic monitoring to exclude other diagnostic conditions.		
10	Specified or unspecified sleep-wake disorders can never be diagnosed in children or adolescents.		

Matching Exercise

1. A temporary diagnosis used when insufficient information is available. [ ]
2. A category used for sleep disturbances that do not meet full criteria but cause significant distress. [ ]
3. A condition characterized by excessive daytime sleepiness without meeting full diagnostic criteria. [ ]
4. A distinguishing feature of "Specified" Sleep-Wake Disorders. [ ]
5. A treatment goal for Other Specified Insomnia Disorder. [ ]
6. A population where Unspecified categories are frequently used. [ ]

Descriptions:

- A. Detailed explanation of how criteria are not fully met
- B. Other Specified Hypersomnolence Disorder
- C. Unspecified Sleep-Wake Disorder
- D. Improving sleep quality and reducing impairments
- E. Emergency settings or limited clinical information
- F. Significant distress despite subthreshold symptoms

Case Study

A 30-year-old woman presents with significant daytime fatigue and difficulty maintaining a consistent sleep schedule. She reports frequently waking up feeling unrefreshed, despite spending adequate time in bed. The patient denies loud snoring, restless legs, or frequent nighttime awakenings. Her symptoms do not meet criteria for Insomnia Disorder, Hypersomnolence Disorder, or a circadian rhythm disorder. She has a history of mild anxiety but no other medical conditions.

1. Which category would be most appropriate for this patient?
   - A. Other Specified Sleep-Wake Disorder
   - B. Unspecified Sleep-Wake Disorder
   - C. Other Specified Insomnia Disorder
   - D. Non-24-Hour Sleep-Wake Disorder
2. What is the most appropriate treatment approach for this patient?
   - A. Behavioral therapy focusing on consistent sleep-wake patterns
   - B. Long-term use of hypnotic medications to improve sleep duration
   - C. Referral for polysomnography to rule out obstructive sleep apnea
   - D. Pharmacological treatment with stimulants to reduce daytime fatigue
3. What complication should be monitored during treatment?
   - A. Worsening of mild anxiety due to inconsistent sleep
   - B. Development of dependence on sleep medications
   - C. Progression to a diagnosed circadian rhythm disorder
   - D. Onset of restless legs syndrome due to inadequate sleep hygiene

Answers

Multiple Choice Questions:
1. A
2. A
3. A
4. A
5. A
6. A
7. C

True/False Questions:
1. True
2. False
3. True
4. False
5. True
6. True
7. True
8. True
9. False
10. False

Matching Exercise:
1. C
2. F
3. B
4. A
5. D
6. E

Case Study Answers and Explanations:
1. A - Explanation: The patient's symptoms suggest a subthreshold presentation, fitting the "Other Specified Sleep-Wake Disorder" category.
2. A - Explanation: Behavioral therapy addressing sleep-wake patterns is a first-line approach for subthreshold sleep disorders.
3. A - Explanation: Anxiety may worsen with persistent sleep disturbances and requires monitoring.

Sexual Dysfunctions

This category includes conditions that significantly affect the sexual response or the ability to experience pleasure, causing personal distress and often leading to relationship difficulties. Although the reasons can be physical, psychological, or a mix of both, it is important to remember that sexuality is shaped by cultural, emotional, and situational factors. For this reason, any assessment calls for careful consideration of both clinical history and environmental influences.

Well-known difficulties include challenges in achieving or maintaining adequate arousal (such as Erectile Disorder or Female Sexual Interest/Arousal Disorder), reduced or absent desire (Male Hypoactive Sexual Desire Disorder), and orgasm problems (Delayed Ejaculation, Female Orgasmic Disorder, Premature [Early] Ejaculation). Another issue is Genito-Pelvic Pain/Penetration Disorder, in which the sexual experience becomes painful or unfeasible due to involuntary muscle contractions, burning sensations, or other physical symptoms interfering with intercourse.

When diagnosing a Sexual Dysfunction, it is important to determine whether the problem has been present from the start (lifelong) or appeared after a period of what could be considered "typical" functioning. It is also essential to note if the issue occurs in all circumstances (generalized) or only in certain situations or with specific partners (situational). Another key point involves symptom duration: these difficulties typically need to persist for at least six months and cause marked distress to meet diagnostic criteria.

A thorough clinical evaluation looks into sexual history, beliefs, and relationship factors. Sexual dysfunctions often appear alongside other conditions (anxiety, depression, couples' problems) or medical issues (endocrine disorders, cardiac conditions) that can influence performance. It is also important to rule out whether medications or substance use may be affecting desire, arousal, or orgasm.

Many individuals benefit from a combination of medical assistance (for instance, medication for erectile issues or hormonal regulation) and psychotherapy. Sex therapy can help identify and alter unhelpful thinking patterns, lower performance anxiety, and improve partner communication. In some situations, a physical therapist specialized in the pelvic area may be helpful, especially when pain or involuntary muscle contractions are the main symptoms.

Overall, evaluating these concerns calls for an integrated approach that acknowledges the biological, psychological, and social dimensions. Physical, emotional, and relational elements interact in complex ways, so understanding them can guide a treatment strategy aimed at restoring or improving sexual well-being, with positive effects on intimacy, relationships, and self-esteem.

Delayed Ejaculation

Multiple Choice Questions

1. A 40-year-old man reports difficulty achieving ejaculation during intercourse but not during masturbation. His partner has been critical of his performance. Which finding suggests a mixed etiology?
    - A. Normal ejaculation during masturbation and relationship strain
    - B. Difficulty ejaculating in all contexts and a history of diabetes
    - C. Onset of symptoms after starting an SSRI
    - D. Absence of sexual arousal
2. What differentiates situational from lifelong Delayed Ejaculation?
    - A. Symptoms occur only with specific partners
    - B. Difficulties occur in all sexual activities
    - C. Symptoms resolve under reduced stress
    - D. Lifelong symptoms begin during puberty
3. Which medical condition is most likely to cause Delayed Ejaculation via nerve damage?
    - A. Diabetes mellitus
    - B. Hypertension treated with beta-blockers
    - C. Hypothyroidism
    - D. Chronic obstructive pulmonary disease
4. A patient's Delayed Ejaculation began after starting an antidepressant. What is the best management strategy?
    - A. Switch to bupropion
    - B. Start testosterone therapy
    - C. Use desensitization techniques
    - D. Prescribe phosphodiesterase inhibitors
5. A 50-year-old man has Delayed Ejaculation. Which factors suggest a persistent mixed etiology?
    - A. Performance anxiety, diabetes, and SSRI use
    - B. Alcohol use, prostate surgery, and high testosterone
    - C. Low libido, unrelated medical issues, and no anxiety
    - D. Stressful job, regular sexual activity, and no medical conditions
6. A 28-year-old man has delayed ejaculation only during intercourse. Symptoms worsen with stress. Which intervention is best?
    - A. Cognitive-behavioral therapy
    - B. Testosterone therapy
    - C. Referral to a urologist
    - D. Sedative medications
7. How do SSRIs contribute to Delayed Ejaculation?
    - A. Increased serotonin in the ejaculatory reflex pathway
    - B. Reduced testosterone production
    - C. Decreased dopamine in the brain
    - D. Inhibited nitric oxide synthesis

True/False Questions

		T	F
1	Persistent adequate sexual arousal is necessary for a diagnosis of Delayed Ejaculation, yet it can coexist with other clinical conditions that affect orgasm.		
2	Delayed Ejaculation can manifest situationally, for instance occurring during intercourse but not during masturbation.		
3	An individual with Delayed Ejaculation never reaches orgasm under any circumstances, including masturbation.		
4	According to the DSM-5, the use of certain medications such as SSRIs does not influence the development of Delayed Ejaculation in any way.		
5	The DSM-5 requires that symptoms of Delayed Ejaculation be present for at least six months before a diagnosis is made.		
6	In the DSM-5, there is no distinction between Delayed Ejaculation and male anorgasmia, as they refer to the same diagnosis.		
7	Psychological factors, such as performance anxiety or relationship conflicts, may contribute to Delayed Ejaculation.		
8	Delayed Ejaculation can involve recurrent difficulty achieving orgasm despite generally adequate sexual desire and arousal.		
9	When assessing Delayed Ejaculation, it is advisable to rule out possible neurological conditions and adverse effects of certain medications.		
10	According to the DSM-5, a diagnosis of Delayed Ejaculation can be made even if the problem does not cause clinically significant distress or negative relationship consequences.		

Matching Exercise

1. A common pharmacological cause of acquired Delayed Ejaculation. [ ]
2. A psychological therapy for performance anxiety in Delayed Ejaculation. [ ]
3. A distinguishing feature of lifelong Delayed Ejaculation. [ ]
4. A medical condition associated with peripheral nerve damage contributing to Delayed Ejaculation. [ ]
5. A sexual dysfunction often comorbid with Delayed Ejaculation. [ ]
6. A primary treatment approach for SSRI-induced Delayed Ejaculation. [ ]

Descriptions:

- A. Selective serotonin reuptake inhibitors (SSRIs)
- B. Cognitive-behavioral therapy
- C. Symptoms present in all sexual contexts, including masturbation
- D. Diabetes mellitus
- E. Switching to bupropion
- F. Erectile dysfunction

Case Study

A 45-year-old man presents with complaints of persistent difficulty achieving ejaculation during intercourse, which began two years ago. He reports no difficulty achieving an erection or experiencing pleasure during sexual activity. His medical history includes type 2 diabetes and long-term SSRI use for depression. He reports no issues ejaculating during masturbation and denies any changes in his libido.

1. Which factor most strongly suggests a mixed etiology for his Delayed Ejaculation?
    - A. Long-term SSRI use and type 2 diabetes
    - B. Normal ejaculation during masturbation
    - C. No changes in libido or sexual arousal
    - D. Persistence of symptoms for two years
2. What is the most appropriate next step in managing this patient's condition?
    - A. Adjusting the SSRI dosage or switching to bupropion
    - B. Initiating testosterone therapy to enhance libido
    - C. Prescribing phosphodiesterase inhibitors to improve performance
    - D. Referral for psychotherapy to address relationship dynamics
3. Which complication should be closely monitored if Delayed Ejaculation remains untreated?
    - A. Increased relationship strain and reduced sexual satisfaction
    - B. Development of premature ejaculation during masturbation
    - C. Onset of generalized sexual aversion disorder
    - D. Chronic fatigue due to nocturnal emissions

Answers

Multiple Choice Questions:
1. A
2. A
3. A
4. A
5. A
6. A
7. A

True/False Questions:
1. True
2. True
3. False
4. False
5. True
6. False
7. True
8. True
9. True
10. False

Matching Exercise:
1. A
2. B
3. C
4. D
5. F
6. E

Case Study Answers and Explanations:
1. A - Explanation: The combination of SSRI use and diabetes suggests a mixed etiology, affecting both neurological and pharmacological pathways.
2. A - Explanation: Switching to bupropion is effective in mitigating sexual side effects caused by SSRIs.
3. A - Explanation: Relationship strain is a common complication of untreated Delayed Ejaculation and can worsen over time.

Erectile Disorder

Multiple Choice Questions

1. A 45-year-old man reports difficulty achieving and maintaining an erection during intercourse. Which finding would most strongly suggest a psychogenic cause?
    - A. Normal nocturnal and morning erections
    - B. Progressive worsening of symptoms over several years
    - C. Erectile dysfunction in all contexts, including masturbation
    - D. Absence of a specific stressor or emotional trigger
2. A 55-year-old patient with poorly controlled diabetes presents with erectile dysfunction. Which of the following mechanisms is most likely contributing to his symptoms?
    - A. Endothelial dysfunction and reduced blood flow to penile arteries
    - B. Increased sympathetic nervous system activity
    - C. Hyperstimulation of the parasympathetic nervous system
    - D. Elevated testosterone levels
3. A patient with Erectile Disorder reports minimal improvement with phosphodiesterase inhibitors. Which action would be the most appropriate next step?
    - A. Assess testosterone levels to rule out hormonal imbalances
    - B. Switch to a different class of erectile dysfunction medication
    - C. Recommend cognitive-behavioral therapy to address anxiety
    - D. Increase the dose of phosphodiesterase inhibitors
4. Which diagnostic tool is most appropriate for distinguishing between organic and psychogenic Erectile Disorder?
    - A. Nocturnal penile tumescence (NPT) testing
    - B. Polysomnography
    - C. Blood glucose monitoring
    - D. CT angiography of the pelvis
5. A 40-year-old man with Erectile Disorder is newly diagnosed with moderate hypertension. Which of the following medications is least likely to exacerbate his condition?
    - A. Angiotensin II receptor blockers (ARBs)
    - B. Beta-blockers
    - C. Thiazide diuretics
    - D. Calcium channel blockers
6. Which therapeutic intervention is most effective for a patient with psychogenic Erectile Disorder?
    - A. Cognitive-behavioral therapy focusing on performance anxiety
    - B. Phosphodiesterase inhibitors without further interventions
    - C. Testosterone replacement therapy
    - D. Long-term use of benzodiazepines to reduce stress
7. Which symptom would differentiate lifelong Erectile Disorder from acquired Erectile Disorder?
    - A. Inability to achieve erection since the onset of puberty
    - B. Progressive difficulty with erections due to a new medical condition
    - C. Difficulty maintaining erections only with a specific partner
    - D. Normal erectile function during masturbation but not with a partner

True/False Questions

		T	F
1	In the DSM-5, erectile difficulties (obtaining, maintaining, or significantly reduced rigidity) must occur in about 75% of sexual encounters for at least six months.		
2	Normal erections during sleep or masturbation do not rule out an Erectile Disorder if there is clinically significant distress.		
3	A markedly reduced sexual desire is always a mandatory requirement for an Erectile Disorder diagnosis in the DSM-5.		
4	The DSM-5 includes decreased erectile rigidity among the criteria for Erectile Disorder, not just a total inability to achieve or maintain an erection.		
5	According to the DSM-5, age is not considered a risk factor for Erectile Disorder and does not increase its likelihood.		
6	The DSM-5 allows specifying whether Erectile Disorder is generalized or situational, as well as whether it is lifelong or acquired.		
7	Taking certain antidepressants or other substances can influence the onset or persistence of Erectile Disorder.		
8	Performance anxiety can contribute to Erectile Disorder even if spontaneous erections are intact in other situations.		
9	If a patient never shows nocturnal erections, the DSM-5 automatically excludes any psychological cause for Erectile Disorder.		
10	Under the DSM-5, Erectile Disorder requires clinically significant distress and no better explanation by another condition or substance use.		

Matching Exercise

1. Difficulty achieving erection despite normal nocturnal erections. [ ]
2. A pharmacological treatment for Erectile Disorder. [ ]
3. A common medical comorbidity associated with Erectile Disorder. [ ]
4. A psychological intervention for psychogenic Erectile Disorder. [ ]
5. A diagnostic test for evaluating vascular causes of Erectile Disorder. [ ]
6. A factor differentiating lifelong from acquired Erectile Disorder. [ ]

Descriptions:

- A. Cardiovascular disease
- B. Phosphodiesterase inhibitors
- C. Nocturnal penile tumescence testing
- D. Performance anxiety
- E. Lifelong symptoms present in all sexual contexts
- F. Penile Doppler ultrasound

Case Study

A 60-year-old man presents with progressive difficulty achieving erections over the past year. He has a history of hypertension and hyperlipidemia but denies smoking or alcohol use. His symptoms persist during partnered activity and masturbation. Physical examination reveals diminished pedal pulses, and blood tests show normal testosterone levels.

1. Which factor most strongly suggests an organic cause for this patient's Erectile Disorder?
   - A. History of hypertension and hyperlipidemia
   - B. Absence of improvement during masturbation
   - C. Normal testosterone levels despite symptoms
   - D. Presence of diminished pedal pulses
2. What is the most appropriate next diagnostic step?
   - A. Penile Doppler ultrasound to assess vascular flow
   - B. Nocturnal penile tumescence testing to evaluate erectile function
   - C. Serum testosterone re-assessment after lifestyle modifications
   - D. Referral for polysomnography to rule out secondary sleep disorders
3. What treatment would most benefit this patient?
   - A. Phosphodiesterase inhibitors and management of cardiovascular risk factors
   - B. Testosterone replacement therapy to improve libido
   - C. Cognitive-behavioral therapy to address psychological stressors
   - D. Surgical penile implant for long-term symptom resolution

Answers

Multiple Choice Questions:
1. A
2. A
3. A
4. A
5. A
6. A
7. A

True/False Questions:
1. True
2. True
3. False
4. True
5. False
6. True
7. True
8. True
9. False
10. True

Matching Exercise:
1. D
2. B
3. A
4. D
5. F
6. E

Case Study Answers and Explanations:
1. D - Explanation: Diminished pedal pulses suggest vascular insufficiency, a common cause of organic Erectile Disorder.
2. A - Explanation: Penile Doppler ultrasound assesses vascular flow and helps confirm vascular causes.
3. A - Explanation: Phosphodiesterase inhibitors, combined with management of cardiovascular risk factors, address the underlying cause.

Female Orgasmic Disorder

Multiple Choice Questions

1. A 32-year-old woman reports difficulty achieving orgasm during intercourse but can achieve orgasm through masturbation. Which finding would most strongly suggest a situational cause?
    - A. Orgasm achieved during non-partnered activity but not with her partner
    - B. Lifelong inability to achieve orgasm in all contexts
    - C. History of pelvic trauma
    - D. Lack of sexual desire
2. Which medical condition is most likely to cause secondary Female Orgasmic Disorder?
    - A. Diabetes mellitus with nerve sensitivity issues
    - B. Hypothyroidism causing low libido
    - C. Generalized anxiety disorder
    - D. Irritable bowel syndrome
3. A 40-year-old woman reports difficulty achieving orgasm after starting an SSRI for depression. What is the most appropriate management strategy?
    - A. Switching to bupropion
    - B. Discontinuing all antidepressants
    - C. Prescribing hormonal therapy
    - D. Initiating phosphodiesterase inhibitors
4. Which psychological factor most commonly contributes to Female Orgasmic Disorder?
    - A. Performance anxiety and fear of judgment
    - B. History of untreated hypothyroidism
    - C. Long-term use of hormonal contraceptives
    - D. Sedentary lifestyle
5. What distinguishes lifelong from acquired Female Orgasmic Disorder?
    - A. Lifelong symptoms occur in all contexts, including masturbation
    - B. Acquired symptoms are limited to specific situations
    - C. Lifelong symptoms improve with psychological therapy alone
    - D. Acquired symptoms are primarily due to hormonal issues
6. Which intervention is most appropriate for treating situational Female Orgasmic Disorder?
    - A. Psychotherapy to address relationship dynamics
    - B. Prescription of sildenafil to improve arousal
    - C. Cognitive-behavioral therapy focused on body image
    - D. Use of topical estrogen creams
7. A patient presents with difficulty achieving orgasm and reports low sexual satisfaction despite adequate stimulation. What is the most likely psychological factor?
    - A. Anxiety related to sexual performance
    - B. Cardiovascular disease
    - C. Hormonal contraceptive use
    - D. Long-term physical inactivity

True/False Questions

		T	F
1	In the DSM-5, Female Orgasmic Disorder also includes reduced orgasmic intensity, not just the complete absence of orgasm.		
2	A woman may be diagnosed with Female Orgasmic Disorder even if she rarely achieves orgasm, provided all other diagnostic criteria are met.		
3	Female Orgasmic Disorder can be diagnosed even without subjective distress.		
4	According to the DSM-5, potential medical or pharmacological causes must be ruled out prior to confirming Female Orgasmic Disorder.		
5	In the DSM-5, age has no impact whatsoever on Female Orgasmic Disorder.		
6	The DSM-5 differentiates Female Orgasmic Disorder as generalized or situational, and as lifelong or acquired.		
7	Low sexual desire automatically precludes a diagnosis of Female Orgasmic Disorder.		
8	Psychological factors, such as performance anxiety, may contribute to Female Orgasmic Disorder even when no obvious organic causes are identified.		
9	If orgasm is absent only under certain circumstances, the DSM-5 allows a situational classification of Female Orgasmic Disorder.		
10	According to the DSM-5, adequate stimulation (including clitoral) can be crucial in distinguishing Female Orgasmic Disorder from normal orgasmic functioning.		

Matching Exercise

1. Persistent difficulty achieving orgasm despite adequate stimulation. [ ]
2. A pharmacological treatment commonly associated with Female Orgasmic Disorder. [ ]
3. A psychological intervention for addressing performance anxiety. [ ]
4. A medical condition that may contribute to Female Orgasmic Disorder. [ ]
5. A distinguishing feature of lifelong Female Orgasmic Disorder. [ ]
6. A primary treatment approach for situational Female Orgasmic Disorder. [ ]

Descriptions:

- A. SSRIs
- B. Cognitive-behavioral therapy
- C. Diabetes mellitus
- D. Persistent symptoms in all sexual contexts
- E. Persistent difficulty achieving orgasm
- F. Psychotherapy addressing relationship dynamics

Case Study

A 38-year-old woman reports difficulty achieving orgasm during intercourse for the past year. She denies experiencing pain or lack of sexual desire but describes tension with her partner regarding communication during sex. She has no medical conditions but recently started an SSRI for depression. She is able to achieve orgasm through masturbation but not during partnered activity.

1. Which factor most strongly suggests a situational component to her Female Orgasmic Disorder?
    - A. Tension with her partner regarding sexual communication
    - B. Recent initiation of SSRI treatment
    - C. Ability to achieve orgasm during masturbation
    - D. Lack of pain or reduced sexual desire
2. What is the most appropriate therapeutic approach for this patient?
    - A. Psychotherapy to address relationship dynamics and communication issues
    - B. Discontinuation of the SSRI and initiation of alternative antidepressants
    - C. Hormonal therapy to enhance sexual response
    - D. Prescription of sildenafil to improve orgasmic function
3. Which complication should be monitored if her SSRI treatment is continued?
    - A. Worsening sexual dysfunction and decreased satisfaction
    - B. Increased risk of cardiovascular complications
    - C. Onset of dyspareunia
    - D. Development of nocturnal emissions

Answers

Multiple Choice Questions:
1. A
2. A
3. A
4. A
5. A
6. A
7. A

True/False Questions:
1. True
2. True
3. False
4. True
5. False
6. True
7. False
8. True
9. True
10. True

Matching Exercise:
1. E
2. A
3. B
4. C
5. D
6. F

Case Study Answers and Explanations:
1. A - Explanation: Tension regarding communication during sex strongly suggests a situational component.
2. A - Explanation: Psychotherapy addressing relationship dynamics and communication issues is the first-line intervention.
3. A - Explanation: SSRIs are a common cause of sexual dysfunction, and monitoring for worsening symptoms is essential.

Female Sexual Interest/Arousal Disorder

Multiple Choice Questions

1. Which of the following findings would most strongly suggest a diagnosis of Female Sexual Interest/Arousal Disorder?
   - A. Persistent absence of sexual fantasies and reduced interest in sexual activity for at least six months
   - B. Difficulty achieving orgasm despite adequate stimulation
   - C. Pain during intercourse without identifiable physical causes
   - D. Sexual disinterest during periods of high stress
2. A 35-year-old woman reports decreased sexual desire for the past year. Which of the following factors would suggest a psychological rather than physiological etiology?
   - A. Symptoms vary based on relationship satisfaction
   - B. Consistently reduced sexual desire across all contexts
   - C. History of diabetes with peripheral neuropathy
   - D. Persistent difficulty achieving orgasm during intercourse
3. Which comorbid condition is most commonly associated with Female Sexual Interest/Arousal Disorder?
   - A. Major depressive disorder
   - B. Chronic pain syndrome
   - C. Hyperthyroidism
   - D. Irritable bowel syndrome
4. Which of the following is a known pharmacological contributor to Female Sexual Interest/Arousal Disorder?
   - A. Selective serotonin reuptake inhibitors (SSRIs)
   - B. Proton pump inhibitors (PPIs)
   - C. Antihistamines
   - D. Nonsteroidal anti-inflammatory drugs (NSAIDs)
5. What distinguishes lifelong Female Sexual Interest/Arousal Disorder from the acquired form?
   - A. Lifelong symptoms are present in all sexual contexts, including masturbation
   - B. Acquired symptoms are primarily linked to hormonal changes
   - C. Lifelong symptoms improve significantly with hormonal therapy
   - D. Acquired symptoms occur only during partnered sexual activity
6. A 40-year-old woman reports reduced sexual desire and arousal after starting an SSRI for depression. What is the most appropriate intervention?
   - A. Switching to bupropion
   - B. Prescribing sildenafil
   - C. Initiating hormone replacement therapy
   - D. Discontinuing antidepressants entirely
7. Which of the following therapeutic approaches is most appropriate for a patient with situational Female Sexual Interest/Arousal Disorder?
   - A. Cognitive-behavioral therapy focusing on body image and relationship dynamics
   - B. Hormonal therapy to enhance sexual function
   - C. Prescription of phosphodiesterase inhibitors
   - D. Use of topical estrogen creams

True/False Questions

		T	F
1	The DSM-5 merges reduced sexual interest and reduced arousal into one diagnosis called Female Sexual Interest/Arousal Disorder.		
2	Decreased frequency of sexual fantasies is one possible criterion for Female Sexual Interest/Arousal Disorder.		
3	According to the DSM-5, symptoms of low sexual desire or arousal must persist for at least six months before a diagnosis is made.		
4	If sexual interest is diminished only with a particular partner, the DSM-5 does not allow a diagnosis of Female Sexual Interest/Arousal Disorder.		
5	Reduced genital or non-genital sensations during sexual activity can indicate Female Sexual Interest/Arousal Disorder.		
6	The DSM-5 excludes psychological factors like anxiety or depression from playing any role in diagnosing Female Sexual Interest/Arousal Disorder.		
7	Under the DSM-5, ruling out medical causes is not required before diagnosing Female Sexual Interest/Arousal Disorder.		
8	The DSM-5 includes a situational subtype of Female Sexual Interest/Arousal Disorder, applying when reduced desire or arousal occurs only in specific contexts.		
9	If sexual desire is low only during penetration but remains adequate with other forms of stimulation, the DSM-5 does not consider the diagnosis valid.		
10	According to the DSM-5, personal or relational distress is a key criterion for Female Sexual Interest/Arousal Disorder.		

Matching Exercise

1. Persistent difficulty experiencing sexual desire or arousal. [ ]
2. A pharmacological cause of reduced sexual interest. [ ]
3. A psychological intervention for situational Female Sexual Interest/Arousal Disorder. [ ]
4. A diagnostic step for evaluating Female Sexual Interest/Arousal Disorder. [ ]
5. A distinguishing feature of lifelong Female Sexual Interest/Arousal Disorder. [ ]
6. A common comorbid condition associated with this disorder. [ ]

Descriptions:

- A. Selective serotonin reuptake inhibitors (SSRIs)
- B. Cognitive-behavioral therapy
- C. Major depressive disorder
- D. Lifelong symptoms in all sexual contexts
- E. Comprehensive sexual history
- F. Persistent difficulty in sexual desire or arousal

Case Study

A 37-year-old woman reports reduced sexual desire and difficulty maintaining arousal for the past year. She denies pain during intercourse but mentions that her relationship with her partner has become strained due to lack of intimacy. She recently started taking an SSRI for anxiety. She expresses significant distress about her symptoms.

1. Which factor most strongly suggests an acquired form of Female Sexual Interest/Arousal Disorder?
   - A. Recent initiation of SSRI treatment
   - B. Tension with her partner
   - C. Persistence of symptoms for the past year
   - D. Lack of pain during intercourse
2. What is the most appropriate first-line intervention for this patient?
   - A. Switching to an antidepressant with fewer sexual side effects
   - B. Hormonal therapy to enhance libido
   - C. Cognitive-behavioral therapy focusing on relationship dynamics
   - D. Prescription of sildenafil to improve arousal
3. Which complication should be monitored if her SSRI treatment is continued without adjustment?
   - A. Persistent sexual dysfunction and decreased relationship satisfaction
   - B. Onset of dyspareunia due to hormonal changes
   - C. Increased risk of nocturnal emissions
   - D. Cardiovascular symptoms due to anxiety

Answers

Multiple Choice Questions:
1. A
2. A
3. A
4. A
5. A
6. A
7. A

True/False Questions:
1. True
2. True
3. True
4. False
5. True
6. False
7. False
8. True
9. False
10. True

Matching Exercise:
1. F
2. A
3. B
4. E
5. D
6. C

Case Study Answers and Explanations:
1. A - Explanation: The onset of symptoms following SSRI use strongly suggests an acquired condition.
2. A - Explanation: Switching to an antidepressant with fewer sexual side effects is a first-line intervention.
3. A - Explanation: Persistent sexual dysfunction can exacerbate relationship strain and overall distress.

Genito-Pelvic Pain/Penetration Disorder

Multiple Choice Questions

1. A 30-year-old woman reports persistent pain and involuntary tensing of pelvic muscles during intercourse. Which finding supports a diagnosis of Genito-Pelvic Pain/Penetration Disorder?
   - A. Persistent symptoms not explained by a medical condition
   - B. Pain only during initial intercourse attempts
   - C. Lack of sexual desire with muscle tension
   - D. Temporary pain postpartum
2. Which feature differentiates Genito-Pelvic Pain/Penetration Disorder from dyspareunia due to a medical condition?
   - A. Symptoms worsen with anticipatory anxiety
   - B. Pain is only vulvar in origin
   - C. Clear medical cause, e.g., endometriosis
   - D. Relief with over-the-counter pain relievers
3. Which psychological factor is most likely to exacerbate this disorder?
   - A. Avoidance behaviors related to sexual activity
   - B. History of infrequent sexual activity
   - C. Use of hormonal contraception
   - D. Grief unrelated to sexual experiences
4. A patient denies gynecological conditions but reports pain during intercourse. Which diagnostic step is most appropriate?
   - A. Comprehensive sexual and psychosocial history
   - B. Imaging to rule out structural abnormalities
   - C. Trial of antidepressants
   - D. Physical exam only
5. Which treatment is most effective for pelvic muscle tension?
   - A. Pelvic floor physical therapy
   - B. Hormonal therapy
   - C. Surgery for anatomical abnormalities
   - D. Antidepressants
6. A 28-year-old woman avoids intercourse due to pain. What is the goal of CBT?
   - A. Reduce anxiety and avoidance behaviors
   - B. Improve lubrication through behavior changes
   - C. Resolve partner conflicts
   - D. Address past trauma
7. Which feature suggests a multifactorial etiology?
   - A. Physical pain, muscle tension, and psychological distress
   - B. Pain only at the vaginal opening
   - C. Symptoms after a medical procedure
   - D. Persistence despite physical therapy

True/False Questions

		T	F
1	The DSM-5 includes anticipatory anxiety about pain and pelvic muscle tension among the symptoms of Genito-Pelvic Pain/Penetration Disorder.		
2	Involuntary pelvic floor muscle contraction automatically rules out Genito-Pelvic Pain/Penetration Disorder, implying a purely organic cause.		
3	The DSM-5 specifies that pain or penetration difficulties must persist for at least six months, either recurrently or continuously, before diagnosing the disorder.		
4	Significant psychological distress, such as fear of experiencing pain, is one of the necessary elements for this diagnosis in the DSM-5.		
5	Under the DSM-5, one may specify whether the condition is situational or generalized, depending on the contexts in which pain or penetration difficulties arise.		
6	According to the DSM-5, physical examination is irrelevant: the mere report of pain is sufficient to make the diagnosis.		
7	The DSM-5 confines the disorder solely to sexual intercourse, excluding issues related to tampon insertion or other vaginally inserted objects.		
8	Psychological factors, such as past trauma or anxiety, can contribute to the development of Genito-Pelvic Pain/Penetration Disorder even without organic causes.		
9	Genito-Pelvic Pain/Penetration Disorder can never coexist with other sexual dysfunctions, according to DSM-5 criteria.		
10	If a woman reports chronic pain during penetration, the DSM-5 does not require any emotional or relational distress to make the diagnosis.		

Matching Exercise

1. Persistent muscle tension causing penetration difficulties. [ ]
2. A psychological intervention for reducing fear and avoidance behaviors. [ ]
3. A first-line physical treatment for pelvic muscle tension. [ ]
4. A history often associated with the development of this disorder. [ ]
5. A distinguishing feature suggesting a multifactorial etiology. [ ]
6. A diagnostic step for evaluating psychological contributions to symptoms. [ ]

Descriptions:

- A. Pelvic floor physical therapy
- B. Cognitive-behavioral therapy
- C. History of sexual trauma
- D. Muscle tension combined with psychological distress
- E. Comprehensive sexual and psychosocial history
- F. Pelvic muscle tension

Case Study

A 34-year-old woman reports persistent pain during intercourse and difficulty with vaginal penetration for the past two years. She denies any history of gynecological conditions but reports significant anxiety about sexual activity. Her partner expresses frustration, which has caused strain in their relationship. A gynecological exam reveals involuntary pelvic muscle contractions but no structural abnormalities.

1. Which feature of this case most strongly suggests a diagnosis of Genito-Pelvic Pain/Penetration Disorder?
    - A. Involuntary pelvic muscle contractions without structural abnormalities
    - B. Persistent pain during intercourse for two years
    - C. Anxiety about sexual activity
    - D. Relationship strain due to symptoms
2. What is the most appropriate first-line treatment for this patient?
    - A. Pelvic floor physical therapy to address muscle tension
    - B. Hormonal therapy to improve lubrication
    - C. Referral for surgical evaluation of pelvic structures
    - D. Long-term use of antidepressants to manage anxiety
3. Which complication should be monitored during treatment?
    - A. Persistent avoidance of sexual activity due to unresolved anxiety
    - B. Development of dyspareunia caused by lubrication issues
    - C. Progression to chronic pelvic inflammatory disease
    - D. Increased risk of urinary tract infections

Answers

Multiple Choice Questions:
1. A
2. A
3. A
4. A
5. A
6. A
7. A

True/False Questions:
1. True
2. False
3. True
4. True
5. True
6. False
7. False
8. True
9. False
10. False

Matching Exercise:
1. F
2. B
3. A
4. C
5. D
6. E

Case Study Answers and Explanations:
1. A - Explanation: Involuntary pelvic muscle contractions without structural abnormalities strongly suggest this disorder.
2. A - Explanation: Pelvic floor physical therapy is effective for addressing muscle tension.
3. A - Explanation: Avoidance behaviors can worsen symptoms and lead to additional psychological distress.

Male Hypoactive Sexual Desire Disorder

Multiple Choice Questions

1. A 40-year-old man reports a lack of sexual desire for the past year. Which feature is required to confirm a diagnosis of Male Hypoactive Sexual Desire Disorder?
    - A. Clinically significant distress about his lack of desire
    - B. Erectile dysfunction accompanying low libido
    - C. Normal testosterone levels
    - D. Low sexual desire occurring only during stressful periods
2. Which of the following medical conditions is most commonly associated with Male Hypoactive Sexual Desire Disorder?
    - A. Hypogonadism
    - B. Irritable bowel syndrome
    - C. Chronic kidney disease
    - D. Asthma
3. A patient with Male Hypoactive Sexual Desire Disorder reports distress about his low libido but no physical symptoms. Which psychological factor is most likely contributing?
    - A. Performance anxiety
    - B. Untreated hypothyroidism
    - C. Relationship dissatisfaction
    - D. History of cardiovascular disease
4. Which pharmacological treatment is most likely to exacerbate Male Hypoactive Sexual Desire Disorder?
    - A. Selective serotonin reuptake inhibitors (SSRIs)
    - B. Angiotensin-converting enzyme (ACE) inhibitors
    - C. Beta-blockers
    - D. Proton pump inhibitors (PPIs)
5. What distinguishes lifelong Male Hypoactive Sexual Desire Disorder from the acquired form?
    - A. Lifelong symptoms are present in all sexual contexts
    - B. Acquired symptoms improve with testosterone therapy
    - C. Lifelong symptoms are limited to partnered sexual activity
    - D. Acquired symptoms are unrelated to psychological factors
6. A patient with low sexual desire reports improvement in libido with testosterone therapy. What does this suggest about the etiology of his condition?
    - A. A primary hormonal imbalance
    - B. Relationship-related psychological factors
    - C. Medication-induced sexual dysfunction
    - D. A situational stressor
7. Which therapeutic approach is most appropriate for a patient with psychological contributors to Male Hypoactive Sexual Desire Disorder?
    - A. Cognitive-behavioral therapy focusing on performance anxiety
    - B. Testosterone replacement therapy
    - C. Antidepressants to address low mood
    - D. Surgical correction of anatomical abnormalities

True/False Questions

		T	F
1	According to the DSM-5, Male Hypoactive Sexual Desire Disorder involves a marked absence of sexual fantasies or desire for sexual activity persisting for at least six months.		
2	The DSM-5 allows specifying whether the reduced sexual desire is generalized or situational, depending on the context or partner.		
3	Having low sexual desire alone is sufficient for the diagnosis, even if it causes no subjective distress or relationship problems.		
4	Before diagnosing, the DSM-5 requires ruling out the possibility that reduced desire is solely due to medications, substances, or other medical conditions.		
5	Psychological factors such as stress, anxiety, or relationship dissatisfaction can substantially contribute to Male Hypoactive Sexual Desire Disorder.		
6	A finding of hypogonadism necessarily rules out Male Hypoactive Sexual Desire Disorder, as it constitutes a purely organic cause.		
7	The DSM-5 only diagnoses Male Hypoactive Sexual Desire Disorder if a man's sexual desire decreases progressively with age, in a gradual manner.		
8	The DSM-5 distinguishes between lifelong and acquired onset for Male Hypoactive Sexual Desire Disorder.		
9	This disorder can coexist with other sexual dysfunctions (e.g., Erectile Disorder), influencing the overall clinical picture.		
10	The DSM-5 requires that low sexual desire cause either personal distress or interpersonal difficulties for the diagnosis.		

Matching Exercise

1. Persistent lack of sexual desire in all contexts. [ ]
2. A pharmacological cause of reduced sexual desire. [ ]
3. A psychological intervention for addressing relationship dissatisfaction. [ ]
4. A diagnostic step for evaluating Male Hypoactive Sexual Desire Disorder. [ ]
5. A distinguishing feature of lifelong Male Hypoactive Sexual Desire Disorder. [ ]
6. A medical condition associated with reduced testosterone production. [ ]

Descriptions:

- A. Hypogonadism
- B. SSRIs
- C. Lifelong symptoms in all sexual contexts
- D. Cognitive-behavioral therapy
- E. Comprehensive sexual history
- F. Persistent lack of sexual desire

Case Study

A 38-year-old man reports a lack of sexual desire for the past two years, causing strain in his marriage. He denies erectile dysfunction or difficulty achieving orgasm. He reports increased work-related stress and dissatisfaction with his relationship. Blood tests show normal testosterone levels. The patient expresses significant distress about his symptoms.

1. Which factor most strongly suggests a psychological contributor to his condition?
   - A. Work-related stress and relationship dissatisfaction
   - B. Normal testosterone levels
   - C. Persistence of symptoms for two years
   - D. Lack of erectile dysfunction
2. What is the most appropriate therapeutic approach for this patient?
   - A. Cognitive-behavioral therapy focusing on relationship dynamics
   - B. Testosterone replacement therapy
   - C. Antidepressants to address mood issues
   - D. Referral for urological evaluation
3. Which complication should be monitored if his symptoms remain untreated?
   - A. Increased relationship strain and reduced marital satisfaction
   - B. Development of erectile dysfunction
   - C. Onset of hormonal imbalances
   - D. Progression to generalized anxiety disorder

Answers

Multiple Choice Questions:
1. A
2. A
3. C
4. A
5. A
6. A
7. A

True/False Questions:
1. True
2. True
3. False
4. True
5. True
6. False
7. False
8. True
9. True
10. True

Matching Exercise:
1. F
2. B
3. D
4. E
5. C
6. A

Case Study Answers and Explanations:
1. A - Explanation: Work-related stress and relationship dissatisfaction are strong psychological contributors.
2. A - Explanation: Cognitive-behavioral therapy is effective in addressing psychological and relational factors.
3. A - Explanation: Relationship strain can worsen without appropriate intervention, reducing overall marital satisfaction.

Premature Ejaculation

Multiple Choice Questions

1. A 32-year-old man reports ejaculating within one minute of penetration consistently for the past six months, causing significant distress. Which additional finding is required to confirm a diagnosis of Premature Ejaculation?
    - A. Lack of control over the timing of ejaculation
    - B. Absence of sexual desire
    - C. Difficulty achieving an erection during intercourse
    - D. Ejaculation occurring only with a specific partner
2. Which of the following distinguishes lifelong Premature Ejaculation from the acquired form?
    - A. Symptoms have been present since the onset of sexual activity
    - B. Ejaculation time is influenced by psychological factors
    - C. Symptoms occur only during partnered sexual activity
    - D. Symptoms improve with the use of topical anesthetics
3. Which medical condition is most likely to contribute to acquired Premature Ejaculation?
    - A. Prostatitis
    - B. Diabetes mellitus
    - C. Obstructive sleep apnea
    - D. Hypothyroidism
4. A patient with Premature Ejaculation reports that symptoms occur exclusively with his current partner. What does this suggest about the etiology?
    - A. Psychological factors related to relationship dynamics
    - B. A hormonal imbalance requiring testosterone therapy
    - C. Organic causes due to a medical condition
    - D. Use of medications affecting ejaculatory latency
5. What is the most appropriate first-line pharmacological treatment for Premature Ejaculation?
    - A. Selective serotonin reuptake inhibitors (SSRIs)
    - B. Testosterone replacement therapy
    - C. Phosphodiesterase inhibitors
    - D. Antipsychotic medications
6. A 40-year-old man presents with lifelong Premature Ejaculation. Which behavioral intervention is most effective?
    - A. The stop-start technique to delay ejaculation
    - B. Regular use of topical anesthetics
    - C. Cognitive-behavioral therapy for performance anxiety
    - D. Avoidance of sexual activity to reduce stress
7. Which diagnostic tool is most appropriate for evaluating potential medical contributors to Premature Ejaculation?
    - A. Comprehensive sexual and medical history
    - B. Serum testosterone level testing
    - C. Penile Doppler ultrasound
    - D. Nocturnal penile tumescence (NPT) testing

True/False Questions

		T	F
1	Clinical studies suggest that coexisting erectile dysfunction in the presence of Premature Ejaculation can complicate diagnosis and require a distinct therapeutic approach.		
2	According to the DSM-5, symptomatology must be present for at least six months in order to diagnose persistent Premature Ejaculation.		
3	The DSM-5 states that ejaculation must occur within the first 30 seconds of vaginal penetration to be considered premature.		
4	In the DSM-5 classification, there is a distinction between “lifelong” and “acquired” Premature Ejaculation.		
5	If tactile stimulation is minimal and there are no relationship difficulties, Premature Ejaculation cannot be diagnosed according to the DSM-5.		
6	Intravaginal ejaculatory latency time (IELT) is considered a key parameter for diagnosing Premature Ejaculation in the DSM-5.		
7	A specific alteration in serotonergic activity has been linked to the onset of Premature Ejaculation.		
8	The DSM-5 guidelines allow for a diagnosis of Premature Ejaculation without considering the psychological distress associated with the disorder.		
9	According to the DSM-5, symptoms must appear in most or nearly all sexual encounters to meet the criteria for Premature Ejaculation.		
10	In the DSM-5 criteria, relationship dynamics and performance anxiety can significantly affect the clinical course of Premature Ejaculation.		

Matching Exercise

1. Persistent ejaculation within one minute of penetration. [ ]
2. A pharmacological treatment used to increase ejaculatory latency. [ ]
3. A behavioral technique for managing Premature Ejaculation. [ ]
4. A medical condition associated with acquired Premature Ejaculation. [ ]
5. A distinguishing feature of lifelong Premature Ejaculation. [ ]
6. A diagnostic step for evaluating the underlying cause. [ ]

Descriptions:

- A. Prostatitis
- B. SSRIs
- C. Lifelong symptoms present since the onset of sexual activity
- D. Comprehensive sexual and medical history
- E. Stop-start technique
- F. Ejaculation within one minute

Case Study

A 35-year-old man reports ejaculating within 30 seconds of penetration consistently over the past year, causing significant distress and relationship strain. He denies a history of this issue in prior relationships and states that his symptoms began following a period of high stress at work. He has no medical conditions and denies any medication use.

1. Which factor most strongly suggests an acquired form of Premature Ejaculation?
   - A. Onset of symptoms following high stress
   - B. Persistence of symptoms for one year
   - C. Relationship strain due to symptoms
   - D. Lack of prior history of Premature Ejaculation
2. What is the most appropriate initial intervention for this patient?
   - A. Cognitive-behavioral therapy focusing on performance anxiety
   - B. Immediate initiation of SSRIs
   - C. Testosterone therapy to improve ejaculatory control
   - D. Referral for urological evaluation
3. Which complication should be monitored if his symptoms remain untreated?
   - A. Increased relationship strain and reduced intimacy
   - B. Progression to Erectile Dysfunction
   - C. Onset of nocturnal emissions
   - D. Development of prostate-related complications

Answers

Multiple Choice Questions:
1. A
2. A
3. A
4. A
5. A
6. A
7. A

True/False Questions:
1. True
2. True
3. False
4. True
5. False
6. True
7. True
8. False
9. True
10. True

Matching Exercise:
1. F
2. B
3. E
4. A
5. C
6. D

Case Study Answers and Explanations:
1. A - Explanation: The onset of symptoms following a period of high stress strongly suggests an acquired form.
2. A - Explanation: Cognitive-behavioral therapy addresses performance anxiety and stress-related factors.
3. A - Explanation: Relationship strain is a common complication of untreated Premature Ejaculation.

Other Sexual Dysfunctions

Multiple Choice Questions

1. When is the "Other Specified Sexual Dysfunction" category most appropriate?
    - A. When the patient presents with sexual dysfunction symptoms that do not fully meet criteria for a specific disorder but cause significant distress
    - B. When the symptoms are secondary to a known medical condition
    - C. When the sexual dysfunction is associated exclusively with a psychiatric disorder
    - D. When there is complete absence of distress about the symptoms
2. Which example best illustrates "Other Specified Sexual Dysfunction"?
    - A. A man with delayed ejaculation that occurs only during specific sexual activities
    - B. A woman with pain during intercourse due to an anatomical abnormality
    - C. A man with premature ejaculation despite treatment with SSRIs
    - D. A woman with consistent difficulty achieving orgasm due to past trauma
3. Which scenario justifies the use of the "Unspecified Sexual Dysfunction" category?
    - A. A patient in an emergency setting presents with significant sexual dysfunction but insufficient information is available to determine the cause
    - B. A patient meets criteria for Female Sexual Interest/Arousal Disorder but declines treatment
    - C. A patient with erectile dysfunction fails to respond to phosphodiesterase inhibitors
    - D. A patient reports episodic sexual distress unrelated to performance
4. Which clinical presentation would most likely fall under the "Specified" category rather than "Unspecified"?
    - A. A clear but subthreshold presentation of delayed ejaculation causing distress
    - B. Generalized sexual dissatisfaction without identifiable triggers
    - C. Sexual dysfunction exclusively related to substance use
    - D. Episodic anorgasmia during high-stress periods
5. Which therapeutic goal is most relevant for a patient with "Other Specified Sexual Dysfunction"?
    - A. Reducing distress and improving sexual satisfaction
    - B. Eliminating symptoms entirely within one month
    - C. Avoiding pharmacological treatment options
    - D. Focusing solely on medical causes without addressing psychological factors
6. Which distinguishing feature separates the "Unspecified" category from "Specified Sexual Dysfunction"?
    - A. Lack of a detailed explanation for why criteria are not fully met in the "Unspecified" category
    - B. Symptoms are less severe in the "Specified" category
    - C. The "Unspecified" category is used only in research contexts
    - D. The "Specified" category always requires comorbid conditions
7. A patient with significant sexual dysfunction symptoms refuses further diagnostic testing. Which category would be most appropriate?
    - A. Unspecified Sexual Dysfunction
    - B. Other Specified Sexual Dysfunction
    - C. Erectile Disorder
    - D. Hypoactive Sexual Desire Disorder

True/False Questions

		T	F
1	According to the DSM-5, in the case of Substance/Medication-Induced Sexual Dysfunction, the dysfunction must manifest during or immediately after intoxication or withdrawal, or as a side effect of a medication.		
2	The DSM-5 removed Sexual Aversion Disorder, which was included in previous editions, although it is still mentioned historically in the literature.		
3	To diagnose Female Orgasmic Disorder, the DSM-5 requires a total absence of orgasm under any circumstance, including self-stimulation, for at least 12 months.		
4	In the DSM-5, vaginismus and dyspareunia have been consolidated into a single diagnosis called "Genito-Pelvic Pain/Penetration Disorder."		
5	In the DSM-5, diagnosing Male Hypoactive Sexual Desire Disorder requires only one recorded episode of low desire, regardless of personal, relational, or cultural factors.		
6	According to the DSM-5, diagnosing Female Sexual Interest/Arousal Disorder merely requires finding reduced subjective desire, without the need to consider physical arousal or relational factors.		
7	The DSM-5 specifies whether a Sexual Dysfunction is generalized or situational and whether it is "lifelong" or acquired.		
8	In the DSM-5, a Sexual Dysfunction diagnosis should be ruled out if it is primarily due to severe relationship distress, another medical condition, or the effects of substances or medications.		
9	The DSM-5 acknowledges the importance of cultural context in identifying Sexual Dysfunctions but recognizes that significant personal distress may still warrant a diagnosis.		
10	In the DSM-5, the presence of clinically significant distress or interpersonal difficulties is a key criterion for diagnosing a Sexual Dysfunction.		

Matching Exercise

1. A temporary diagnosis when insufficient information is available. [ ]
2. A distinguishing feature of the Specified category. [ ]
3. A goal of treatment for both Specified and Unspecified Sexual Dysfunctions. [ ]
4. A condition that can contribute to both Specified and Unspecified Sexual Dysfunctions. [ ]
5. A therapeutic approach commonly used for Specified Sexual Dysfunctions. [ ]
6. A clinical scenario suitable for the Unspecified category. [ ]

Descriptions:

- A. Lack of detailed explanation of subthreshold symptoms
- B. Substance-induced sexual dysfunction
- C. Improving sexual satisfaction and reducing distress
- D. Comprehensive sexual history and psychological assessment
- E. Use in emergency settings
- F. Explanation of why criteria are not met

Case Study

A 45-year-old woman reports episodes of sexual dissatisfaction and difficulty maintaining arousal, which occur only during high-stress periods. She denies pain during intercourse or lack of desire but expresses frustration with her inability to enjoy sexual activity consistently. The patient has no medical conditions and declines further diagnostic testing. She reports significant distress about her symptoms.

1. Which category would be most appropriate for this patient?
    - A. Other Specified Sexual Dysfunction
    - B. Unspecified Sexual Dysfunction
    - C. Female Sexual Interest/Arousal Disorder
    - D. Generalized Anxiety Disorder
2. What is the most appropriate first-line therapeutic approach for this patient?
    - A. Cognitive-behavioral therapy to address psychological factors
    - B. Hormonal therapy to improve arousal
    - C. Prescription of phosphodiesterase inhibitors
    - D. Surgical evaluation for anatomical abnormalities
3. Which complication should be monitored if her symptoms remain untreated?
    - A. Increased relationship strain and reduced intimacy
    - B. Development of chronic dyspareunia
    - C. Onset of hormonal imbalances
    - D. Progression to a generalized sexual dysfunction

Answers

Multiple Choice Questions:
1. A
2. A
3. A
4. A
5. A
6. A
7. A

True/False Questions:
1. True
2. True
3. False
4. True
5. False
6. False
7. True
8. True
9. True
10. True

Matching Exercise:
1. E
2. F
3. C
4. B
5. D
6. A

Case Study Answers and Explanations:
1. A - Explanation: The patient's symptoms and lack of further diagnostic testing fit the Specified category.
2. A - Explanation: Cognitive-behavioral therapy addresses psychological factors contributing to situational symptoms.
3. A - Explanation: Relationship strain is a common complication if symptoms remain untreated.

Your Impact on the Clinical Community

"Knowledge shared is knowledge multiplied." – Robert Noyce

Imagine helping someone you've never met—without spending a dime or a minute more than you can spare. If that sounds like something you'd do, here's a simple way to make it happen.

This workbook was designed to improve clinical skills and test knowledge through engaging exercises and real-world case studies. If you've found value in its pages so far, your perspective can make a difference to someone else.

Leaving a review is one of the easiest ways to support a community of clinicians striving for excellence. Think of a student preparing for their exams, or a seasoned professional refreshing their skills. Your review could be the nudge they need to pick up this resource and enhance their practice.

Your feedback—whether it's about what you loved, what challenged you, or what could be improved—is deeply appreciated. Each review helps guide others toward tools they need to grow in their clinical work.

Scan to leave a review on Amazon

Thank you for taking a moment to share your experience. Your voice matters!

Gender Dysphoria

This area focuses on the distress that some individuals experience when there is a clear discrepancy between the gender they perceive themselves to be and the sex they were assigned at birth. It is not simply a matter of expressing gender differently; rather, the incongruence creates significant discomfort that can affect day-to-day activities, social interactions, and psychological balance.

Gender Dysphoria may emerge at various stages of life. Some children show signs early on, such as rejecting their physical traits or expressing a strong desire to be another gender. In other cases, recognition of this gap becomes more intense during adolescence or adulthood, as individuals reflect on their identity and how they wish to express it. Preferences related to clothing, interests, or play may be involved, but most importantly, there is an internal conviction of not matching the assigned sex.

Evaluating Gender Dysphoria involves distinguishing genuine distress from other forms of gender variance that do not necessarily lead to a profound sense of discomfort. This requires carefully observing how much distress is present, how it affects the person's everyday life, and how long it has persisted. A diagnosis typically calls for ongoing distress, not just temporary moments of confusion or exploration. It is also crucial to consider family or cultural contexts that could heighten the sense of incongruence or limit the person's freedom to express themselves.

Clinically, support may include psychological counseling, psychoeducation, and, where appropriate, gender affirmation procedures. In certain cases, people may opt for hormonal treatments or surgery. However, these decisions generally follow a thorough assessment and a multidisciplinary approach, involving mental health professionals as well as specialists in gender issues and endocrinology.

Research indicates that social, family, and medical support can reduce distress and enhance overall well-being, while stigma and discrimination may intensify depression, anxiety, or social withdrawal. Consequently, it is vital to promote objective, nonjudgmental information and encourage a deeper understanding of each individual's identity journey.

If left unrecognized or unaddressed, Gender Dysphoria can lead to further emotional challenges, such as anxiety, depression, or relationship difficulties. Tailored interventions that account for each person's circumstances can help alleviate discomfort and foster informed choices regarding gender identity. The ultimate goal is to support self-acceptance and a sense of alignment between one's internal perception and daily life.

Gender Dysphoria

Multiple Choice Questions

1. A 16-year-old adolescent reports persistent distress about their assigned gender, expressing a desire to live as a different gender. Which additional finding supports a diagnosis of Gender Dysphoria?
    - A. A strong desire to be treated as a different gender
    - B. Temporary feelings of discomfort with assigned gender during puberty
    - C. Symptoms resolving spontaneously without intervention
    - D. Distress limited to societal stigma without internal conflict
2. Which of the following clinical features is most characteristic of Gender Dysphoria in children?
    - A. Strong preference for toys, games, or activities stereotypically associated with another gender
    - B. Difficulty forming friendships with peers of their assigned gender
    - C. Temporary exploration of clothing or roles associated with another gender
    - D. Recurrent nightmares about gendered roles
3. Which of the following best differentiates Gender Dysphoria from non-distressing gender nonconformity?
    - A. Significant emotional distress or functional impairment due to incongruence with assigned gender
    - B. A preference for roles and clothing typically associated with another gender
    - C. Experimentation with gender expression during adolescence
    - D. Absence of societal support for gender exploration
4. Which therapeutic approach is most appropriate for addressing distress associated with Gender Dysphoria in adolescents?
    - A. Affirmative therapy to explore gender identity and support social transition
    - B. Behavioral therapy aimed at reinforcing alignment with assigned gender roles
    - C. Pharmacological intervention to manage emotional distress exclusively
    - D. Avoidance of intervention to minimize external stigmatization
5. A 10-year-old child reports consistent identification with a different gender and distress about their assigned gender. What is the most appropriate next step?
    - A. A comprehensive psychosocial assessment to evaluate the child's gender identity and support needs
    - B. Immediate initiation of gender-affirming hormone therapy
    - C. Referral for surgical consultation to address physical incongruence
    - D. Recommendation of no intervention until the child reaches adulthood
6. Which factor most strongly suggests a stable gender identity requiring medical or social transition support?
    - A. Persistent and consistent identification with a different gender over time
    - B. Temporary experimentation with gender roles during adolescence
    - C. Increased conflict with parents about gender expression
    - D. A history of anxiety unrelated to gender concerns
7. Which of the following complications is most commonly associated with untreated Gender Dysphoria?
    - A. Increased risk of depression and suicidal ideation
    - B. Development of psychotic symptoms unrelated to gender
    - C. Chronic physical illness due to stress hormones
    - D. Obsessive-compulsive symptoms targeting body image

True/False Questions

		T	F
1	The diagnostic criteria for Gender Dysphoria in children necessarily require a manifestation of discomfort or aversion toward the sex assigned at birth.		
2	The diagnosis of Gender Dysphoria in adults requires the presence of at least six specific characteristics, according to the DSM-5.		
3	Persistent identification with a gender different from the one assigned at birth is one of the main criteria for the diagnosis of Gender Dysphoria.		
4	In children, the desire to belong to another gender must be clearly verbalized for at least six months to meet the diagnostic criteria.		
5	The intensity of clinically significant distress varies depending on the individual's cultural and social context.		
6	Gender Dysphoria can be diagnosed regardless of whether the individual has started a physical or social transition process.		
7	The presence of psychological comorbidities, such as depression and anxiety, is common in individuals with Gender Dysphoria but is not a diagnostic criterion.		
8	In the DSM-5, the diagnostic focus of Gender Dysphoria is more on psychological distress than on gender identity itself.		
9	The DSM-5 provides different criteria for diagnosing Gender Dysphoria in children compared to adults and adolescents.		
10	To be diagnosed, Gender Dysphoria must necessarily include an explicit desire to undergo medical transition interventions.		

Matching Exercise

1. A strong desire to live and be treated as a different gender. [ ]
2. A reversible intervention supporting gender exploration. [ ]
3. A common mental health challenge associated with untreated Gender Dysphoria. [ ]
4. A therapeutic approach to address distress and support gender identity. [ ]
5. A distinguishing feature of Gender Dysphoria in adolescents. [ ]
6. A diagnostic step to assess Gender Dysphoria in children. [ ]

Descriptions:

- A. Persistent and consistent identification with a different gender
- B. Affirmative therapy
- C. Depression and suicidal ideation
- D. Comprehensive psychosocial assessment
- E. Social transition
- F. A strong desire to change physical characteristics

Case Study

A 14-year-old adolescent assigned male at birth reports feeling distressed about their body and consistently identifies as female. They express a desire to socially transition by changing their name and pronouns and report discomfort with male physical characteristics. Their parents are supportive but worried about the impact of societal stigma. The adolescent denies any suicidal ideation but expresses frustration about delays in accessing gender-affirming care.

1. Which feature most strongly supports a diagnosis of Gender Dysphoria?
    - A. Persistent identification as female and distress about assigned male gender
    - B. Desire to change name and pronouns
    - C. Parental concerns about societal stigma
    - D. Frustration about delays in accessing care
2. What is the most appropriate next step for this adolescent?
    - A. Referral for a comprehensive psychosocial evaluation and discussion of social transition
    - B. Immediate initiation of puberty blockers to halt physical changes
    - C. Surgical consultation for gender-affirming procedures
    - D. Recommendation of family therapy to address parental concerns
3. Which complication should be monitored if the adolescent's Gender Dysphoria is left untreated?
    - A. Increased risk of depression and social withdrawal
    - B. Development of physical illness related to stress hormones
    - C. Onset of obsessive-compulsive symptoms unrelated to gender
    - D. Chronic conflict with parents about medical care

Answers

Multiple Choice Questions:

1. A
2. A
3. A
4. A
5. A
6. A
7. A

True/False Questions:

1. True
2. False
3. True
4. True
5. True
6. True
7. True
8. True
9. True
10. False

Matching Exercise:

1. A
2. E
3. C
4. B
5. F
6. D

Case Study Answers and Explanations:

1. A - Explanation: Persistent identification as a different gender and distress are key criteria for Gender Dysphoria.
2. A - Explanation: A psychosocial evaluation and discussion of social transition are essential first steps.
3. A - Explanation: Depression and social withdrawal are common risks associated with untreated Gender Dysphoria.

Gender-Related Disorders

Multiple Choice Questions

1. When is the "Other Specified Gender-Related Disorder" category most appropriate?
    - A. When the patient presents with significant distress about gender identity that does not meet full criteria for Gender Dysphoria
    - B. When symptoms are exclusively associated with societal stigma
    - C. When there is no evidence of functional impairment despite gender-related distress
    - D. When symptoms resolve spontaneously without intervention
2. Which scenario best illustrates "Other Specified Gender-Related Disorder"?
    - A. A patient with intermittent distress about gender identity without persistent feelings of incongruence
    - B. A patient who meets full criteria for Gender Dysphoria but declines treatment
    - C. A patient with gender-related distress limited to dissatisfaction with specific gender roles
    - D. A patient experiencing no distress despite exploring gender roles
3. When is the "Unspecified Gender-Related Disorder" category used?
    - A. When insufficient information is available to make a more specific diagnosis
    - B. When the patient declines gender-affirming interventions despite persistent distress
    - C. When the patient exhibits gender nonconformity without any associated distress
    - D. When symptoms align closely with another psychiatric diagnosis
4. Which of the following presentations would likely fall under the "Specified" category rather than the "Unspecified"?
    - A. Subthreshold symptoms of Gender Dysphoria causing distress and impairment
    - B. Temporary exploration of gender roles without distress
    - C. Gender nonconformity occurring exclusively during adolescence
    - D. Symptoms of gender-related distress that resolve without treatment
5. Which treatment goal is most relevant for patients with "Other Specified Gender-Related Disorder"?
    - A. Reducing distress and improving overall functioning
    - B. Encouraging alignment with assigned gender roles
    - C. Focusing exclusively on medical interventions
    - D. Avoiding discussions about gender identity to minimize distress
6. Which of the following best differentiates the "Specified" category from the "Unspecified" category?
    - A. "Specified" includes a clear explanation for why criteria are not met, while "Unspecified" does not.
    - B. "Unspecified" requires comorbid psychiatric conditions for diagnosis.
    - C. "Specified" is used only in research contexts.
    - D. "Unspecified" applies only to children and adolescents.
7. A patient presents with intermittent gender-related distress but refuses further evaluation. Which category would be most appropriate?
    - A. Unspecified Gender-Related Disorder
    - B. Other Specified Gender-Related Disorder
    - C. Gender Dysphoria
    - D. Generalized Anxiety Disorder

True/False Questions

		T	F
1	Gender dysphoria can only be diagnosed in children if they meet at least six criteria, including the desire to belong to the opposite gender.		
2	In the diagnostic criteria for gender dysphoria in adults, clinically significant distress is not required.		
3	An increase in the incidence of gender dysphoria diagnoses has been observed more frequently in adolescent females compared to males.		
4	Gender dysphoria is necessarily associated with other psychopathological conditions such as depression or anxiety.		
5	According to the DSM-5, a diagnosis of gender dysphoria cannot be made in the presence of sexual development disorders.		
6	The diagnosis of gender dysphoria in children requires a minimum duration of six months for symptoms.		
7	The presence of gender nonconforming behavior is sufficient to diagnose gender dysphoria in the DSM-5.		
8	In the DSM-5, the incongruence between assigned sex and gender identity is an essential element for the diagnosis of gender dysphoria.		
9	Medical transition (e.g., hormone therapies or surgical interventions) is a mandatory component for the diagnosis of gender dysphoria in the DSM-5.		
10	Adults with gender dysphoria may not perceive any physical incongruence but only social rejection of their assigned gender role.		

Matching Exercise

1. A temporary diagnosis due to insufficient clinical information. [ ]
2. A distinguishing feature of the Specified category. [ ]
3. A goal of treatment for patients in both categories. [ ]
4. A clinical scenario suitable for the Unspecified category. [ ]
5. A step in evaluating subthreshold presentations of Gender Dysphoria. [ ]
6. A potential complication of untreated distress in these categories. [ ]

Descriptions:

- A. Lack of detailed explanation for subthreshold symptoms
- B. Reducing distress and improving functioning
- C. Increased risk of depression or anxiety
- D. Comprehensive psychosocial assessment
- E. Subthreshold distress about gender identity
- F. Use in settings where full evaluation is not feasible

Case Study

A 20-year-old patient reports intermittent distress about their gender identity but denies consistent incongruence with their assigned gender. They experience occasional discomfort in gendered social settings but state that the distress is not persistent. They decline further evaluation or discussion about gender-affirming interventions.

1. Which category would be most appropriate for this patient?
   - A. Other Specified Gender-Related Disorder
   - B. Unspecified Gender-Related Disorder
   - C. Gender Dysphoria
   - D. Adjustment Disorder
2. What is the most appropriate therapeutic approach for this patient?
   - A. Supportive therapy to explore gender identity and address situational distress
   - B. Immediate referral for gender-affirming medical interventions
   - C. Cognitive-behavioral therapy focused on anxiety management
   - D. Avoiding further discussion to minimize distress
3. Which complication should be monitored if the patient's symptoms remain untreated?
   - A. Increased risk of depression and social withdrawal
   - B. Development of obsessive-compulsive symptoms related to body image
   - C. Progression to generalized anxiety disorder
   - D. Onset of severe functional impairment

Answers

Multiple Choice Questions:
1. A
2. A
3. A
4. A
5. A
6. A
7. A

True/False Questions:
1. True
2. False
3. True
4. False
5. False
6. True
7. False
8. True
9. False
10. True

Matching Exercise:
1. F
2. A
3. B
4. E
5. D
6. C

Case Study Answers and Explanations:
1. A - Explanation: The patient's symptoms fit the "Other Specified Gender-Related Disorder" category due to intermittent distress.
2. A - Explanation: Supportive therapy helps explore identity and address situational distress.
3. A - Explanation: Depression and social withdrawal are common complications of untreated distress.

Disruptive, Impulse-Control, and Conduct Disorders

This group covers conditions in which individuals show substantial difficulty regulating impulses and behaviors, with negative outcomes for both the affected person and those around them. A common element is the tendency to act in a rash or aggressive way without giving adequate thought to the consequences, often defying social rules or infringing on the rights of others. Contributing factors may stem from biological, relational, or environmental influences, or a combination of several aspects.

A well-known example is Oppositional Defiant Disorder (ODD), marked by a pattern of defiance and hostility toward authority figures, including arguing, disobedience, and frequent irritability. It typically appears in childhood or early adolescence, and, if not recognized and addressed, can develop into more serious rule-breaking behaviors. Intermittent Explosive Disorder, on the other hand, is characterized by disproportionate outbursts of anger relative to the triggering situation. These episodes may involve sudden verbal or physical aggression that can lead to property damage or ruptured relationships.

Conduct Disorder is another significant condition in which individuals persistently violate social norms and the rights of others. Manifestations may include aggression toward people or animals, destruction of property, deceitfulness, or theft. When these behaviors become entrenched and enduring, they can lead to long-term social and legal problems, emphasizing the need for timely intervention. Additional disorders in this category, such as Pyromania (deliberate fire-setting) or Kleptomania (the irresistible urge to steal objects of minimal personal value), highlight the impaired impulse control at the core of these conditions.

From a diagnostic standpoint, it is important to differentiate these patterns from one-off behaviors triggered by conflict or short-term rebellion, by evaluating their frequency, intensity, and underlying motivations. Clinicians must also rule out psychotic disorders, substance abuse, or neurological problems that could fuel aggression or loss of self-control. The individual's cultural and relational context should also be considered: what might be seen as "disruptive" in one society may take on a different meaning in another.

Treatment often involves behavioral interventions, psychological support, and sometimes collaboration with the family or school environment. Particular attention is placed on preventing repeat offenses and building prosocial skills—key elements in managing impulsivity and channeling a person's energy in more constructive directions. In this regard, early detection of a disruptive behavior disorder can be crucial, providing the chance to address family dynamics, emotional factors, and relationship issues that perpetuate aggression or antisocial conduct.

Oppositional Defiant Disorder

Multiple Choice Questions

1. Which of the following is a diagnostic criterion for Oppositional Defiant Disorder?
    - A. Repetitive behaviors that violate the rights of others.
    - B. Persistent anger, irritability, and hostile behavior toward authority figures.
    - C. Difficulty concentrating and excessive impulsivity.
    - D. Persistent fear in social situations.
2. To diagnose Oppositional Defiant Disorder, symptoms must be present:
    - A. In at least one social setting (e.g., school or home).
    - B. In two or more different social settings.
    - C. Only at home.
    - D. Only in school settings.
3. Which of the following behaviors is typical of Oppositional Defiant Disorder?
    - A. Repeated compulsions.
    - B. Marked social withdrawal.
    - C. Frequent arguments with adults or authority figures.
    - D. Psychotic episodes.
4. To be diagnosed as Oppositional Defiant Disorder, symptoms must last at least:
    - A. 1 month.
    - B. 6 months.
    - C. 3 months.
    - D. 12 months.
5. What is an important aspect of evaluating Oppositional Defiant Disorder?
    - A. The presence of psychotic symptoms.
    - B. The frequency and intensity of problematic behaviors compared to peers.
    - C. The response to antipsychotic medications.
    - D. The presence of motor tics.
6. Which of the following is a risk factor for Oppositional Defiant Disorder?
    - A. Head trauma.
    - B. Emotional abuse or an unstable family environment.
    - C. Avoidant attachment style.
    - D. Cognitive deficits.
7. Oppositional Defiant Disorder is most commonly diagnosed in:
    - A. Infants.
    - B. Preschool and school-age children.
    - C. Adolescents with depression.
    - D. Adults with antisocial personality disorder.

True/False Questions

		T	F
1	To diagnose Oppositional Defiant Disorder (ODD) in children, symptoms must appear in at least two settings (e.g., home and school).		
2	Children with ODD frequently exhibit aggressive behavior toward people and animals.		
3	In the DSM-5, ODD is divided into three severity categories based on the number of settings where symptoms are observed.		
4	The minimum duration of symptoms to diagnose ODD is six months.		
5	ODD symptoms must cause clinically significant distress to the child or those around them.		
6	The DSM-5 specifies that ODD cannot coexist with Attention-Deficit/Hyperactivity Disorder (ADHD).		
7	Difficulties in emotional regulation are a core feature of ODD in the DSM-5.		
8	ODD is frequently diagnosed in adults, although it is more common in children and adolescents.		
9	The oppositional behaviors of ODD can be directed at both authority figures and peers.		
10	ODD symptoms must be persistent and cannot be attributed to a temporary reaction to a specific stressor.		

Matching Exercise

1. Persistent anger and irritability. [ ]
2. Frequent arguments with adults or authority figures. [ ]
3. Vindictive or spiteful behavior. [ ]
4. Symptoms present for at least 6 months. [ ]
5. Frequency and intensity of symptoms above age norms. [ ]
6. Unstable family environment as a risk factor. [ ]

Descriptions:

- A. Required duration for diagnosis.
- B. Emotions commonly exhibited by children with this disorder.
- C. A key feature of Oppositional Defiant Disorder.
- D. Environmental factor increasing risk of onset.
- E. Hostile or aggressive behavior.
- F. Distinction from peers.

Case Study

Marco, a 9-year-old boy, lives in an unstable family environment with frequent parental conflicts. At school, he exhibits oppositional behavior toward teachers, frequently argues with peers, and often refuses to follow rules. His mother reports that he is irritable and often seeks revenge when he feels treated unfairly. These behaviors have been occurring both at home and school for over six months.

1. Which of the following best supports a diagnosis of Oppositional Defiant Disorder for Marco?
    - A. The unstable family environment.
    - B. The duration of symptoms.
    - C. The presence of psychotic episodes.
    - D. Parental conflicts.
2. Which intervention would be most appropriate as a first step in Marco's treatment?
    - A. Antipsychotic medication.
    - B. Family therapy and behavior management.
    - C. School isolation.
    - D. Testing for cognitive deficits.
3. Which symptom is NOT typical of Oppositional Defiant Disorder?
    - A. Persistent anger.
    - B. Vindictive behavior.
    - C. Sleep disturbances.
    - D. Disobedience toward adults.

Answers

Multiple Choice Questions:

1. B
2. A
3. C
4. B
5. B
6. B
7. B

True/False Questions:

1. False
2. False
3. True
4. True
5. True
6. False
7. True
8. False
9. True
10. True

Matching Exercise:

1. B
2. C
3. E
4. A
5. F
6. D

Case Study Answers and Explanations:

1. B - Explanation: The duration of symptoms is a key criterion for diagnosis.
2. B - Explanation: Family therapy is crucial to improving Marco's environment and managing his behavior.
3. C - Explanation: Sleep disturbances are not characteristic of Oppositional Defiant Disorder.

Intermittent Explosive Disorder

Multiple Choice Questions

1. Which of the following behaviors is characteristic of Intermittent Explosive Disorder?
    - A. Persistent defiance toward authority figures.
    - B. Verbal or physical outbursts that are disproportionate to the situation.
    - C. Repeated episodes of theft or deceit.
    - D. Avoidance of social interactions.
2. How frequently must outbursts occur to meet the diagnostic criteria for Intermittent Explosive Disorder?
    - A. At least once a week for three months.
    - B. At least three times a month for six months.
    - C. At least twice a month for one year.
    - D. There is no set frequency requirement.
3. Which of the following is NOT a criterion for Intermittent Explosive Disorder?
    - A. The outbursts are impulsive and not premeditated.
    - B. The aggressive episodes cause significant distress or impairment.
    - C. The aggressive episodes occur exclusively during a psychotic episode.
    - D. The aggression is disproportionate to any provocation.
4. Which neurotransmitter is most commonly implicated in the pathophysiology of Intermittent Explosive Disorder?
    - A. Dopamine.
    - B. Serotonin.
    - C. Glutamate.
    - D. Acetylcholine.
5. A diagnosis of Intermittent Explosive Disorder can only be made if:
    - A. The individual is older than 6 years.
    - B. The aggressive episodes involve physical harm to others.
    - C. The behavior occurs across multiple contexts (e.g., home, school, work).
    - D. There is a history of trauma.
6. Which of the following conditions must be ruled out before diagnosing Intermittent Explosive Disorder?
    - A. Generalized Anxiety Disorder.
    - B. Conduct Disorder.
    - C. Specific Phobia.
    - D. Obsessive-Compulsive Disorder.
7. What type of intervention is considered first-line treatment for Intermittent Explosive Disorder?
    - A. Antipsychotic medication.
    - B. Cognitive-behavioral therapy.
    - C. Electroconvulsive therapy.
    - D. Psychoanalytic therapy.

True/False Questions

		T	F
1	To diagnose IED, aggressive outbursts must be planned and premeditated.		
2	Aggressive outbursts in IED can be verbal or physical, but they must not cause material damage.		
3	To meet the DSM-5 criteria for IED, the frequency of verbal aggressive episodes must be at least twice a week for three months.		
4	In the DSM-5, IED cannot be diagnosed in children under six years old.		
5	IED requires that aggressive behavior is not better explained by another mental disorder or general medical condition.		
6	Episodes of IED must cause clinically significant distress or functional impairment to be diagnosable.		
7	The DSM-5 includes criteria to distinguish between impulsive and predatory aggression in IED.		
8	IED is considered a rare disorder, with a prevalence below 1% in the general population.		
9	The intensity of aggressive reactions in IED is disproportionate to the provocation or triggering stressor.		
10	The diagnosis of IED requires at least three episodes of physical aggression causing damage to people or things within one year.		

Matching Exercise

1. Outbursts that are impulsive and disproportionate to the situation. [ ]
2. Episodes cause significant distress or functional impairment. [ ]
3. Dysfunction in the amygdala and prefrontal cortex. [ ]
4. Aggressive episodes that occur without premeditation. [ ]
5. Diagnosed only in individuals older than 6 years. [ ]
6. First-line treatment is cognitive-behavioral therapy. [ ]

Descriptions:

- A. Neural basis of the disorder.
- B. A diagnostic criterion for Intermittent Explosive Disorder.
- C. Distinction from deliberate aggression.
- D. A developmental consideration for diagnosis.
- E. The most effective therapeutic intervention.
- F. Impact on emotional and social functioning.

Case Study

Ethan, a 15-year-old male, is referred to therapy after several instances of explosive aggression at school and home. These outbursts often involve yelling, breaking objects, and occasional physical aggression toward peers. Ethan reports feeling intense remorse afterward but says he "can't stop" when angered. His parents note that he has been easily angered since childhood and has no history of substance abuse or psychosis. The episodes occur roughly twice a week and have been ongoing for more than a year. Ethan's academic performance and relationships have been severely affected.

1. Which feature most strongly supports a diagnosis of Intermittent Explosive Disorder for Ethan?
    - A. The frequency of his outbursts.
    - B. The physical aggression involved in the episodes.
    - C. The remorse he feels after each episode.
    - D. His age at the onset of symptoms.
2. Which of the following differential diagnoses should be most carefully considered in Ethan's case?
    - A. Conduct Disorder.
    - B. Bipolar Disorder.
    - C. Generalized Anxiety Disorder.
    - D. Specific Phobia.
3. Which treatment plan would be most appropriate for Ethan?
    - A. Family therapy with parental training.
    - B. Antipsychotic medication.
    - C. Cognitive-behavioral therapy with anger management techniques.
    - D. Inpatient hospitalization.

Answers

Multiple Choice Questions:
1. B
2. A
3. C
4. B
5. A
6. B
7. B

True/False Questions:
1. False
2. False
3. True
4. True
5. True
6. True
7. False
8. False
9. True
10. False

Matching Exercise:
1. B
2. F
3. A
4. C
5. D
6. E

Case Study Answers and Explanations:
1. A - Explanation: The frequency of outbursts meets the diagnostic criteria for Intermittent Explosive Disorder.
2. A - Explanation: Conduct Disorder must be ruled out, as it can present with similar aggressive behaviors.
3. C - Explanation: Cognitive-behavioral therapy is evidence-based and includes anger management strategies tailored to Ethan's needs.

Conduct Disorder

Multiple Choice Questions

1. Which of the following behaviors is most characteristic of Conduct Disorder?
   - A. Frequent arguments with authority figures.
   - B. Repeated violation of societal norms and the rights of others.
   - C. Persistent irritability without aggressive actions.
   - D. Avoidance of social interactions.
2. What is required for a diagnosis of Conduct Disorder in terms of the duration of symptoms?
   - A. Persistent symptoms for at least 3 months.
   - B. Persistent symptoms for at least 6 months.
   - C. Persistent symptoms for at least 12 months.
   - D. Persistent symptoms for at least 18 months.
3. Which subtype of Conduct Disorder is associated with an earlier onset and a worse prognosis?
   - A. Childhood-onset type.
   - B. Adolescent-onset type.
   - C. Late-adulthood onset type.
   - D. Situational-onset type.
4. Which of the following is NOT a diagnostic criterion for Conduct Disorder?
   - A. Aggression toward people and animals.
   - B. Deliberate destruction of property.
   - C. Persistent defiance toward authority figures.
   - D. Deceitfulness or theft.
5. Which neurobiological factor is commonly associated with Conduct Disorder?
   - A. Reduced activity in the prefrontal cortex.
   - B. Increased dopamine transmission.
   - C. Elevated levels of norepinephrine.
   - D. Hyperactivity in the hippocampus.
6. Which comorbid disorder is most frequently observed in individuals with Conduct Disorder?
   - A. Autism Spectrum Disorder.
   - B. Attention-Deficit/Hyperactivity Disorder (ADHD).
   - C. Obsessive-Compulsive Disorder.
   - D. Schizophrenia.
7. Which intervention is considered most effective for the treatment of Conduct Disorder?
   - A. Individual psychoanalysis.
   - B. Multisystemic therapy (MST).
   - C. Pharmacological treatment only.
   - D. Restrictive inpatient care.

True/False Questions

		T	F
1	Conduct Disorder (CD) requires the presence of at least three problematic behaviors in the past 12 months and at least one in the past six months.		
2	The DSM-5 distinguishes between childhood-onset, adolescent-onset, and unspecified subtypes of CD.		
3	To diagnose CD, behaviors must necessarily include physical aggression toward people or animals.		
4	Conduct Disorder can only be diagnosed in individuals over the age of 10.		
5	The presence of limited prosocial emotions is an optional specifier in the DSM-5 for CD.		
6	The DSM-5 considers CD as an independent condition that cannot coexist with Oppositional Defiant Disorder (ODD).		
7	Individuals with CD with the "limited prosocial emotions" specifier often show guilt and remorse for their behaviors.		
8	Criteria for CD include acts of vandalism, such as destroying others' property, among relevant behaviors.		
9	The diagnosis of CD requires that problematic behaviors cause significant functional impairment in social, school, or work contexts.		
10	The onset of CD is more frequently associated with genetic factors than environmental ones.		

Matching Exercise

1. Repeated violation of societal norms. [ ]
2. Aggression toward people and animals. [ ]
3. Destruction of property. [ ]
4. Peer rejection and social isolation as risk factors. [ ]
5. Reduced activity in the prefrontal cortex. [ ]
6. Multisystemic therapy as a treatment. [ ]

Descriptions:

- A. A hallmark symptom of Conduct Disorder.
- B. Neurobiological factor associated with poor impulse control.
- C. Deliberate damage to physical objects.
- D. Environmental risk factors for developing Conduct Disorder.
- E. Evidence-based therapeutic approach targeting multiple domains.
- F. Persistent disregard for societal rules and expectations.

Case Study

Sophia, a 13-year-old female, has been reported to display aggressive behaviors, such as bullying peers and initiating physical fights. She has also been caught stealing from local stores and vandalizing school property. Sophia often blames others for her actions and shows little remorse. Her teachers note a decline in academic performance and increased truancy. At home, her parents describe her as defiant and disrespectful, refusing to follow household rules. Sophia's behaviors have persisted for over a year, causing significant problems at school and home.

1. Which feature most strongly supports a diagnosis of Conduct Disorder in Sophia?
   - A. The duration of her behaviors.
   - B. Her defiance toward authority figures.
   - C. Her academic struggles.
   - D. Her lack of remorse.
2. Which of the following differential diagnoses should be considered for Sophia?
   - A. Oppositional Defiant Disorder.
   - B. Bipolar Disorder.
   - C. Intermittent Explosive Disorder.
   - D. Generalized Anxiety Disorder.
3. What is the most appropriate treatment recommendation for Sophia?
   - A. Pharmacological treatment with antipsychotics.
   - B. Cognitive-behavioral therapy with a focus on anger management.
   - C. Multisystemic therapy involving family, school, and community interventions.
   - D. Placement in a residential treatment center.

Answers

Multiple Choice Questions:
1. B
2. C
3. A
4. C
5. A
6. B
7. B

True/False Questions:
1. True
2. True
3. False
4. False
5. True
6. False
7. False
8. True
9. True
10. False

Matching Exercise:
1. F
2. A
3. C
4. D
5. B
6. E

Case Study Answers and Explanations:
1. A - Explanation: The behaviors have persisted for over a year, meeting the duration criterion for Conduct Disorder.
2. A - Explanation: Oppositional Defiant Disorder shares some overlapping features but lacks the severity of rule violations seen in Conduct Disorder.
3. C - Explanation: Multisystemic therapy is the most effective intervention, addressing Sophia's needs across different environments.

Pyromania

Multiple Choice Questions

1. Which of the following is a defining feature of Pyromania?
    - A. Deliberate fire-setting to gain financial benefits.
    - B. An uncontrollable fascination with fire and fire-related paraphernalia.
    - C. Fire-setting during psychotic episodes with hallucinations.
    - D. Fire-setting to express anger or revenge.
2. For a diagnosis of Pyromania, the individual must:
    - A. Have a history of Conduct Disorder in childhood.
    - B. Experience pleasure, gratification, or relief when setting fires.
    - C. Use fire-setting as a means to intimidate others.
    - D. Have no history of previous fire-setting incidents.
3. Which of the following scenarios would NOT meet the criteria for Pyromania?
    - A. A person setting fires out of curiosity about fire behavior.
    - B. A person setting fires due to a strong urge despite knowing the risks.
    - C. A person setting fires to collect insurance money.
    - D. A person setting fires and experiencing intense satisfaction during the act.
4. What distinguishes Pyromania from other forms of fire-setting behavior?
    - A. It is always associated with criminal behavior.
    - B. The fire-setting is intentional and motivated by psychological gratification rather than external incentives.
    - C. It occurs exclusively in individuals with substance use disorders.
    - D. It requires the presence of comorbid mood disorders.
5. Pyromania is classified as:
    - A. A dissociative disorder.
    - B. A personality disorder.
    - C. A disorder of impulse control.
    - D. A psychotic disorder.
6. Which of the following is a common risk factor for Pyromania?
    - A. Exposure to trauma or abuse during childhood.
    - B. Family history of bipolar disorder.
    - C. Low cognitive abilities or intellectual disabilities.
    - D. High socioeconomic status.
7. What is the most effective treatment approach for individuals diagnosed with Pyromania?
    - A. Antipsychotic medication.
    - B. Cognitive-behavioral therapy focusing on impulse control.
    - C. Long-term inpatient psychiatric care.
    - D. Electroconvulsive therapy.

True/False Questions

		T	F
1	Pyromania is characterized by an impulsive and uncontrollable desire to set fires, without any secondary gain or personal benefit.		
2	In the DSM-5, the diagnosis of pyromania requires that the individual has set fires on at least five separate occasions.		
3	Fire-setting in pyromania is preceded by increasing affective tension or arousal.		
4	Pyromania can be diagnosed in individuals who set fires for revenge or to cover up a crime.		
5	The diagnosis of pyromania requires that the behavior is not better explained by conduct disorder, a manic episode, or substance intoxication.		
6	Pyromania is more frequently diagnosed in adolescents than in adults.		
7	Individuals with pyromania experience pleasure, gratification, or relief when witnessing the consequences of their fires.		
8	The DSM-5 includes pyromania under the category of impulse-control and conduct disorders.		
9	Setting fires for economic gain is included in the diagnostic criteria for pyromania.		
10	Pyromania is a very rare condition, with an estimated prevalence of less than 1% in the general population.		

Matching Exercise

1. Deliberate and recurrent fire-setting. [ ]
2. Emotional gratification or relief experienced during fire-setting. [ ]
3. Fascination with fire and fire-related paraphernalia. [ ]
4. Risk factor: childhood exposure to trauma or abuse. [ ]
5. Impulse control disorder classification. [ ]
6. Effective treatment: cognitive-behavioral therapy. [ ]

Descriptions:

- A. An intrinsic characteristic of Pyromania.
- B. A common psychological feature of the disorder.
- C. Evidence-based intervention for managing symptoms.
- D. Environmental influence linked to the development of Pyromania.
- E. Diagnostic category under the DSM-5.
- F. Behavior central to the diagnostic criteria.

Case Study

Ryan, a 17-year-old male, has a history of setting multiple small fires in his neighborhood without any apparent external motivation, such as revenge or financial gain. He describes feeling an overwhelming urge to set fires and reports intense satisfaction and relief afterward. Ryan often spends time collecting lighters, matches, and other fire-related objects, which he keeps hidden. Despite the repeated incidents, he shows little concern for the consequences of his actions. His family reports that he was exposed to significant neglect during childhood.

1. Which feature most strongly supports a diagnosis of Pyromania in Ryan's case?
   - A. His fascination with fire-related objects.
   - B. The absence of external motivations for fire-setting.
   - C. His age and gender.
   - D. His lack of concern for consequences.
2. Which of the following differential diagnoses should be considered for Ryan?
   - A. Conduct Disorder.
   - B. Bipolar Disorder.
   - C. Obsessive-Compulsive Disorder.
   - D. Intermittent Explosive Disorder.
3. What is the most appropriate intervention for Ryan?
   - A. Family therapy to address past neglect.
   - B. Cognitive-behavioral therapy with a focus on impulse control strategies.
   - C. Medication to reduce his fascination with fire.
   - D. Placement in a juvenile detention facility to prevent further incidents.

Answers

Multiple Choice Questions:

1. B
2. B
3. C
4. B
5. C
6. A
7. B

True/False Questions:

1. True
2. False
3. True
4. False
5. True
6. False
7. True
8. True
9. False
10. True

Matching Exercise:

1. F
2. B
3. A
4. D
5. E
6. C

Case Study Answers and Explanations:

1. B - Explanation: The absence of external motivations aligns with the diagnostic criteria for Pyromania.
2. A - Explanation: Conduct Disorder often involves fire-setting but is associated with broader patterns of rule violations and antisocial behavior.
3. B - Explanation: Cognitive-behavioral therapy is the most effective approach for addressing Ryan's impulse control issues.

Kleptomania

Multiple Choice Questions

1. Which of the following is a core feature of Kleptomania?
    - A. Persistent preoccupation with stealing valuable items for personal gain.
    - B. Recurrent failure to resist impulses to steal objects of little or no monetary value.
    - C. Stealing as a means to cope with feelings of anger or revenge.
    - D. Engaging in theft exclusively during manic episodes.
2. What distinguishes Kleptomania from ordinary theft or shoplifting?
    - A. It involves stealing items of significant monetary value.
    - B. The individual experiences guilt and remorse before the act.
    - C. The act of stealing is impulsive and not motivated by personal or financial gain.
    - D. The stolen items are always discarded after the act.
3. Which of the following is NOT a diagnostic criterion for Kleptomania?
    - A. A sense of tension before the theft.
    - B. Pleasure or relief after committing the theft.
    - C. Stealing to meet financial obligations.
    - D. The inability to resist the impulse to steal.
4. Kleptomania is most commonly associated with which of the following comorbid conditions?
    - A. Bipolar Disorder.
    - B. Obsessive-Compulsive Disorder.
    - C. Antisocial Personality Disorder.
    - D. Specific Phobia.
5. Which gender is Kleptomania more commonly diagnosed in?
    - A. Males.
    - B. Females.
    - C. It is equally common in both genders.
    - D. No significant gender differences have been reported.
6. What is the primary treatment approach for Kleptomania?
    - A. Long-term incarceration.
    - B. Psychoanalysis focused on early childhood trauma.
    - C. Cognitive-behavioral therapy with exposure and response prevention techniques.
    - D. Electroconvulsive therapy.
7. Which neurotransmitter imbalance is hypothesized to play a role in Kleptomania?
    - A. Dopamine.
    - B. Serotonin.
    - C. Norepinephrine.
    - D. GABA.

True/False Questions

		T	F
1	In the DSM-5, kleptomania is included under the obsessive-compulsive spectrum disorders and not under impulse-control disorders.		
2	Individuals with kleptomania are often unaware of the legal consequences of their actions.		
3	The diagnosis of kleptomania requires that theft occur without preceding tension or emotional arousal.		
4	Episodes of kleptomania can be episodic or chronic, but they are never associated with spontaneous remission periods.		
5	Kleptomania is frequently associated with mood disorders, such as major depression or bipolar disorder, according to the DSM-5.		
6	Impulsive theft in kleptomania can be considered a manifestation of antisocial personality disorder when the behavior occurs in adult individuals.		
7	In the DSM-5, kleptomania is excluded if the theft is explained as a response to a delusion or hallucination.		
8	Individuals with kleptomania often target high-value items, even if they do not need them.		
9	The DSM-5 specifies that kleptomania-related theft is rarely premeditated and does not involve accomplices.		
10	Kleptomania is more frequently diagnosed in clinical settings compared to the general population, with a significantly higher rate among psychiatric patients.		

Matching Exercise

1. Recurrent failure to resist the impulse to steal. [ ]
2. Sense of relief or gratification after stealing. [ ]
3. Objects stolen have little or no monetary value. [ ]
4. Cognitive-behavioral therapy as a treatment. [ ]
5. Serotonin imbalance hypothesized in pathophysiology. [ ]
6. Female predominance in diagnosis. [ ]

Descriptions:

- A. Effective intervention for managing symptoms of Kleptomania.
- B. A hallmark feature of the disorder.
- C. Psychological response following the act of theft.
- D. Neurotransmitter implicated in impulse control disorders.
- E. Typical characteristic of items targeted in theft.
- F. Gender-related observation in Kleptomania prevalence.

Case Study

Emma, a 32-year-old woman, has been caught multiple times stealing small items, such as pens, notepads, and inexpensive trinkets, from stores and workplaces. She reports feeling a buildup of tension before each theft and describes a sense of relief and satisfaction immediately afterward. Emma denies needing the items for personal use or financial reasons and often discards them after the act. She expresses guilt but feels unable to resist the impulse to steal. Emma also reports a history of anxiety and occasional obsessive thoughts.

1. Which feature most strongly supports a diagnosis of Kleptomania in Emma's case?
    - A. Her history of anxiety.
    - B. Her repeated thefts of inexpensive items.
    - C. The tension she feels before and relief she experiences after stealing.
    - D. Her guilt over the thefts.
2. Which differential diagnosis should be most carefully considered in Emma's case?
    - A. Bipolar Disorder.
    - B. Obsessive-Compulsive Disorder.
    - C. Antisocial Personality Disorder.
    - D. Intermittent Explosive Disorder.
3. What treatment plan would be most appropriate for Emma?
    - A. Incarceration to prevent future thefts.
    - B. Exposure and response prevention techniques through CBT.
    - C. Long-term psychoanalysis to explore underlying conflicts.
    - D. Antipsychotic medication.

Answers

Multiple Choice Questions:

1. B
2. C
3. C
4. B
5. B
6. C
7. B

True/False Questions:

1. False
2. False
3. False
4. False
5. True
6. False
7. True
8. False
9. True
10. True

Matching Exercise:

1. B
2. C
3. E
4. A
5. D
6. F

Case Study Answers and Explanations:

1. C - Explanation: The tension before and relief after stealing are key diagnostic features of Kleptomania.
2. B - Explanation: Obsessive-Compulsive Disorder shares some overlapping features, such as repetitive behaviors driven by anxiety.
3. B - Explanation: Cognitive-behavioral therapy with exposure and response prevention is an evidence-based treatment for Kleptomania.

Other Disruptive, Impulse-Control, and Conduct Disorder

Multiple Choice Questions

1. Which of the following best describes a Specified Disruptive, Impulse-Control, and Conduct Disorder?
    - A. A diagnosis given when symptoms meet the criteria for more than one disorder in the category.
    - B. A disorder where the symptoms clearly meet criteria for a specific diagnosis within the DSM-5.
    - C. A disorder characterized by symptoms of impulse control issues that do not fully meet criteria for any specific disorder.
    - D. A diagnosis used for individuals under the age of 12 only.
2. An example of a Specified Disruptive, Impulse-Control, and Conduct Disorder might include:
    - A. Persistent episodes of stealing without guilt or remorse.
    - B. Impulsive aggressive outbursts that do not meet the frequency for Intermittent Explosive Disorder.
    - C. Severe and recurrent physical aggression directed only toward animals.
    - D. Persistent irritability that occurs exclusively during manic episodes.
3. Unspecified Disruptive, Impulse-Control, and Conduct Disorder is most appropriate when:
    - A. The symptoms are better explained by a depressive or psychotic disorder.
    - B. Symptoms of disruptive behavior do not fit neatly into existing DSM-5 diagnostic criteria.
    - C. The individual refuses to disclose information necessary for diagnosis.
    - D. A comorbid condition prevents accurate classification of symptoms.
4. Which of the following features is most commonly associated with disorders in this category?
    - A. Pervasive fear of abandonment.
    - B. Difficulty regulating emotions and impulsive behaviors.
    - C. Persistent cognitive deficits.
    - D. Recurrent hallucinations or delusions.
5. Which intervention is considered the most appropriate first-line treatment for disorders in this category?
    - A. Long-term psychodynamic therapy.
    - B. Cognitive-behavioral therapy with a focus on emotion regulation.
    - C. Pharmacological treatment with antipsychotics.
    - D. Incarceration or residential care.
6. Which of the following risk factors increases the likelihood of developing a Specified or Unspecified Disruptive, Impulse-Control, and Conduct Disorder?
    - A. Living in a high socioeconomic status environment.
    - B. History of trauma or inconsistent parental discipline.
    - C. Presence of a neurodevelopmental disorder such as Autism Spectrum Disorder.
    - D. Lack of exposure to peer interactions during childhood.
7. Which of the following comorbidities is most commonly associated with these disorders?
    - A. Substance use disorders.
    - B. Post-traumatic stress disorder.
    - C. Specific phobia.
    - D. Schizophrenia.

True/False Questions

		T	F
1	The category "Other Disruptive, Impulse-Control, and Conduct Disorders" only includes behaviors not fitting other specific diagnoses.		
2	Symptoms may result from a general medical condition if they show uncontrollable impulses.		
3	For this diagnosis, the DSM-5 requires symptoms to cause significant distress in at least two settings.		
4	Planned aggressive behaviors cannot be included in this category.		
5	The category may include traits similar to those of personality disorders like borderline.		
6	A history of disruptive behaviors since childhood is necessary for this diagnosis.		
7	All symptoms must be present for at least six months to qualify for this category.		
8	These disorders can be diagnosed even with a major neurocognitive disorder.		
9	The category includes outbursts that don't meet criteria for Intermittent Explosive Disorder.		
10	Substance abuse is often associated with these diagnoses, per the DSM-5.		

Matching Exercise

1. Impulsive aggression not meeting frequency criteria for Intermittent Explosive Disorder. [ ]
2. Symptoms of disruptive behavior not fully meeting any DSM-5 criteria. [ ]
3. Emotional dysregulation and impulsivity as core features. [ ]
4. Cognitive-behavioral therapy as a treatment approach. [ ]
5. History of trauma or inconsistent parental discipline as a risk factor. [ ]
6. Significant impairment in social or occupational functioning. [ ]

Descriptions:

- A. A defining characteristic of the disorders in this category.
- B. Environmental influence increasing risk.
- C. Evidence-based therapeutic intervention.
- D. Impulsive behaviors outside specific diagnostic thresholds.
- E. Impairment caused by disruptive behaviors.
- F. Appropriate diagnosis when criteria for specific disorders are not fully met.

Case Study

Jacob, a 14-year-old boy, has a history of aggressive outbursts, including yelling and throwing objects, but the frequency and severity of these behaviors do not meet the diagnostic criteria for Intermittent Explosive Disorder. His teachers describe him as impulsive and easily frustrated, and his parents report inconsistent discipline at home. Jacob struggles with maintaining friendships and is frequently suspended from school for disruptive behavior. Despite this, he does not meet full criteria for any specific disruptive or conduct disorder.

1. Which feature most strongly supports a diagnosis of a Specified or Unspecified Disruptive, Impulse-Control, and Conduct Disorder in Jacob's case?
   - A. His inability to maintain friendships.
   - B. His aggressive outbursts that fall below the threshold for other disorders.
   - C. His history of inconsistent discipline.
   - D. His difficulty in school performance.
2. Which of the following interventions would be most appropriate for Jacob?
   - A. Long-term incarceration in a juvenile facility.
   - B. Cognitive-behavioral therapy focusing on emotion regulation.
   - C. Antipsychotic medication to control aggression.
   - D. Psychoanalysis to explore childhood trauma.
3. Which differential diagnosis should be ruled out before diagnosing Jacob?
   - A. Obsessive-Compulsive Disorder.
   - B. Generalized Anxiety Disorder.
   - C. Intermittent Explosive Disorder.
   - D. Specific Phobia.

Answers

Multiple Choice Questions:

1. C
2. B
3. B
4. B
5. B
6. B
7. A

True/False Questions:

1. True
2. False
3. False
4. True
5. True
6. False
7. False
8. True
9. True
10. True

Matching Exercise:

1. D
2. F
3. A
4. C
5. B
6. E

Case Study Answers and Explanations:

1. B - Explanation: Aggressive outbursts that do not meet criteria for other disorders align with this diagnosis.
2. B - Explanation: CBT focusing on emotion regulation is an effective and evidence-based intervention.
3. C - Explanation: Intermittent Explosive Disorder must be ruled out due to similar behavioral patterns.

Substance-Related and Addictive Disorders

This category covers all conditions where the use of alcohol, drugs, or other substances becomes problematic, impairing personal, social, or occupational functioning. Alongside Substance Use Disorders—which involve regular, uncontrolled use (leading to tolerance, withdrawal, and inability to cut back despite physical or psychological harm)—the DSM-5-TR also includes Substance-Induced Disorders, which occur during or after substance ingestion (for example, intoxication or withdrawal).

A variety of substances are addressed, from alcohol and opioids to cannabis and sedatives, hypnotics, or anxiolytics, as well as stimulants like cocaine or amphetamines, and emerging "designer drugs." Each substance may yield a distinct set of symptoms, yet they often share features such as loss of control over quantity or frequency of use, a strong craving, a reduction in other activities (work, relationships, leisure), and continued use despite negative outcomes.

Another crucial element is the psychological and/or physical dependence involved. Tolerance means higher amounts of the substance are needed to achieve the same effect, while withdrawal causes a range of physical or psychological symptoms (agitation, tremors, anxiety, pain) once usage is cut back or stopped. In more severe scenarios—chronic alcohol abuse, for instance—withdrawal can lead to life-threatening complications (such as delirium tremens).

In addition to substance-related problems, the DSM-5-TR also includes Gambling Disorder, recognizing that betting can trigger responses similar to those seen in alcohol or drug misuse. Individuals may chase losses, wagering increasing sums of money, and find it very difficult to quit despite serious financial or relational consequences.

Diagnosis considers the severity of the problem (mild, moderate, or severe), based on the number of criteria met. Clinicians examine how frequently and how much the person uses the substance, as well as how deeply this behavior disrupts the individual's life. They must also check for any comorbid psychiatric conditions—such as depression or personality disorders—since complications or relapses are more likely when multiple issues overlap.

Treatment often involves individual or group psychotherapy, detoxification, or rehabilitation in specialized settings, possibly including medication (for example, opioid agonists or anticraving drugs for alcohol). Family involvement and participation in support groups, such as Alcoholics Anonymous or Narcotics Anonymous, frequently play a major part in recovery.

Prevention is also a significant factor, relying on awareness campaigns and early interventions for young people or those facing vulnerability (economic hardship, a family history of substance-related disorders). Limiting easy access to substances, promoting healthier lifestyles, and ensuring the availability of support services are all measures that can help reduce the prevalence of these disorders and support positive change.

Alcohol-Related Disorders

Multiple Choice Questions

1. Which of the following is a diagnostic criterion for Alcohol Use Disorder?
    - A. Alcohol consumption limited to social occasions.
    - B. A persistent desire or unsuccessful efforts to cut down or control alcohol use.
    - C. Alcohol consumption exclusively during stressful events.
    - D. Physical symptoms limited to mild headaches after drinking.
2. Tolerance in Alcohol Use Disorder is defined as:
    - A. Drinking alcohol in social settings.
    - B. A need for markedly increased amounts of alcohol to achieve the desired effect.
    - C. Avoiding withdrawal symptoms by not drinking alcohol.
    - D. Developing severe allergic reactions to alcohol.
3. Which of the following symptoms is characteristic of alcohol withdrawal?
    - A. Persistent euphoria.
    - B. Hallucinations, tremors, and autonomic hyperactivity.
    - C. Sudden improvement in cognitive function.
    - D. Excessive need for sleep.
4. Alcohol-Induced Major Neurocognitive Disorder is most commonly associated with:
    - A. Liver dysfunction.
    - B. Vitamin B1 (thiamine) deficiency.
    - C. Dehydration after prolonged alcohol use.
    - D. Increased dopamine levels.
5. Which of the following is a key feature of alcohol intoxication?
    - A. Hyperactivity and excessive speech.
    - B. Slurred speech, incoordination, and impaired memory or attention.
    - C. Significant weight loss.
    - D. Increased sensitivity to sound and light.
6. Which of the following treatments is commonly used to manage alcohol withdrawal symptoms?
    - A. Antipsychotic medications.
    - B. Benzodiazepines to reduce the risk of seizures.
    - C. Stimulants to counteract fatigue.
    - D. Beta-blockers for anxiety management.
7. What is the most effective long-term treatment for Alcohol Use Disorder?
    - A. Acute medical detoxification alone.
    - B. Long-term inpatient psychiatric care.
    - C. A combination of psychotherapy and pharmacological interventions.
    - D. Avoidance of social situations involving alcohol.

True/False Questions

		T	F
1	The DSM-5 no longer distinguishes between "alcohol abuse" and "alcohol dependence," but instead uses the term "Alcohol Use Disorder" with an additional severity specifier.		
2	According to DSM-5 criteria, alcohol withdrawal cannot include tactile hallucinations.		
3	Craving was introduced as an additional diagnostic criterion for Alcohol Use Disorder in the DSM-5.		
4	The DSM-5 requires that, to diagnose Alcohol Use Disorder, the patient must never have experienced severe intoxication.		
5	Severe alcohol intoxication may include perceptual disturbances or transient psychotic symptoms.		
6	The DSM-5 defines Alcohol Use Disorder as pathological exclusively when tolerance and withdrawal are present.		
7	It is possible to diagnose Alcohol Use Disorder even when binge drinking occurs intermittently, if functional impairment criteria are met.		
8	In the DSM-5, there is no way to specify whether Alcohol Use Disorder is mild, moderate, or severe.		
9	During sustained remission (at least 12 months of abstinence), partially meeting diagnostic criteria is not allowed, even if there is a significant reduction in drinking frequency.		
10	In manuals prior to the DSM-5, "abuse" and "dependence" were separate diagnoses, whereas they are now combined into a single Alcohol Use Disorder diagnosis with varying levels of severity.		

Matching Exercise

1. Recurrent alcohol use despite negative consequences. [ ]
2. Increased need for alcohol to achieve intoxication. [ ]
3. Tremors, hallucinations, and autonomic hyperactivity. [ ]
4. Slurred speech and impaired motor coordination. [ ]
5. Vitamin deficiency leading to cognitive impairment. [ ]
6. Combination of therapy and medication for treatment. [ ]

Descriptions:

- A. A hallmark symptom of alcohol withdrawal.
- B. Alcohol intoxication-related impairments.
- C. A long-term treatment approach.
- D. A defining feature of Alcohol Use Disorder.
- E. Tolerance as part of diagnostic criteria.
- F. Thiamine deficiency causing Wernicke-Korsakoff Syndrome.

Case Study

Michael, a 45-year-old male, reports drinking 6–8 beers daily for the past five years. He has tried to reduce his drinking multiple times but finds it difficult to stop. Recently, he has been experiencing tremors and sweating in the mornings, which subside after consuming alcohol. Michael's partner has expressed concerns about his behavior, including missing work and forgetting important commitments. Despite these consequences, Michael continues to drink. He denies any current hallucinations but admits to occasional confusion during the day.

1. Which feature most strongly supports a diagnosis of Alcohol Use Disorder in Michael's case?
    - A. His inability to stop drinking despite efforts.
    - B. The specific type of alcohol he consumes.
    - C. His denial of hallucinations.
    - D. His confusion during the day.
2. Which of the following treatments would be most appropriate for Michael's withdrawal symptoms?
    - A. Antidepressants to improve his mood.
    - B. Benzodiazepines to prevent seizures and manage symptoms.
    - C. Antipsychotics to control confusion.
    - D. Stimulants to improve his focus.
3. What long-term treatment plan would be most appropriate for Michael?
    - A. Detoxification alone to manage his symptoms.
    - B. Cognitive-behavioral therapy and medications like naltrexone.
    - C. Long-term isolation from alcohol-related environments.
    - D. Surgery to repair alcohol-induced damage.

Answers

Multiple Choice Questions:

1. B
2. B
3. B
4. B
5. B
6. B
7. C

True/False Questions:

1. True
2. False
3. True
4. False
5. True
6. False
7. True
8. False
9. False
10. True

Matching Exercise:

1. D
2. E
3. A
4. B
5. F
6. C

Case Study Answers and Explanations:

1. A - Explanation: Michael's repeated inability to stop drinking despite efforts and negative consequences is a key feature of Alcohol Use Disorder.
2. B - Explanation: Benzodiazepines are the first-line treatment for managing alcohol withdrawal symptoms and preventing complications like seizures.
3. B - Explanation: Cognitive-behavioral therapy combined with medications like naltrexone is effective for long-term treatment of Alcohol Use Disorder.

Caffeine-Related Disorders

Multiple Choice Questions

1. Which of the following is a diagnostic criterion for Caffeine Intoxication?
    - A. Persistent fatigue and drowsiness.
    - B. Recent consumption of caffeine and five or more associated symptoms such as restlessness or tachycardia.
    - C. Hallucinations and delusions.
    - D. Symptoms occurring exclusively during alcohol withdrawal.
2. Which of the following symptoms is most commonly associated with Caffeine Withdrawal?
    - A. Increased heart rate and euphoria.
    - B. Headache, fatigue, and depressed mood.
    - C. Hallucinations and hyperactivity.
    - D. Elevated blood pressure and aggression.
3. Caffeine Use Disorder is:
    - A. Not formally recognized as a diagnosis in the DSM-5 but can be clinically significant.
    - B. Defined as the excessive use of caffeine to the point of causing psychosis.
    - C. Diagnosed when caffeine use interferes with occupational or social functioning for more than a year.
    - D. A common comorbidity in psychotic disorders.
4. Which of the following doses of caffeine is most likely to cause symptoms of intoxication in a non-tolerant adult?
    - A. 50 mg.
    - B. 100 mg.
    - C. 250 mg or more.
    - D. 500 mg only.
5. Which of the following treatment strategies is recommended for managing Caffeine Withdrawal?
    - A. Gradual reduction of caffeine intake.
    - B. Immediate cessation of caffeine use without substitution.
    - C. Administration of benzodiazepines to manage anxiety.
    - D. Increased physical activity to combat fatigue.
6. What is the primary mechanism of action of caffeine in the brain?
    - A. Inhibition of serotonin reuptake.
    - B. Blocking adenosine receptors, leading to increased arousal.
    - C. Enhancing dopamine synthesis.
    - D. Increasing GABAergic activity.
7. Which of the following symptoms is NOT commonly associated with excessive caffeine consumption?
    - A. Restlessness.
    - B. Insomnia.
    - C. Bradycardia.
    - D. Gastrointestinal upset.

True/False Questions

		T	F
1	The DSM-5 includes Caffeine Use Disorder as an official diagnosis with fully validated criteria.		
2	Caffeine is listed in the DSM-5 among the substances that can cause intoxication and withdrawal.		
3	Headache is one of the most common symptoms of caffeine withdrawal, according to the DSM-5.		
4	A single intake of 100 mg of caffeine already fulfills the diagnostic requirement for caffeine intoxication, regardless of individual tolerance.		
5	The DSM-5 formally recognizes caffeine withdrawal as a distinct diagnostic category.		
6	For caffeine withdrawal, according to the DSM-5, the presence of two symptoms among fatigue, headache, difficulty concentrating, and irritability is sufficient.		
7	High caffeine consumption can contribute to the diagnosis of Substance-Induced Insomnia if the criteria for a primary sleep disorder are not met.		
8	According to the DSM-5, excessive caffeine intake does not affect the severity of a pre-existing Anxiety Disorder.		
9	The presence of cardiac conditions is not considered in the evaluation of possible caffeine intoxication.		
10	Caffeine Use Disorder is listed in Section III of the DSM-5 as a condition requiring further research, but it does not have fully approved diagnostic criteria.		

Matching Exercise

1. Consumption of over 250 mg of caffeine leading to restlessness and tachycardia. [ ]
2. Symptoms such as headache, and depressed mood after cessation of caffeine use. [ ]
3. Blocking adenosine receptors in the brain, leading to increased arousal. [ ]
4. The most widely consumed psychoactive substance globally. [ ]
5. Gradual reduction in consumption as a treatment strategy. [ ]
6. Insomnia, nervousness, and psychomotor agitation. [ ]

Descriptions:

- A. Primary mechanism of action of caffeine.
- B. A common feature of Caffeine Intoxication.
- C. A key feature of Caffeine Withdrawal.
- D. A safe and effective approach to manage withdrawal symptoms.
- E. A defining characteristic of caffeine as a substance.
- F. A diagnostic criterion for Caffeine Intoxication.

Case Study

Lily, a 28-year-old woman, reports experiencing headaches, fatigue, and a depressed mood every time she stops drinking coffee. She typically consumes 6–7 cups of coffee daily but has been trying to cut back. When she doesn't drink coffee, Lily finds it hard to concentrate at work and feels irritable. She denies any other substance use or significant medical issues.

1. Which feature most strongly supports a diagnosis of Caffeine Withdrawal in Lily's case?
   - A. Her irritability and difficulty concentrating.
   - B. Her consumption of 6–7 cups of coffee daily.
   - C. The presence of headaches and fatigue when she stops drinking coffee.
   - D. Her lack of medical issues or other substance use.
2. What would be the most appropriate recommendation to help Lily manage her symptoms?
   - A. Immediate cessation of caffeine intake.
   - B. Gradual reduction in caffeine consumption over time.
   - C. Substituting caffeine with an alternative stimulant.
   - D. Taking antidepressant medication to improve her mood.
3. Which of the following differential diagnoses should be considered in Lily's case?
   - A. Generalized Anxiety Disorder.
   - B. Obsessive-Compulsive Disorder.
   - C. Major Depressive Disorder.
   - D. None, as her symptoms align clearly with Caffeine Withdrawal.

Answers

Multiple Choice Questions:
1. B
2. B
3. A
4. C
5. A
6. B
7. C

True/False Questions:
1. False
2. True
3. True
4. False
5. True
6. False
7. True
8. False
9. False
10. True

Matching Exercise:
1. F
2. C
3. A
4. E
5. D
6. B

Case Study Answers and Explanations:
1. C - Explanation: The presence of headaches and fatigue upon cessation of caffeine is a hallmark feature of Caffeine Withdrawal.
2. B - Explanation: Gradual reduction in caffeine intake is the recommended approach to minimize withdrawal symptoms.
3. D - Explanation: Her symptoms are classic for Caffeine Withdrawal, and no other differential diagnosis is necessary.

Cannabis-Related Disorders

Multiple Choice Questions

1. Which of the following is a diagnostic criterion for Cannabis Use Disorder?
    - A. Continued use of cannabis despite persistent social or interpersonal problems caused by its effects.
    - B. Infrequent cannabis use limited to medical purposes.
    - C. Temporary cravings for cannabis without recurrent use.
    - D. Exclusive use of cannabis during episodes of depression.
2. Cannabis Intoxication is characterized by:
    - A. Increased energy and hyperactivity.
    - B. Impaired motor coordination, euphoria, and anxiety.
    - C. Severe withdrawal symptoms after a single use.
    - D. Persistent auditory hallucinations.
3. Which of the following symptoms is most commonly associated with Cannabis Withdrawal?
    - A. Excessive sweating and seizures.
    - B. Irritability, sleep disturbances, and decreased appetite.
    - C. Psychosis and agitation.
    - D. Chronic fatigue and hypersomnia.
4. Which of the following medical conditions is Cannabis-Induced Psychosis most likely associated with?
    - A. Persistent depression due to substance abuse.
    - B. Acute intoxication in individuals predisposed to psychosis.
    - C. Long-term cannabis use without intoxication.
    - D. Minor withdrawal symptoms in healthy individuals.
5. Which of the following is a primary feature of Cannabis Hyperemesis Syndrome?
    - A. Cyclical vomiting relieved by hot showers or baths.
    - B. Persistent nausea relieved only by cessation of cannabis use.
    - C. Weight loss due to prolonged cannabis withdrawal.
    - D. Severe dehydration following a single use of cannabis.
6. Which neurotransmitter system is most directly affected by cannabis use?
    - A. Dopamine.
    - B. Serotonin.
    - C. Endocannabinoid.
    - D. Glutamate.
7. What is the most effective approach for managing Cannabis Use Disorder?
    - A. Gradual tapering of cannabis use.
    - B. Cognitive-behavioral therapy and motivational interviewing.
    - C. Pharmacological interventions with antipsychotics.
    - D. Electroconvulsive therapy.

True/False Questions

		T	F
1	According to the DSM-5-TR, a minimum duration of two consecutive days of symptoms is required to diagnose cannabis withdrawal.		
2	Significant changes in heart rate and blood pressure can occur during cannabis intoxication.		
3	The DSM-5-TR provides specific criteria to differentiate a primary psychotic episode from a cannabis-induced psychotic disorder, partly based on the absence of symptoms outside of substance use.		
4	Irritability is the sole manifestation required to meet the DSM-5-TR criteria for cannabis withdrawal.		
5	Cannabis use does not meet the criteria for a Sedative Use Disorder, even though some compounds have relaxing effects.		
6	The severity levels of Cannabis Use Disorder are determined by the number of criteria met, in a manner similar to other substance use disorders.		
7	The DSM-5-TR uses the same ICD-10-CM coding for Cannabis Use Disorder that was present in the DSM-IV, with no significant modifications.		
8	The DSM-5-TR equates some liver-related complications from cannabis use with those commonly seen in Alcohol Use Disorder, specifying similar criteria for hepatic damage.		
9	To define early remission of Cannabis Use Disorder, the DSM-5-TR specifies a period of at least three months (but less than 12) with no diagnostic criteria met, aside from craving.		
10	The DSM-5-TR officially includes "cannabis-induced sleep disorder" as a standalone category, separate from other sleep disturbances associated with substance use.		

Matching Exercise

1. Continued use despite social or interpersonal problems. [ ]
2. Impaired motor coordination and anxiety. [ ]
3. Cyclical vomiting relieved by hot showers. [ ]
4. Irritability and decreased appetite after cessation. [ ]
5. Endocannabinoid system's role in cannabis effects. [ ]
6. Cognitive-behavioral therapy as a treatment approach. [ ]

Descriptions:

- A. Cannabis Hyperemesis Syndrome.
- B. Cannabis Use Disorder.
- C. Common symptoms of Cannabis Withdrawal.
- D. System affected by cannabis.
- E. Intoxication symptoms.
- F. Evidence-based intervention for managing use.

Case Study

Alex, a 25-year-old male, has been using cannabis daily for the past three years. Recently, he has started experiencing difficulty sleeping, irritability, and decreased appetite when he tries to stop. He also reports that his cannabis use has caused arguments with his family and negatively impacted his work performance. Despite these issues, Alex continues to use cannabis, feeling unable to stop.

1. Which feature most strongly supports a diagnosis of Cannabis Use Disorder in Alex's case?
   - A. His daily cannabis use for three years.
   - B. The conflicts with his family caused by cannabis use.
   - C. His inability to stop using despite negative consequences.
   - D. The decreased appetite he experiences when he stops using cannabis.
2. What is the most appropriate first-line treatment for Alex's condition?
   - A. Immediate detoxification in a medical setting.
   - B. Cognitive-behavioral therapy and motivational interviewing.
   - C. Pharmacological treatment with antipsychotic medication.
   - D. Substitution of cannabis with a less harmful substance.
3. Which differential diagnosis should be ruled out in Alex's case?
   - A. Generalized Anxiety Disorder.
   - B. Cannabis-Induced Psychosis.
   - C. Cannabis Hyperemesis Syndrome.
   - D. Substance-Induced Mood Disorder.

Answers

Multiple Choice Questions:

1. A
2. B
3. B
4. B
5. A
6. C
7. B

True/False Answers

1. False
2. True
3. True
4. False
5. True
6. True
7. False
8. False
9. True
10. False

Matching Exercise:

1. B
2. E
3. A
4. C
5. D
6. F

Case Study Answers and Explanations:

1. C - Explanation: Continued use despite negative consequences is a key feature of Cannabis Use Disorder.
2. B - Explanation: Cognitive-behavioral therapy and motivational interviewing are effective evidence-based treatments.
3. D - Explanation: Substance-Induced Mood Disorder should be ruled out, as it can present with overlapping symptoms.

Hallucinogen-Related Disorders

Multiple Choice Questions

1. Which of the following is a key feature of Hallucinogen Persisting Perception Disorder (HPPD)?
    - A. Flashbacks involving re-experiencing previous perceptual distortions long after substance use.
    - B. Continuous hallucinations only during periods of active substance use.
    - C. Delusions and auditory hallucinations occurring with polysubstance abuse.
    - D. Persistent euphoria and heightened sensory perception.
2. Lysergic acid diethylamide (LSD) intoxication is most commonly associated with:
    - A. Auditory hallucinations and paranoia.
    - B. Visual distortions, altered time perception, and synesthesia.
    - C. Severe depressive episodes and loss of motor coordination.
    - D. Tremors, hyperactivity, and gastrointestinal upset.
3. Which of the following is a distinguishing feature of Phencyclidine (PCP) intoxication?
    - A. Marked aggression, dissociation, and nystagmus.
    - B. Heightened tactile sensitivity and paranoia.
    - C. Rapid speech and persistent fear of dying.
    - D. Extreme sedation and respiratory depression.
4. Hallucinogen Use Disorder is diagnosed when:
    - A. The individual uses hallucinogens daily for at least 12 months.
    - B. The use of hallucinogens causes significant impairment in social or occupational functioning.
    - C. The individual experiences withdrawal symptoms upon cessation of hallucinogen use.
    - D. Hallucinogens are used in combination with stimulants.
5. Which neurotransmitter system is primarily affected by classic hallucinogens like LSD?
    - A. Dopaminergic.
    - B. Serotonergic.
    - C. Glutamatergic.
    - D. GABAergic.
6. Which of the following conditions should be considered as a differential diagnosis for Hallucinogen Persisting Perception Disorder (HPPD)?
    - A. Generalized Anxiety Disorder.
    - B. Temporal Lobe Epilepsy.
    - C. Borderline Personality Disorder.
    - D. Post-Traumatic Stress Disorder.
7. Which of the following is an evidence-based treatment for managing Hallucinogen Persisting Perception Disorder?
    - A. High-dose benzodiazepines.
    - B. Antipsychotics and mood stabilizers.
    - C. Cognitive-behavioral therapy and symptomatic pharmacotherapy.
    - D. Detoxification and abstinence without further intervention.

True/False Questions

		T	F
1	The DSM-5-TR recognizes a pronounced withdrawal syndrome with physical symptoms for classic hallucinogens (e.g., LSD, psilocybin), comparable to that of opioids.		
2	Disorders related to PCP are often addressed separately from classic hallucinogens in the DSM-5-TR, due to its dissociative properties and potential psychomotor symptoms.		
3	Hallucinogen Persisting Perception Disorder (HPPD) requires continued use of hallucinogens in order for symptoms to persist without significant breaks.		
4	The DSM-5-TR includes altered time perception and visual distortions among the criteria for hallucinogen intoxication.		
5	One criterion for Hallucinogen Use Disorder is the inability to cut down or control use, similar to other substance use disorders.		
6	In the DSM-5-TR, a diagnosis of Hallucinogen Use Disorder mandates the presence of persistent daily craving.		
7	The DSM-5-TR provides different codes for early remission and sustained remission for Hallucinogen Use Disorder.		
8	Tactile hallucinations alone are sufficient to diagnose a Hallucinogen-Induced Psychotic Disorder, regardless of other changes or contextual factors.		
9	The DSM-5-TR clarifies that some intoxication symptoms, such as paranoid ideation or persecutory delusions, can be more common with dissociative hallucinogens like PCP.		
10	The term "Flashback" officially replaces the Hallucinogen Persisting Perception Disorder definition in the DSM-5-TR, as it is considered more precise.		

Matching Exercise

1. Re-experiencing perceptual distortions long after substance use. [ ]
2. Visual distortions and altered perception of time. [ ]
3. Dissociation and aggression during intoxication. [ ]
4. Significant social or occupational impairment due to hallucinogen use. [ ]
5. Synesthesia and heightened sensory experiences. [ ]
6. Cognitive-behavioral therapy for persistent perceptual disturbances. [ ]

Descriptions:

- A. Hallucinogen Persisting Perception Disorder (HPPD).
- B. LSD intoxication.
- C. PCP intoxication.
- D. Hallucinogen Use Disorder.
- E. Symptom of classic hallucinogen intoxication.
- F. Evidence-based treatment for perceptual disturbances.

Case Study

Daniel, a 29-year-old man, reports experiencing visual distortions and heightened colors for several months after using LSD. He describes these episodes as occurring randomly and interfering with his ability to concentrate at work. Daniel denies current drug use but feels anxious and worried about these "flashbacks." He also reports mild sleep disturbances and has difficulty focusing on his daily activities.

1. Which feature most strongly supports a diagnosis of Hallucinogen Persisting Perception Disorder (HPPD) in Daniel's case?
    - A. His history of LSD use.
    - B. His visual distortions and random "flashbacks."
    - C. His sleep disturbances.
    - D. His anxiety about the episodes.
2. What would be the most appropriate intervention for Daniel?
    - A. High-dose antipsychotic medication.
    - B. Cognitive-behavioral therapy and symptomatic pharmacotherapy.
    - C. Immediate detoxification in a medical setting.
    - D. Psychodynamic therapy focused on his substance use history.
3. Which differential diagnosis should be ruled out in Daniel's case?
    - A. Bipolar Disorder.
    - B. Temporal Lobe Epilepsy.
    - C. Obsessive-Compulsive Disorder.
    - D. Post-Traumatic Stress Disorder.

Answers

Multiple Choice Questions:
1. A
2. B
3. A
4. B
5. B
6. B
7. C

True/False Questions:
1. False
2. True
3. False
4. True
5. True
6. False
7. True
8. False
9. True
10. False

Matching Exercise:
1. A
2. B
3. C
4. D
5. E
6. F

Case Study Answers and Explanations:
1. B - Explanation: Random "flashbacks" involving perceptual distortions are a hallmark feature of HPPD.
2. B - Explanation: Cognitive-behavioral therapy and pharmacotherapy can address both the perceptual disturbances and associated anxiety.
3. B - Explanation: Temporal Lobe Epilepsy can present with visual distortions and must be ruled out before diagnosing HPPD.

Inhalant-Related Disorders

Multiple Choice Questions

1. A 15-year-old boy presents with slurred speech, unsteady gait, and euphoria after being found in a garage. Which of the following substances is most likely responsible for his symptoms?
    - A. Lysergic acid diethylamide (LSD).
    - B. Toluene, a common solvent in paint thinners.
    - C. Cocaine.
    - D. Methamphetamine.
2. Inhalant Use Disorder is most accurately diagnosed when:
    - A. The individual uses inhalants exclusively for recreational purposes.
    - B. Repeated use of inhalants leads to significant impairment or distress in multiple domains of functioning.
    - C. Withdrawal symptoms are present after cessation of inhalant use.
    - D. The individual reports a single episode of intoxication.
3. Which of the following neurological complications is commonly associated with chronic inhalant use?
    - A. Permanent cerebellar damage causing ataxia.
    - B. Increased seizure threshold due to CNS excitation.
    - C. Development of auditory hallucinations.
    - D. Long-term improvement in memory and executive functioning.
4. Inhalant intoxication can mimic which of the following medical conditions?
    - A. Alcohol intoxication.
    - B. Schizophrenia.
    - C. Parkinson's disease.
    - D. Hypothyroidism.
5. Which of the following is a key difference between Inhalant Intoxication and Hallucinogen Intoxication?
    - A. Inhalant intoxication rarely affects motor coordination.
    - B. Inhalant intoxication includes signs such as dizziness and slurred speech, while hallucinogens primarily alter perception and cognition.
    - C. Hallucinogens typically result in respiratory depression, while inhalants do not.
    - D. Hallucinogens lead to long-term cognitive deficits, while inhalants do not.
6. Which cardiac complication is most closely associated with inhalant intoxication?
    - A. Bradycardia due to central nervous system suppression.
    - B. Arrhythmias, commonly referred to as "sudden sniffing death syndrome."
    - C. Acute myocardial infarction due to vasospasm.
    - D. Pulmonary hypertension.
7. Inhalant intoxication typically causes which of the following effects?
    - A. Hyperactivity and increased focus.
    - B. Sedation and slowed speech.
    - C. Euphoria, dizziness, and impaired judgment.
    - D. Increased appetite and improved concentration.

True/False Questions

		T	F
1	According to the DSM-5-TR, an Inhalant Use Disorder can be diagnosed even without regular use, provided there is significant harm and impairment in functioning.		
2	Chronic inhalant use can lead to peripheral neuropathy.		
3	Inhalant intoxication may present with signs similar to alcohol intoxication, such as slurred speech and ataxia.		
4	The DSM-5-TR excludes craving for inhalants as a criterion for Inhalant Use Disorder.		
5	Compared to the DSM-IV, the DSM-5-TR changed the criteria for Inhalant Use Disorder by removing specific subtypes based on the type of solvent used.		
6	Prolonged inhalation of volatile solvents can result in permanent liver and kidney damage.		
7	Aerosol sprays, paint, and spray deodorants are categorized as inhalants in the DSM-5-TR when misused.		
8	Excessive inhalant use does not lead to long-lasting cognitive deficits if discontinued before adulthood.		
9	The DSM-5-TR acknowledges the possibility of an Inhalant-Induced Psychotic Disorder, although it is considered rare, particularly when delusions or strong paranoid ideation are present.		
10	A clearly defined inhalant withdrawal syndrome with its own diagnostic code is described in the DSM-5-TR.		

Matching Exercise

1. Dizziness, slurred speech, and unsteady gait. [ ]
2. Chronic use associated with cerebellar degeneration. [ ]
3. Sudden cardiac arrhythmia caused by inhalants. [ ]
4. Impulsive behaviors during episodes of intoxication. [ ]
5. Socioeconomic factors increasing risk of use. [ ]
6. Cognitive-behavioral therapy as an intervention. [ ]

Descriptions:

- A. Symptom of inhalant intoxication.
- B. Commonly associated with "sudden sniffing death syndrome."
- C. Behavioral response linked to acute intoxication.
- D. Long-term neurological consequence of chronic use.
- E. A contributing factor to inhalant use in vulnerable populations.
- F. Evidence-based treatment for reducing inhalant use.

Case Study

Lisa, a 17-year-old girl, presents with tremors, dizziness, and complaints of weakness. Her mother reports finding multiple empty cans of aerosol spray in her room. Lisa admits to inhaling the substance several times a week for the past year. She describes feeling "high" and disconnected after each use. Recently, Lisa has been struggling with memory issues and coordination, which have affected her school performance.

1. Which symptom in Lisa's case is most consistent with chronic inhalant use?
   - A. Dizziness and weakness.
   - B. Complaints of "feeling high."
   - C. Memory issues and coordination problems.
   - D. Her frequency of use over the past year.
2. Which of the following complications is Lisa at risk for if she continues inhalant use?
   - A. Chronic obstructive pulmonary disease (COPD).
   - B. Cerebellar degeneration and irreversible neurological damage.
   - C. Increased susceptibility to mood disorders.
   - D. Development of acute psychosis.
3. Which intervention would be most appropriate as a first step in Lisa's treatment plan?
   - A. Long-term residential treatment.
   - B. Immediate medical detoxification.
   - C. Cognitive-behavioral therapy focused on impulse control and decision-making.
   - D. Prescription of benzodiazepines to manage withdrawal.

Answers

Multiple Choice Questions:

1. B
2. B
3. A
4. A
5. B
6. B
7. C

True/False Questions:

1. False
2. True
3. True
4. False
5. False
6. True
7. True
8. False
9. True
10. False

Matching Exercise:

1. A
2. D
3. B
4. C
5. E
6. F

Case Study Answers and Explanations:

1. C - Explanation: Memory issues and coordination problems are hallmarks of chronic inhalant use.
2. B - Explanation: Chronic inhalant use can lead to permanent cerebellar damage and other neurological complications.
3. C - Explanation: Cognitive-behavioral therapy is a well-established intervention for addressing the behavioral and psychological aspects of inhalant use.

Opioid-Related Disorders

Multiple Choice Questions

1. A 34-year-old man is brought to the emergency room after being found unresponsive. Physical exam reveals pinpoint pupils, bradypnea, and cyanosis. Which of the following is the most appropriate initial intervention?
    - A. Administer naloxone.
    - B. Initiate CPR.
    - C. Perform a CT scan of the head.
    - D. Provide high-dose benzodiazepines.
2. A 26-year-old woman reports using increasing amounts of heroin over the past year to achieve the same "high." Which of the following best explains this phenomenon?
    - A. Tolerance.
    - B. Dependence.
    - C. Withdrawal.
    - D. Reinforcement.
3. Which of the following symptoms is least characteristic of opioid withdrawal?
    - A. Rhinorrhea and lacrimation.
    - B. Mydriasis.
    - C. Diarrhea and abdominal cramping.
    - D. Respiratory depression.
4. Which of the following is a distinguishing feature of opioid intoxication compared to alcohol intoxication?
    - A. Slurred speech.
    - B. Impaired coordination.
    - C. Miosis.
    - D. Aggression.
5. A patient with a history of opioid use disorder is started on methadone therapy. What is the primary rationale for this treatment?
    - A. Methadone eliminates withdrawal symptoms and cravings.
    - B. Methadone blocks opioid receptors, preventing intoxication.
    - C. Methadone accelerates detoxification.
    - D. Methadone prevents relapse by causing severe side effects when combined with opioids.
6. Which neurotransmitter system is primarily involved in the reinforcing effects of opioids?
    - A. Dopaminergic.
    - B. Serotonergic.
    - C. Glutamatergic.
    - D. GABAergic.
7. A patient who abruptly discontinues high-dose opioid use is most at risk for which life-threatening complication?
    - A. Respiratory depression.
    - B. Seizures.
    - C. Cardiac arrhythmias.
    - D. None; opioid withdrawal is typically non-life-threatening.

True/False Questions

		T	F
1	According to the DSM-5-TR, an Opioid Use Disorder can be diagnosed even in cases of therapeutic opioid use, provided that compulsive drug-seeking behaviors are present.		
2	The presence of delirium is always required to diagnose opioid intoxication in the DSM-5-TR.		
3	The DSM-5-TR uses the number of criteria met to specify the severity of Opioid Use Disorder, as it does for most Substance Use Disorders.		
4	If an individual takes a prescribed opioid according to medical instructions, without misuse or deviation, Opioid Use Disorder cannot be diagnosed, even if tolerance and withdrawal are present.		
5	Craving for opioids, first introduced in the DSM-5, remains a diagnostic criterion in the DSM-5-TR.		
6	The DSM-5-TR states that persistent hallucinations weeks after last opioid use qualify as an Opioid-Induced Psychotic Disorder.		
7	To diagnose opioid withdrawal, the DSM-5-TR requires at least three symptoms, such as tearing, insomnia, and gastrointestinal disturbances.		
8	The DSM-5-TR distinguishes between early remission and sustained remission for Opioid Use Disorder, based on how long the individual has not met diagnostic criteria (aside from craving).		
9	Sedation is not considered one of the typical signs of opioid intoxication in the DSM-5-TR.		
10	The DSM-5-TR includes Opioid-Induced Mood Disorder as a distinct diagnosis, which must be differentiated from a primary depressive episode.		

Matching Exercise

1. Pinpoint pupils, respiratory depression, and sedation. [ ]
2. Rhinorrhea, mydriasis, and muscle aches. [ ]
3. Medication combining buprenorphine and naloxone. [ ]
4. Long-acting opioid agonist used in maintenance therapy. [ ]
5. Increased dopamine release in the reward system. [ ]
6. Needle-sharing practices leading to infectious complications. [ ]

Descriptions:

- A. Features of opioid intoxication.
- B. Symptoms of opioid withdrawal.
- C. Risk factor for hepatitis C and HIV.
- D. Mechanism of opioid reinforcement.
- E. Suboxone.
- F. Methadone.

Case Study

Jason, a 29-year-old man, has been using intravenous heroin daily for three years. He seeks help at a clinic, reporting that he wants to quit but fears withdrawal symptoms. He describes past withdrawal episodes as "the worst pain ever," with diarrhea, abdominal cramping, sweating, and muscle aches. Jason also admits to sharing needles, and his recent blood tests reveal positive hepatitis C antibodies.

1. Which of the following is the most appropriate first step in Jason's treatment?
   - A. Begin methadone therapy for maintenance.
   - B. Administer naloxone to prevent further intoxication.
   - C. Prescribe benzodiazepines for symptom management.
   - D. Schedule Jason for immediate detoxification in an inpatient setting.
2. Jason expresses interest in a medication that he can take at home to manage cravings. Which of the following would be most appropriate?
   - A. Naltrexone.
   - B. Buprenorphine/naloxone (Suboxone).
   - C. High-dose methadone.
   - D. Immediate-release morphine.
3. Which complication is Jason most at risk for due to his history of intravenous drug use?
   - A. Alcohol withdrawal seizures.
   - B. Sudden sniffing death syndrome.
   - C. Infective endocarditis.
   - D. Wernicke-Korsakoff syndrome.

Answers

Multiple Choice Questions:

1. A
2. A
3. D
4. C
5. A
6. A
7. D

True/False Questions:

1. True
2. False
3. True
4. True
5. True
6. False
7. False
8. True
9. False
10. False

Matching Exercise:

1. A
2. B
3. E
4. F
5. D
6. C

Case Study Answers and Explanations:

1. A - Explanation: Methadone therapy is an evidence-based option for maintenance and withdrawal prevention.
2. B - Explanation: Suboxone is a preferred outpatient medication due to its safety and efficacy.
3. C - Explanation: Intravenous drug use increases the risk of infective endocarditis and other infections.

Sedative, Hypnotic, or Anxiolytic-Related Disorders

Multiple Choice Questions

1. A 40-year-old woman presents with confusion, slurred speech, and difficulty walking. Her history reveals prolonged use of diazepam for anxiety. Which of the following symptoms would most strongly suggest sedative intoxication?
    - A. Tachycardia.
    - B. Miosis.
    - C. Slurred speech and unsteady gait.
    - D. Mydriasis and hallucinations.
2. Which of the following is the primary mechanism of action of benzodiazepines?
    - A. Inhibition of serotonin reuptake.
    - B. Enhancement of GABA activity at GABA-A receptors.
    - C. Blocking NMDA receptors.
    - D. Dopamine receptor antagonism.
3. A 28-year-old man stops taking alprazolam abruptly after 8 months of use. Which of the following symptoms is most concerning during benzodiazepine withdrawal?
    - A. Diarrhea and abdominal cramps.
    - B. Generalized seizures.
    - C. Persistent euphoria.
    - D. Excessive appetite.
4. Which of the following distinguishes sedative intoxication from opioid intoxication?
    - A. Presence of respiratory depression.
    - B. Slurred speech and impaired coordination.
    - C. Miosis.
    - D. Lack of pinpoint pupils in sedative intoxication.
5. A patient reports using high doses of barbiturates for sleep for several years. Which of the following is a major risk associated with barbiturate withdrawal?
    - A. Psychotic symptoms.
    - B. Life-threatening seizures.
    - C. Persistent fatigue.
    - D. Chronic diarrhea.
6. Which of the following is the most effective treatment for benzodiazepine withdrawal in a clinical setting?
    - A. Immediate discontinuation of the drug.
    - B. Gradual tapering of the benzodiazepine dose.
    - C. Substitution with an opioid agonist.
    - D. High-dose antipsychotic therapy.
7. Long-term use of sedatives is most likely to lead to which cognitive complication?
    - A. Reversible short-term memory loss.
    - B. Persistent executive function impairment.
    - C. Enhanced cognitive performance during withdrawal.
    - D. Development of psychotic features.

True/False Questions

		T	F
1	In the DSM-5-TR, tolerance and withdrawal are not counted as criteria for Sedative, Hypnotic, or Anxiolytic Use Disorder if the substance is taken exactly as prescribed and no misuse is present.		
2	Sedation and psychomotor impairment are listed among the possible symptoms of sedative, hypnotic, or anxiolytic intoxication in the DSM-5-TR.		
3	According to the DSM-5-TR, a minimum of 12 continuous months of use is required before diagnosing Sedative, Hypnotic, or Anxiolytic Use Disorder.		
4	Craving for sedatives, hypnotics, or anxiolytics is explicitly included among the diagnostic criteria in the DSM-5-TR.		
5	Benzodiazepine withdrawal in the DSM-5-TR may encompass a wide range of symptoms, from mild insomnia to seizures and delirium.		
6	The DSM-5-TR does not allow for early or sustained remission of Sedative, Hypnotic, or Anxiolytic Use Disorder.		
7	In the DSM-5-TR, the effects of sedative, hypnotic, or anxiolytic overdose are never distinguished from those of opioids, as they present entirely identical symptoms.		
8	A presentation of sedative, hypnotic, or anxiolytic intoxication may include paradoxical agitation, although it is less common than sedation.		
9	Sedative-, Hypnotic-, or Anxiolytic-Induced Psychotic Disorder is considered one of the most frequent substance-induced psychoses, and the DSM-5-TR lists it among the most common diagnoses.		
10	Even in cases of improper use, the development of tolerance is not included among the diagnostic criteria for Sedative, Hypnotic, or Anxiolytic Use Disorder in the DSM-5-TR.		

Matching Exercise

1. Confusion, slurred speech, and unsteady gait. [ ]
2. Enhancement of GABA-A receptor activity. [ ]
3. Gradual tapering to prevent withdrawal seizures. [ ]
4. Flumazenil as a reversal agent. [ ]
5. Seizures and psychosis during withdrawal. [ ]
6. Cognitive-behavioral therapy for relapse prevention. [ ]

Descriptions:

- A. Key symptoms of sedative intoxication.
- B. Mechanism of action of benzodiazepines.
- C. Recommended approach to benzodiazepine withdrawal.
- D. Pharmacological treatment for benzodiazepine overdose.
- E. Severe complications of barbiturate withdrawal.
- F. Evidence-based treatment for Sedative Use Disorder.

Case Study

Laura, a 36-year-old woman, has been using lorazepam daily for 3 years to manage anxiety. She reports needing higher doses to achieve the same effect and experiences restlessness, sweating, and tremors when she skips a dose. Recently, she has been having difficulty focusing at work and has had multiple conflicts with coworkers. Laura expresses interest in discontinuing lorazepam but fears the symptoms of withdrawal.

1. Which feature most strongly supports a diagnosis of Sedative Use Disorder in Laura's case?
    - A. Her long-term use of lorazepam for anxiety.
    - B. Her need for increasing doses to achieve the same effect.
    - C. Her conflicts with coworkers.
    - D. Her fear of withdrawal symptoms.
2. Which intervention would be most appropriate to address Laura's concerns?
    - A. Gradual tapering of lorazepam under medical supervision.
    - B. Immediate discontinuation of lorazepam.
    - C. Substitution of lorazepam with an SSRI.
    - D. Long-term inpatient detoxification.
3. What is the most concerning potential complication if Laura abruptly stops taking lorazepam?
    - A. Persistent insomnia.
    - B. Generalized seizures.
    - C. Chronic fatigue.
    - D. Weight loss.

Answers

Multiple Choice Questions:
1. C
2. B
3. B
4. D
5. B
6. B
7. B

True/False Questions:
1. True
2. True
3. False
4. True
5. True
6. False
7. False
8. True
9. False
10. False

Matching Exercise:
1. A
2. B
3. C
4. D
5. E
6. F

Case Study Answers and Explanations:
1. B - Explanation: The need for increasing doses indicates tolerance, a key feature of Sedative Use Disorder.
2. A - Explanation: Gradual tapering is the safest and most effective approach to prevent withdrawal symptoms.
3. B - Explanation: Abrupt discontinuation of lorazepam can lead to life-threatening withdrawal seizures.

Stimulant-Related Disorders

Multiple Choice Questions

1. A 25-year-old man presents with restlessness, insomnia, and increased talkativeness after using a substance. On examination, his pupils are dilated, and his heart rate is elevated. Which of the following substances is most likely responsible for his symptoms?
    - A. Cocaine.
    - B. Alcohol.
    - C. Benzodiazepines.
    - D. Cannabis.
2. Which of the following is a key feature of stimulant intoxication?
    - A. Miosis and bradycardia.
    - B. Increased energy, hyperactivity, and paranoia.
    - C. Hallucinations and respiratory depression.
    - D. Hypothermia and sedation.
3. A 32-year-old woman who frequently uses methamphetamine reports extreme fatigue, depression, and anhedonia after a binge. Which of the following terms best describes her condition?
    - A. Tolerance.
    - B. Withdrawal.
    - C. Intoxication.
    - D. Dependence.
4. Chronic use of cocaine is most likely to cause which of the following complications?
    - A. Peripheral neuropathy.
    - B. Severe respiratory depression.
    - C. Nasal septum perforation.
    - D. Renal failure.
5. A 19-year-old college student uses stimulants to stay awake during exams. Which of the following symptoms would suggest stimulant use disorder rather than casual use?
    - A. Using stimulants only during finals week.
    - B. Repeated inability to stop using stimulants despite negative consequences.
    - C. Mild insomnia after using stimulants.
    - D. Experiencing euphoria during stimulant use.
6. Which neurotransmitter system is most directly affected by stimulants like cocaine and amphetamines?
    - A. Serotonergic.
    - B. Glutamatergic.
    - C. Dopaminergic.
    - D. GABAergic.
7. Which of the following is the most appropriate intervention for managing stimulant withdrawal?
    - A. Immediate detoxification with benzodiazepines.
    - B. Supportive care and management of depressive symptoms.
    - C. Substitution therapy with methadone.
    - D. Administration of flumazenil to reverse withdrawal effects.

True/False Questions

		T	F
1	Methamphetamine use can lead to psychotic symptoms that, according to the DSM-5-TR, must be distinguished from a primary psychotic episode by assessing whether symptoms persist in the absence of the substance.		
2	Craving was removed as a criterion for Stimulant Use Disorder in the transition from the DSM-5 to the DSM-5-TR.		
3	In the DSM-5-TR, stimulant intoxication (e.g., cocaine) may include impulsive behaviors and mood changes, in addition to physiological alterations such as tachycardia and hypertension.		
4	The DSM-5-TR allows for the severity of a Stimulant Use Disorder to be classified by the total number of criteria met, in a manner consistent with other Substance Use Disorders.		
5	A diagnosis of cocaine withdrawal requires the presence of pronounced psychomotor agitation, according to the DSM-5-TR.		
6	A Stimulant-Induced Psychotic Disorder can involve visual or tactile hallucinations, provided these are not attributable to an underlying medical condition.		
7	In the DSM-5-TR, using prescribed stimulant medication for ADHD is considered equivalent to a Stimulant Use Disorder if tolerance and withdrawal develop.		
8	Even without regular use, a single high-dose exposure to stimulants can, in rare instances, result in persistent symptoms that qualify as a Stimulant-Induced Psychotic Disorder.		
9	Amphetamine withdrawal is deemed potentially fatal and requires immediate medical intervention in almost all circumstances, according to the DSM-5-TR.		
10	The DSM-5-TR acknowledges the possibility of both early and sustained remission for Stimulant Use Disorder, as long as diagnostic criteria are not met (aside from craving).		

Matching Exercise

1. Dilated pupils, increased energy, and paranoia. [ ]
2. Depressive symptoms and fatigue following cessation of use. [ ]
3. Nasal septum perforation with chronic use. [ ]
4. Increased dopamine in the reward system. [ ]
5. Psychosis during chronic use. [ ]
6. Supportive care as a treatment for withdrawal. [ ]

Descriptions:

- A. Symptom of stimulant intoxication.
- B. Characteristic of stimulant withdrawal.
- C. Complication of chronic cocaine use.
- D. Mechanism of stimulant action.
- E. Long-term complication of methamphetamine use.
- F. Evidence-based management for withdrawal.

Case Study

Emma, a 30-year-old woman, has been using cocaine daily for the past year. She reports feeling irritable, paranoid, and restless during use. Recently, she has experienced severe fatigue and depressive symptoms during periods when she stops using the drug. Emma also reports significant financial problems and strained relationships due to her inability to control her use.

1. Which feature most strongly supports a diagnosis of Stimulant Use Disorder in Emma's case?
   - A. Her daily use of cocaine.
   - B. Her depressive symptoms during periods of abstinence.
   - C. Her inability to control her use despite negative consequences.
   - D. Her feelings of paranoia during use.
2. Which of the following is the most appropriate first-line intervention for Emma?
   - A. Cognitive-behavioral therapy to address her substance use.
   - B. Immediate detoxification with benzodiazepines.
   - C. Long-term inpatient hospitalization.
   - D. Pharmacological treatment with methadone.
3. Which of the following complications is Emma most at risk for due to her chronic cocaine use?
   - A. Myocardial infarction.
   - B. Cirrhosis of the liver.
   - C. Wernicke-Korsakoff syndrome.
   - D. Acute kidney failure.

Answers

Multiple Choice Questions:

1. A
2. B
3. B
4. C
5. B
6. C
7. B

True/False Questions:

1. True
2. False
3. True
4. True
5. False
6. True
7. False
8. True
9. False
10. True

Matching Exercise:

1. A
2. B
3. C
4. D
5. E
6. F

Case Study Answers and Explanations:

1. C - Explanation: Inability to stop using despite negative consequences is a key feature of Stimulant Use Disorder.
2. A - Explanation: Cognitive-behavioral therapy is evidence-based for addressing stimulant use.
3. A - Explanation: Cocaine use is a major risk factor for myocardial infarction due to its effects on the cardiovascular system.

Tobacco-Related Disorders

Multiple Choice Questions

1. Which of the following is the most commonly reported withdrawal symptom in individuals attempting to quit tobacco?
    - A. Euphoria.
    - B. Anxiety and irritability.
    - C. Excessive sweating.
    - D. Hypersomnia.
2. Which neurotransmitter system is primarily affected by nicotine, the active compound in tobacco?
    - A. Dopaminergic.
    - B. Serotonergic.
    - C. Glutamatergic.
    - D. GABAergic.
3. A 45-year-old man has been smoking one pack of cigarettes daily for 20 years. He attempts to quit but experiences intense cravings and irritability. Which of the following medications would be most appropriate to help him quit?
    - A. Benzodiazepines.
    - B. Varenicline.
    - C. Antipsychotics.
    - D. Lithium.
4. Which of the following is a hallmark feature of Tobacco Use Disorder?
    - A. Persistent use despite awareness of significant health risks.
    - B. Infrequent use limited to social situations.
    - C. Exclusive use of nicotine replacement therapy.
    - D. Intoxication symptoms following use.
5. Which of the following is the primary mechanism of action of varenicline in treating Tobacco Use Disorder?
    - A. Blocking serotonin reuptake.
    - B. Acting as a partial agonist at nicotinic acetylcholine receptors.
    - C. Enhancing dopamine release in the reward system.
    - D. Binding to GABA receptors to reduce cravings.
6. Chronic tobacco use is most strongly associated with which of the following long-term complications?
    - A. Cirrhosis of the liver.
    - B. Chronic obstructive pulmonary disease (COPD).
    - C. Pancreatitis.
    - D. Chronic kidney disease.
7. Which of the following behavioral interventions has been shown to be most effective in helping individuals quit smoking?
    - A. Psychoanalysis.
    - B. Motivational interviewing and behavioral counseling.
    - C. Long-term hospitalization.
    - D. Hypnotherapy alone.

True/False Questions

		T	F
1	The DSM-5-TR recognizes tobacco withdrawal as a distinct diagnosis, featuring symptoms such as irritability, anxiety, and concentration difficulties.		
2	In the DSM-5-TR, a diagnosis of Tobacco Use Disorder requires evidence of physical dependence, including the presence of chronic lung disease.		
3	To determine the severity of Tobacco Use Disorder, the DSM-5-TR uses the number of criteria met, similar to other Substance Use Disorders.		
4	Weight gain during tobacco cessation is formally classified by the DSM-5-TR as a core withdrawal symptom.		
5	Craving for nicotine is included among the criteria that may contribute to the diagnosis of Tobacco Use Disorder in the DSM-5-TR.		
6	According to the DSM-5-TR, there are no specific codes to differentiate between early and sustained remission of Tobacco Use Disorder.		
7	In the DSM-5-TR, using non-combustible forms of tobacco (e.g., chewing tobacco) can still meet criteria for a Tobacco Use Disorder if problematic consumption patterns and difficulty quitting are evident.		
8	The presence of another tobacco-related medical condition (such as a cardiovascular disease) automatically rules out a diagnosis of Tobacco Use Disorder in the DSM-5-TR.		
9	The DSM-5-TR specifies that early remission for Tobacco Use Disorder requires at least three months (but less than 12) without meeting diagnostic criteria, apart from craving.		
10	A typical sign of "tobacco intoxication" is listed among the DSM-5-TR's diagnostic criteria, resembling the intoxication symptoms of other stimulants.		

Matching Exercise

1. Increased appetite, anxiety, and irritability following cessation. [ ]
2. Chronic tobacco use leading to impaired lung function. [ ]
3. First-line pharmacological treatment that acts on nicotinic receptors. [ ]
4. Behavioral therapy that helps individuals explore ambivalence toward quitting. [ ]
5. Nicotine's impact on the reward system. [ ]
6. Long-term risk of cardiovascular diseases. [ ]

Descriptions:

- A. Tobacco withdrawal symptoms.
- B. Chronic obstructive pulmonary disease (COPD).
- C. Varenicline.
- D. Motivational interviewing.
- E. Increased dopamine release.
- F. Common complication of tobacco use.

Case Study

Michael, a 50-year-old man, has smoked two packs of cigarettes daily for 25 years. He reports difficulty concentrating and irritability when attempting to quit in the past. Michael is concerned about his health after being diagnosed with mild COPD. He is willing to try quitting but fears failure due to strong cravings and withdrawal symptoms.

1. Which symptom most strongly indicates nicotine withdrawal in Michael's case?
   - A. Difficulty concentrating.
   - B. Mild COPD.
   - C. His fear of failure.
   - D. His history of two-pack-per-day smoking.
2. Which intervention would be most appropriate as part of Michael's smoking cessation plan?
   - A. Immediate cessation without medication.
   - B. Combination of varenicline and behavioral counseling.
   - C. Long-term inpatient detoxification.
   - D. Use of benzodiazepines to manage withdrawal symptoms.
3. Which of the following health benefits is most likely to occur within a few weeks of Michael quitting smoking?
   - A. Complete reversal of COPD.
   - B. Significant improvement in lung function.
   - C. Elimination of cardiovascular disease risk.
   - D. Total elimination of withdrawal symptoms.

Answers

Multiple Choice Questions:

1. B
2. A
3. B
4. A
5. B
6. B
7. B

True/False Questions:

1. True
2. False
3. True
4. False
5. True
6. False
7. True
8. False
9. True
10. False

Matching Exercise:

1. A
2. B
3. C
4. D
5. E
6. F

Case Study Answers and Explanations:

1. A - Explanation: Difficulty concentrating is a hallmark symptom of nicotine withdrawal.
2. B - Explanation: Varenicline combined with behavioral counseling is a first-line approach for smoking cessation.
3. B - Explanation: Smoking cessation often leads to measurable improvements in lung function within weeks, although COPD is not fully reversible.

Other or Unknown Substance–Related Disorders

Multiple Choice Questions

1. A patient is brought to the emergency department with confusion, agitation, and an unusual odor on their breath. They deny substance use, but their symptoms suggest intoxication. Which of the following is the most appropriate first step in managing this patient?
    - A. Perform a detailed toxicology screen.
    - B. Start naloxone immediately.
    - C. Administer benzodiazepines for sedation.
    - D. Initiate hemodialysis.
2. Which of the following features distinguishes unknown substance intoxication from intoxication by known substances?
    - A. Presence of severe agitation.
    - B. Atypical symptoms not aligning with any common substance category.
    - C. Development of respiratory depression.
    - D. The need for hospitalization.
3. A 22-year-old man presents with hallucinations, hypertension, tachycardia, and agitation after taking an unknown substance at a party. Which of the following is the best immediate intervention?
    - A. Administer antipsychotics to manage hallucinations.
    - B. Provide intravenous fluids and monitor cardiovascular status.
    - C. Begin high-dose corticosteroids.
    - D. Discharge the patient with instructions to avoid future use.
4. In cases of intoxication with unknown substances, which of the following is a priority during initial assessment?
    - A. Identifying the exact substance ingested.
    - B. Stabilizing the patient's vital signs and addressing acute symptoms.
    - C. Determining the patient's psychiatric history.
    - D. Contacting poison control immediately.
5. Which of the following is a common presentation of withdrawal from an unknown substance?
    - A. Predictable symptoms based on known substance classes.
    - B. A wide range of symptoms, including agitation, anxiety, and autonomic instability.
    - C. Absence of any withdrawal symptoms.
    - D. Severe depression with hallucinations.
6. A patient recovering from unknown substance intoxication asks about long-term health risks. Which of the following is the most accurate response?
    - A. "There are no long-term risks if the substance is unknown."
    - B. "It depends on the substance and its potential toxicity to organs."
    - C. "All unknown substances cause irreversible brain damage."
    - D. "You are at risk for addiction regardless of the substance."
7. Which intervention is most appropriate for patients with recurrent use of unknown substances?
    - A. Long-term inpatient rehabilitation without substance identification.
    - B. Cognitive-behavioral therapy focusing on decision-making and harm reduction.
    - C. Pharmacological treatment with a broad-spectrum antidote.
    - D. Immediate detoxification followed by outpatient observation.

True/False Questions

		T	F
1	The DSM-5-TR uses "Other (or Unknown) Substance Use Disorder" if the substance does not fit known categories or cannot be accurately identified.		
2	Lab confirmation is always required to diagnose "Unknown Substance Intoxication."		
3	Persistent, compulsive use alone is enough to diagnose Unknown Substance Use Disorder, regardless of intoxication or withdrawal signs.		
4	The DSM-5-TR strictly distinguishes "designer drugs" from "Other (or Unknown) Substance," allowing no diagnostic overlap.		
5	If an unknown substance produces effects similar to a recognized class (e.g., opioid-like), "Other (or Unknown) Substance Use Disorder" is still used.		
6	Unknown substance withdrawal can be diagnosed without knowing the pharmacology, if there is clinically significant distress when use stops.		
7	The DSM-5-TR mandates reclassification of "Unknown Substance Use Disorder" once the substance is precisely identified.		
8	"Unknown Substance-Induced Psychotic Disorder" can be diagnosed if there is a temporal link between use and symptoms, and no primary psychiatric disorder.		
9	Under the DSM-5-TR, lacking craving for the unknown substance rules out Unknown Substance Use Disorder.		
10	Continuing use of an unidentified substance that impairs functioning can still meet criteria for a Substance Use Disorder, even without an exact name.		

Matching Exercise

1. Stabilization of vital signs and acute symptom management. [ ]
2. Unusual symptoms not aligning with known substance classes. [ ]
3. Contacting poison control for guidance. [ ]
4. Long-term risks dependent on the substance's toxicity. [ ]
5. Cognitive-behavioral therapy for harm reduction. [ ]
6. Autonomic instability during withdrawal. [ ]

Descriptions:

- A. Priority in the acute management of unknown substance intoxication.
- B. A typical feature of withdrawal from unknown substances.
- C. Standard protocol for unknown substance cases.
- D. Symptom presentation unique to unknown substances.
- E. Effective intervention for recurrent use.
- F. Dependent on the specific substance used.

Case Study

Anna, a 19-year-old woman, arrives at the emergency department after collapsing at a party. Witnesses report that she took a substance she believed to be "natural." On examination, she is hypertensive, tachycardic, and agitated, with dilated pupils. She has no significant medical history. Toxicology results are inconclusive, and her symptoms resolve after several hours of supportive care.

1. Which feature most strongly suggests unknown substance intoxication in Anna's case?
    - A. Her belief that the substance was "natural."
    - B. Hypertension and agitation with inconclusive toxicology results.
    - C. Resolution of symptoms within hours.
    - D. Her lack of significant medical history.
2. Which intervention would be most appropriate to address Anna's condition?
    - A. Immediate administration of naloxone.
    - B. Supportive care with monitoring of cardiovascular status.
    - C. High-dose antipsychotics for agitation.
    - D. Long-term inpatient detoxification.
3. Which of the following is the most important next step in Anna's case?
    - A. Repeating the toxicology screen.
    - B. Educating her about the risks of using unknown substances.
    - C. Starting pharmacological treatment for hypertension.
    - D. Discharging her without further follow-up.

Answers

Multiple Choice Questions:

1. A
2. B
3. B
4. B
5. B
6. B
7. B

True/False Questions:

1. True
2. False
3. False
4. False
5. True
6. True
7. False
8. True
9. False
10. True

Matching Exercise:

1. A
2. D
3. C
4. F
5. E
6. B

Case Study Answers and Explanations:

1. B - Explanation: Hypertension, agitation, and inconclusive toxicology results are consistent with unknown substance intoxication.
2. B - Explanation: Supportive care and monitoring are the safest initial approaches for managing unknown substance intoxication.
3. B - Explanation: Educating the patient about the risks of unknown substances is critical for harm reduction and preventing future incidents.

Gambling Disorder

Multiple Choice Questions

1. A 35-year-old man gambles to "chase his losses," hoping to recover spent money. What best explains this behavior in the context of Gambling Disorder?
   - A. A cognitive bias that overestimates future wins.
   - B. A lack of financial insight.
   - C. Avoidance of withdrawal-like symptoms.
   - D. A coping mechanism for mood disorders.
2. A patient with Gambling Disorder has severe depression and suicidal thoughts due to debt. What should be prioritized first?
   - A. Referral for financial counseling.
   - B. Psychiatric evaluation for suicide risk.
   - C. Behavioral strategies to reduce gambling.
   - D. Antidepressants to address mood symptoms.
3. Which scenario best distinguishes Gambling Disorder from non-problematic gambling?
   - A. Gambling occasionally with friends without exceeding a spending limit.
   - B. Gambling with increasing amounts but stopping after large losses.
   - C. Gambling despite being evicted due to unpaid debts.
   - D. Gambling recreationally once a week but feeling mild regret afterward.
4. Gambling Disorder often co-occurs with psychiatric conditions. Which condition is most likely to worsen gambling?
   - A. Generalized Anxiety Disorder.
   - B. Attention-Deficit/Hyperactivity Disorder.
   - C. Bipolar Disorder during mania.
   - D. Specific Phobia.
5. In Gambling Disorder, which neurobiological mechanism most contributes to persistent behaviors?
   - A. Prefrontal cortex activation improving decision-making.
   - B. Mesolimbic dopamine dysregulation linked to reward.
   - C. Increased serotonergic activity driving impulsivity.
   - D. GABAergic inhibition reducing anxiety.
6. A 42-year-old woman blames her gambling on bad luck and believes she is "due for a win." Which cognitive distortion is this?
   - A. Illusion of control.
   - B. Confirmation bias.
   - C. Gambler's fallacy.
   - D. Optimism bias.
7. Which treatment for Gambling Disorder directly addresses distorted thoughts and beliefs?
   - A. Financial budgeting with a counselor.
   - B. Opioid antagonist pharmacological treatment.
   - C. Cognitive restructuring via cognitive-behavioral therapy.
   - D. Referral to self-help groups like Gamblers Anonymous.

True/False Questions

		T	F
1	Under the DSM-5-TR, at least four criteria must be met to diagnose Gambling Disorder.		
2	According to the DSM-5-TR, an active manic episode does not preclude the diagnosis of Gambling Disorder.		
3	The DSM-5-TR introduces gambling withdrawal as an independent criterion, similar to substance withdrawal.		
4	Gambling Disorder can be diagnosed even without severe financial losses, provided there is significant impairment.		
5	The DSM-5-TR allows specification of early or sustained remission for Gambling Disorder, akin to Substance Use Disorders.		
6	Repeated lying to conceal gambling involvement is one of the core diagnostic criteria for Gambling Disorder.		
7	The DSM-5-TR requires a minimum of 24 consecutive months of problematic gambling to make the diagnosis.		
8	In the DSM-5-TR, chasing losses is regarded as a primary criterion for Gambling Disorder.		
9	The DSM-5-TR includes craving as a central symptom when assessing the severity of Gambling Disorder.		
10	If an individual meets the required number of criteria, but symptoms occur only during a manic episode, the DSM-5-TR mandates ruling out Gambling Disorder.		

Matching Exercise

1. "Chasing losses" as a hallmark behavior. [ ]
2. Targeting cognitive distortions through structured therapy. [ ]
3. Activation of the mesolimbic dopamine system. [ ]
4. Co-occurring psychiatric condition exacerbating gambling behaviors. [ ]
5. Gamblers' belief that a "win is due" after a series of losses. [ ]
6. Behavioral strategies to establish financial limits. [ ]

Descriptions:

- A. Gambler's fallacy.
- B. Core feature of Gambling Disorder.
- C. Cognitive-behavioral therapy.
- D. Bipolar Disorder in manic phases.
- E. Neurobiological mechanism in Gambling Disorder.
- F. Financial counseling.

Case Study

Peter, a 37-year-old man, seeks treatment after being confronted by his family about his gambling debts. He reports spending most of his evenings at the casino and has maxed out several credit cards. Peter admits that he feels a sense of control when gambling but often ends up losing more than he can afford. He has tried to stop gambling multiple times but relapses whenever he feels stressed or anxious. Peter denies using drugs or alcohol but has a history of depression.

1. Which aspect of Peter's behavior most strongly supports a diagnosis of Gambling Disorder?
    - A. His attempts to quit gambling but repeated relapses.
    - B. His use of credit cards to fund gambling activities.
    - C. His sense of control when gambling.
    - D. His lack of substance use.
2. Which therapeutic intervention would be most appropriate to address Peter's gambling behaviors?
    - A. Financial counseling alone to resolve his debts.
    - B. Cognitive-behavioral therapy focusing on thought patterns and stress management.
    - C. Long-term inpatient treatment.
    - D. Antidepressant medication without therapy.
3. Peter reports a belief that gambling helps him cope with stress. This belief is best addressed through:
    - A. Cognitive restructuring to challenge this maladaptive belief.
    - B. Medication to reduce his anxiety.
    - C. Immediate abstinence enforced through hospitalization.
    - D. Group therapy without individual intervention.

Answers

Multiple Choice Questions:

1. A
2. B
3. C
4. C
5. B
6. C
7. C

True/False Questions:

1. True
2. True
3. False
4. True
5. True
6. True
7. False
8. True
9. False
10. False

Matching Exercise:

1. B
2. C
3. E
4. D
5. A
6. F

Case Study Answers and Explanations:

1. A - Explanation: Repeated unsuccessful attempts to quit are a hallmark of Gambling Disorder.
2. B - Explanation: Cognitive-behavioral therapy addresses distorted thoughts and helps manage stress triggers.
3. A - Explanation: Cognitive restructuring is essential to challenge the belief that gambling is an effective coping mechanism.

Neurocognitive Disorders

This category encompasses conditions involving a significant decline in cognitive functioning compared to an individual's prior level. The decline can affect one or more domains, such as memory, attention, executive functioning, language, or visuospatial abilities. The DSM-5-TR distinguishes between Major and Mild Neurocognitive Disorders, depending on how these deficits interfere with daily autonomy: in Major Neurocognitive Disorder, the individual requires assistance with day-to-day tasks, whereas in Mild Neurocognitive Disorder, the person can manage most activities but needs extra effort or compensatory strategies.

The causes vary. One of the most common is Alzheimer's Disease, which presents as a progressive decline in memory and other cognitive skills, eventually accompanied by personality changes and altered behavior in later stages. Other forms include Vascular Dementia, often stemming from multiple small infarcts; Dementia with Lewy Bodies, characterized by attention fluctuations, visual hallucinations, and parkinsonian features; and conditions linked to Parkinson's Disease, where motor impairment and progressive cognitive decline coexist. Huntington's Disease, with its choreic movements and psychiatric manifestations, is yet another example.

Not all types of cognitive decline are irreversible, however. Substance- or medication-induced disorders, nutritional deficiencies (such as vitamin B12), or certain endocrine and metabolic problems may produce deficits that are partly reversible or temporary. Traumatic brain injuries and infections (for example, HIV) can also result in various levels of deterioration, influenced by factors like the promptness of diagnosis and appropriate intervention.

Diagnosis requires a detailed clinical and neuropsychological assessment, aimed at pinpointing which cognitive skills are affected, to what extent, and how these difficulties affect everyday functioning. Imaging studies (MRI, CT, PET) can help identify any lesions, areas of atrophy, or metabolic changes that clarify the underlying cause. It is also crucial to rule out other conditions (delirium, primary psychiatric disorders, depression) that might mimic neurocognitive decline.

Management of Neurocognitive Disorders may involve pharmacological treatment (such as cholinesterase inhibitors or memantine) along with psychosocial and environmental measures. Keeping a predictable routine, promoting existing abilities, supporting family members, and planning for ongoing care can make a difference. Cognitive stimulation or occupational therapies may slow down functional decline or boost quality of life. While some conditions are progressive and cannot be cured, early detection and the right support help manage symptoms more effectively and create a safer, more comfortable environment for those affected.

Delirium

Multiple Choice Questions

1. A 78-year-old woman develops acute confusion and agitation after starting a new medication for pain. Which factor best differentiates delirium from a primary psychiatric disorder?
   - A. The presence of disorientation.
   - B. Acute symptom onset.
   - C. The patient's advanced age.
   - D. Absence of hallucinations.
2. A hospitalized patient with delirium secondary to a urinary tract infection becomes increasingly agitated at night. Which intervention would best address this symptom?
   - A. Administer a high-dose antipsychotic.
   - B. Use physical restraints to prevent harm.
   - C. Provide a calm, well-lit environment with reorientation cues.
   - D. Initiate benzodiazepine therapy.
3. Which lab finding is most associated with delirium in a patient with chronic alcohol use?
   - A. Hypokalemia.
   - B. Elevated liver enzymes.
   - C. Thiamine deficiency.
   - D. Hyperglycemia.
4. In evaluating a patient with suspected delirium, which finding suggests an alternative diagnosis such as dementia?
   - A. Gradual progression over months.
   - B. Fluctuating attention levels.
   - C. Agitation worsened by hospitalization.
   - D. Disorganized thinking.
5. Which neurotransmitter alteration is most implicated in delirium?
   - A. Increased serotonin activity.
   - B. Decreased dopamine transmission.
   - C. Reduced acetylcholine levels.
   - D. Enhanced GABA activity.
6. A 72-year-old man with Parkinson's disease presents with confusion and visual hallucinations. Which feature suggests delirium rather than Parkinson's psychosis?
   - A. Fluctuating confusion and inattention.
   - B. Vivid visual hallucinations.
   - C. Long-standing Parkinsonian symptoms.
   - D. Gradual onset of hallucinations.
7. Which strategy is most effective to prevent delirium in hospitalized patients?
   - A. Routine antipsychotics as prophylaxis.
   - B. Early mobilization, hydration, and reorientation.
   - C. Isolation in a quiet room with minimal stimulation.
   - D. Avoidance of all sedatives.

True/False Questions

		T	F
1	The DSM-5-TR describes delirium as a gradual cognitive decline developing over at least two weeks.		
2	Disorganized thinking can appear in delirium, with incoherent speech or abrupt topic shifts.		
3	Under the DSM-5-TR, there is only one category of delirium with no mention of hyperactive or hypoactive forms.		
4	Altered attention and awareness is a central criterion for delirium in the DSM-5-TR.		
5	Delirium is not reversible unless treated with intensive pharmacological intervention, according to the DSM-5-TR.		
6	The DSM-5-TR allows diagnosing substance-induced delirium if symptoms arise during or immediately after intoxication or withdrawal.		
7	The DSM-5-TR requires definitively ruling out any underlying medical condition before diagnosing delirium.		
8	An acute onset and fluctuating course help distinguish delirium from dementia in the DSM-5-TR.		
9	The DSM-5-TR mandates that delirium symptoms last at least one month to meet the diagnostic criteria.		
10	The DSM-5-TR allows specification if delirium is caused by multiple factors, such as concurrent medical conditions and medication use.		

Matching Exercise

1. Acute confusion with disorganized thinking and fluctuating attention. [ ]
2. Deficiency strongly associated with delirium in chronic alcohol users. [ ]
3. Effective prevention strategy for hospitalized patients. [ ]
4. Pathophysiological neurotransmitter alteration in delirium. [ ]
5. Core risk factor for developing delirium. [ ]
6. Hallucination type more commonly associated with delirium. [ ]

Descriptions:

- A. Acetylcholine deficiency.
- B. Advanced age.
- C. Early mobilization and regular reorientation.
- D. Visual hallucinations.
- E. Disorganized thinking with acute onset.
- F. Thiamine deficiency.

Case Study

Mary, a 79-year-old woman with a history of hypertension, is admitted to the hospital for treatment of pneumonia. On her second night in the hospital, she becomes confused, restless, and repeatedly attempts to get out of bed, stating she needs to "catch the train." She is oriented to her name but disoriented to time and place. Physical examination reveals no focal neurological deficits, but she exhibits fluctuating levels of attention. Her family notes that she was cognitively intact before hospitalization.

1. What is the most likely precipitating factor for Mary's delirium?
    - A. Advanced age combined with hospitalization.
    - B. History of hypertension.
    - C. Family history of dementia.
    - D. Use of sedatives prior to hospitalization.
2. Which intervention would be most effective in managing Mary's symptoms?
    - A. Use of antipsychotics to control her agitation.
    - B. Addressing the underlying infection and ensuring a structured environment.
    - C. Immediate transfer to a long-term care facility.
    - D. Administration of high-dose benzodiazepines.
3. Which feature most strongly differentiates Mary's delirium from a neurocognitive disorder?
    - A. Her fluctuating levels of attention.
    - B. Her advanced age.
    - C. Her restlessness and agitation.
    - D. Her disorientation to time and place.

Answers

Multiple Choice Questions:

1. B
2. C
3. C
4. A
5. C
6. A
7. B

True/False Questions:

1. False
2. True
3. False
4. True
5. False
6. True
7. False
8. True
9. False
10. True

Matching Exercise:

1. E
2. F
3. C
4. A
5. B
6. D

Case Study Answers and Explanations:

1. A - Advanced age and hospitalization are significant risk factors for delirium.
2. B - Managing the underlying cause, in this case pneumonia, is the cornerstone of delirium treatment.
3. A - Fluctuating attention is a hallmark of delirium and helps differentiate it from chronic neurocognitive disorders.

Major or Mild Neurocognitive Disorder Due to Alzheimer's Disease

Multiple Choice Questions

1. A 76-year-old woman presents with progressive memory loss and difficulty recalling recent events over the past two years. She remains independent in daily activities but requires reminders for appointments. What stage of Alzheimer's disease is most consistent with her symptoms?
   - A. Preclinical Alzheimer's disease.
   - B. Mild Neurocognitive Disorder due to Alzheimer's disease.
   - C. Major Neurocognitive Disorder due to Alzheimer's disease.
   - D. Advanced Alzheimer's disease.
2. Which of the following is a hallmark pathological feature of Alzheimer's disease?
   - A. Neurofibrillary tangles and amyloid plaques.
   - B. Lewy bodies in the substantia nigra.
   - C. Vascular infarcts in cortical regions.
   - D. Prion protein accumulation in neural tissue.
3. Which of the following differentiates Mild from Major Neurocognitive Disorder due to Alzheimer's disease?
   - A. Major involves only memory loss, while Mild involves multiple cognitive domains.
   - B. Major causes significant impairment in independence, while Mild preserves independence.
   - C. Mild is reversible, while Major is irreversible.
   - D. Mild is characterized by sudden onset, while Major has a gradual progression.
4. Which genetic mutation is most strongly associated with early-onset Alzheimer's disease?
   - A. APOE-ε4.
   - B. PSEN1 (Presenilin 1).
   - C. MAPT (Microtubule-Associated Protein Tau).
   - D. TREM2 (Triggering Receptor Expressed on Myeloid Cells 2).
5. A patient with Alzheimer's disease demonstrates difficulty recalling recent conversations but retains procedural memory such as tying shoes. Which brain region is most likely affected?
   - A. Hippocampus.
   - B. Cerebellum.
   - C. Basal ganglia.
   - D. Occipital cortex.
6. Which pharmacological treatment is most commonly used to slow cognitive decline in Alzheimer's disease?
   - A. Levodopa.
   - B. Donepezil.
   - C. Lithium.
   - D. Risperidone.
7. In patients with advanced Alzheimer's disease, which of the following symptoms is most commonly observed?
   - A. Worsening apathy and social withdrawal.
   - B. Improvement in executive functioning.
   - C. Hallucinations with fluctuating alertness.
   - D. Episodic hyperactivity and mood elevation.

True/False Questions

		T	F
1	According to the DSM-5-TR, a gradual onset and progressive decline in cognitive functions are key for diagnosing Alzheimer's disease.		
2	Biological confirmation (through imaging or genetic tests) is always required to diagnose Neurocognitive Disorder due to Alzheimer's.		
3	The DSM-5-TR allows for a distinction between "Probable" and "Possible" Alzheimer's disease, partly based on genetic evidence or the absence of other pathologies.		
4	The level of impairment in daily activities is the main criterion differentiating Major from Mild Neurocognitive Disorder due to Alzheimer's.		
5	In the DSM-5-TR, memory deficits are only one of several possible cognitive domains affected by Alzheimer's disease.		
6	The DSM-5-TR states that if there is no significant decline in memory, a Mild Neurocognitive Disorder due to Alzheimer's cannot be diagnosed.		
7	Initial personality or behavioral changes, without memory impairment, are considered the typical presentation of Alzheimer's disease in the DSM-5-TR.		
8	The DSM-5-TR allows an Alzheimer's diagnosis even if another medical condition is present, as long as that condition does not fully account for the cognitive decline.		
9	The typical presentation of Alzheimer's disease in the DSM-5-TR primarily involves executive function deficits rather than memory impairment.		
10	According to the DSM-5-TR, a "behavioral" subtype of Alzheimer's is defined by the predominant emergence of psychotic symptoms.		

Matching Exercise

1. Gradual onset and progression of memory loss. [ ]
2. Defining neuropathological feature of Alzheimer's disease. [ ]
3. Most commonly used medication to slow cognitive decline. [ ]
4. Brain region initially affected in Alzheimer's disease. [ ]
5. Genetic mutation associated with early-onset Alzheimer's disease. [ ]
6. Typical symptom of advanced Alzheimer's disease. [ ]

Descriptions:

- A. Amyloid plaques and neurofibrillary tangles.
- B. Donepezil.
- C. Hippocampus.
- D. Apathy and social withdrawal.
- E. Gradual memory loss with progression.
- F. PSEN1 mutation.

Case Study

Mary, a 70-year-old retired teacher, presents with progressive memory difficulties over the past three years. She frequently forgets recent conversations, misplaces objects, and struggles to manage finances. Her family notes increased confusion about dates and places. Physical examination reveals no motor deficits, but neuroimaging shows hippocampal atrophy. Neuropsychological testing confirms impairment in episodic memory and executive functioning, but her basic daily activities remain intact with occasional assistance.

1. What clinical feature in Mary's case supports a diagnosis of Mild rather than Major Neurocognitive Disorder due to Alzheimer's disease?
   - A. Her preserved ability to manage basic daily activities.
   - B. The presence of hippocampal atrophy on imaging.
   - C. Her difficulty managing finances.
   - D. Impairment in episodic memory.
2. Which neuroanatomical finding is most consistent with Mary's symptoms?
   - A. Widespread cortical atrophy.
   - B. Hippocampal atrophy.
   - C. Cerebellar degeneration.
   - D. Subcortical infarcts.
3. Which intervention would be most appropriate for Mary's condition?
   - A. Prescribe donepezil to slow cognitive decline.
   - B. Start antipsychotics to manage behavioral symptoms.
   - C. Recommend long-term inpatient care.
   - D. Perform a genetic test to confirm APOE-ε4 mutation.

Answers

Multiple Choice Questions:
1. B
2. A
3. B
4. B
5. A
6. B
7. A

True/False Questions:
1. True
2. False
3. True
4. True
5. True
6. False
7. False
8. True
9. False
10. False

Matching Exercise:
1. E
2. A
3. B
4. C
5. F
6. D

Case Study Answers and Explanations:
1. A - Explanation: The preservation of basic daily activities suggests Mild rather than Major Neurocognitive Disorder.
2. B - Explanation: Hippocampal atrophy is a hallmark finding in Alzheimer's disease, especially in its early stages.
3. A - Explanation: Donepezil is a first-line pharmacological treatment for slowing cognitive decline in Alzheimer's disease.

Major or Mild Vascular Neurocognitive Disorder

Multiple Choice Questions

1. Which of the following is a key feature of Vascular Neurocognitive Disorder?
    - A. Gradual onset with progressive cognitive decline.
    - B. Sudden onset with a stepwise progression of symptoms.
    - C. Early onset of hallucinations and delusions.
    - D. Rapid improvement in cognitive function following treatment.
2. What is the most common vascular event leading to Vascular Neurocognitive Disorder?
    - A. Hemorrhagic stroke.
    - B. Ischemic stroke.
    - C. Myocardial infarction.
    - D. Subarachnoid hemorrhage.
3. Which neuroimaging finding is most strongly associated with Vascular Neurocognitive Disorder?
    - A. Global cortical atrophy.
    - B. Hippocampal volume loss.
    - C. Multiple infarcts and white matter hyperintensities.
    - D. Thinning of the corpus callosum.
4. In the early stages of Vascular Neurocognitive Disorder, which cognitive domain is typically most affected?
    - A. Episodic memory.
    - B. Language processing.
    - C. Attention and executive functioning.
    - D. Visuospatial abilities.
5. Which of the following conditions is a major risk factor for the development of Vascular Neurocognitive Disorder?
    - A. Parkinson's disease.
    - B. Chronic hypertension.
    - C. Severe vitamin B12 deficiency.
    - D. History of substance use disorder.
6. How does the cognitive decline in Vascular Neurocognitive Disorder typically progress compared to Alzheimer's disease?
    - A. Gradual and steady decline.
    - B. Fluctuating course with significant recovery periods.
    - C. Stepwise decline following vascular events.
    - D. Rapid decline with early hallucinations.
7. Which of the following interventions is the most effective in reducing the risk of progression in Vascular Neurocognitive Disorder?
    - A. Daily use of antipsychotics to manage symptoms.
    - B. Cognitive-behavioral therapy to address memory deficits.
    - C. Aggressive management of vascular risk factors like hypertension.
    - D. High-dose acetylcholinesterase inhibitors.

True/False Questions

		T	F
1	The DSM-5-TR allows Mild Vascular Neurocognitive Disorder to be diagnosed without clearly documented cerebrovascular events if clinical suspicion is strong.		
2	A stepwise decline in cognition following vascular events is typical of Vascular Neurocognitive Disorder.		
3	Multiple infarcts alone, without significant cognitive symptoms, suffice to diagnose Major Vascular Neurocognitive Disorder.		
4	Neuroimaging evidence of vascular pathology is advised but not mandatory for diagnosing Vascular Neurocognitive Disorder.		
5	Subcortical vascular lesions can lead to early deficits in executive function and complex attention.		
6	If cognitive deficits stabilize for a few months, the DSM-5-TR automatically rules out Vascular Neurocognitive Disorder.		
7	A confirmed stroke or TIA is not mandatory if other strong indications point to a vascular basis for cognitive decline.		
8	Under the DSM-5-TR, a gradual, uniform cognitive decline is considered characteristic of Vascular Neurocognitive Disorder.		
9	The DSM-5-TR does not offer "probable" or "possible" specifiers for Vascular Neurocognitive Disorder, providing only a single diagnostic label.		
10	If vascular lesions and Alzheimer's pathology coexist, the DSM-5-TR always rules out Vascular Neurocognitive Disorder.		

Matching Exercise

1. Sudden onset of symptoms with stepwise progression. [ ]
2. Neuroimaging finding characteristic of Vascular Neurocognitive Disorder. [ ]
3. Key risk factor in developing the condition. [ ]
4. Prominent cognitive deficit in the early stages. [ ]
5. First-line treatment approach. [ ]
6. Motor symptom associated with Vascular Neurocognitive Disorder. [ ]

Descriptions:

- A. White matter hyperintensities or multiple infarcts.
- B. Poorly controlled hypertension.
- C. Deficits in attention and executive function.
- D. Stepwise decline.
- E. Managing vascular risk factors.
- F. Hemiparesis or gait disturbances.

Case Study

Michael, a 72-year-old man with a history of hypertension and two prior strokes, presents with progressive difficulty organizing tasks, making decisions, and maintaining focus. His wife reports that his symptoms seem to worsen after each stroke. Neuroimaging reveals multiple cortical and subcortical infarcts. Despite his cognitive challenges, he recalls recent events better than distant ones. He also reports mild weakness on his left side.

1. Which aspect of Michael's presentation most strongly supports the diagnosis of Vascular Neurocognitive Disorder?
   - A. His ability to recall recent events better than distant ones.
   - B. The progressive worsening of symptoms after strokes.
   - C. His history of hypertension.
   - D. The presence of mild left-sided weakness.
2. Which intervention would be most appropriate to prevent further progression of Michael's condition?
   - A. Start donepezil to improve cognitive function.
   - B. Focus on controlling his blood pressure and other vascular risk factors.
   - C. Prescribe antipsychotics to manage his cognitive symptoms.
   - D. Initiate cognitive-behavioral therapy to improve decision-making.
3. Which cognitive deficit in Michael is most characteristic of Vascular Neurocognitive Disorder?
   - A. Episodic memory loss.
   - B. Executive dysfunction.
   - C. Spatial disorientation.
   - D. Rapidly worsening attention deficits.

Answers

Multiple Choice Questions:
1. B
2. C
3. B
4. C
5. A
6. A
7. B

True/False Questions:
1. True
2. True
3. False
4. True
5. True
6. False
7. True
8. False
9. False
10. False

Matching Exercise:
1. D
2. A
3. B
4. C
5. E
6. F

Case Study Answers and Explanations:
1. B - Explanation: A stepwise decline following strokes is a hallmark feature of Vascular Neurocognitive Disorder.
2. B - Explanation: Controlling vascular risk factors, such as hypertension, is essential to prevent further cognitive decline.
3. B - Explanation: Executive dysfunction is a key cognitive deficit in Vascular Neurocognitive Disorder.

Major or Mild Frontotemporal Neurocognitive Disorder

Multiple Choice Questions

1. Which of the following is a hallmark feature of Frontotemporal Neurocognitive Disorder (FTNCD)?
    - A. Memory loss as the first and most prominent symptom.
    - B. Early behavioral and personality changes.
    - C. Visual hallucinations with fluctuating attention.
    - D. Sudden stepwise progression of cognitive decline.
2. Which subtype of FTNCD is characterized by language deficits such as difficulty in word retrieval and speech production?
    - A. Behavioral variant.
    - B. Semantic variant primary progressive aphasia.
    - C. Logopenic variant primary progressive aphasia.
    - D. Nonfluent/agrammatic variant primary progressive aphasia.
3. Which neuroimaging finding is most commonly associated with FTNCD?
    - A. Hippocampal atrophy.
    - B. Atrophy in the frontal and temporal lobes.
    - C. Diffuse white matter hyperintensities.
    - D. Substantia nigra degeneration.
4. Which gene mutation is strongly linked to inherited forms of FTNCD?
    - A. PSEN1.
    - B. MAPT.
    - C. APOE-ε4.
    - D. APP.
5. Which of the following features best differentiates FTNCD from Alzheimer's disease?
    - A. FTNCD typically affects older adults, while Alzheimer's is common in younger patients.
    - B. FTNCD begins with behavioral changes, while Alzheimer's starts with memory loss.
    - C. Alzheimer's disease involves more prominent language deficits than FTNCD.
    - D. FTNCD progresses at a slower rate than Alzheimer's disease.
6. In the behavioral variant of FTNCD, which symptom is most commonly observed?
    - A. Impaired visuospatial skills.
    - B. Early apathy and disinhibition.
    - C. Prominent memory impairment.
    - D. Rapid development of motor symptoms.
7. Which intervention is most appropriate for managing FTNCD?
    - A. Antipsychotic medications for cognitive improvement.
    - B. Behavioral management strategies and caregiver support.
    - C. Cholinesterase inhibitors as first-line therapy.
    - D. High-dose antidepressants to treat core symptoms.

True/False Questions

		T	F
1	The DSM-5-TR mandates the presence of personality or behavioral changes for a Frontotemporal Neurocognitive Disorder diagnosis.		
2	The DSM-5-TR distinguishes a behavioral variant and a language (primary progressive aphasia) variant of Frontotemporal Neurocognitive Disorder.		
3	Memory deficits may be relatively minor in the initial stages, compared to behavioral or language changes.		
4	The DSM-5-TR groups all Frontotemporal Neurocognitive Disorder forms under one single diagnosis without subtypes.		
5	According to the DSM-5-TR, the presence of a known genetic mutation supports a "probable" Frontotemporal Neurocognitive Disorder diagnosis.		
6	The DSM-5-TR states that executive dysfunction is not required to diagnose Frontotemporal Neurocognitive Disorder.		
7	A marked decline in social cognition is viewed as characteristic of Frontotemporal Neurocognitive Disorder.		
8	The DSM-5-TR does not allow specifying whether Frontotemporal Neurocognitive Disorder is Major or Mild.		
9	Sudden onset is a typical feature of Frontotemporal Neurocognitive Disorder.		
10	The language variant of Frontotemporal Neurocognitive Disorder may present with progressive aphasia.		

Matching Exercise

1. Early personality and behavioral changes. [ ]
2. Mutation linked to inherited forms of FTNCD. [ ]
3. Neuroimaging finding in FTNCD. [ ]
4. Subtype involving impaired speech production. [ ]
5. Effective intervention for managing behavioral symptoms. [ ]
6. Symptom differentiating FTNCD from Alzheimer's disease. [ ]

Descriptions:

- A. Frontal and temporal lobe atrophy.
- B. Behavioral management strategies.
- C. Behavioral variant.
- D. MAPT mutation.
- E. Nonfluent/agrammatic variant primary progressive aphasia.
- F. Early apathy and disinhibition.

Case Study

Paul, a 62-year-old retired engineer, is brought to the clinic by his wife due to significant personality changes over the past year. He has become socially inappropriate, makes impulsive decisions, and shows little empathy toward others. He frequently forgets appointments and has difficulty planning daily activities. Physical examination reveals no motor deficits. Neuroimaging shows atrophy in the frontal and temporal lobes.

1. Which feature of Paul's presentation is most characteristic of the behavioral variant of FTNCD?
   - A. Social inappropriateness and impulsivity.
   - B. Forgetfulness and poor planning.
   - C. Atrophy in the frontal and temporal lobes.
   - D. Lack of motor symptoms.
2. Which genetic factor should be considered in Paul's case, given his age and presentation?
   - A. APOE-ε4 mutation.
   - B. MAPT mutation.
   - C. PSEN1 mutation.
   - D. APP mutation.
3. What would be the most effective intervention to manage Paul's symptoms and support his family?
   - A. Initiate cholinesterase inhibitors for cognitive improvement.
   - B. Provide behavioral therapy and caregiver support.
   - C. Recommend inpatient care for advanced neurocognitive symptoms.
   - D. Prescribe antipsychotic medications for immediate symptom control.

Answers

Multiple Choice Questions:

1. B
2. D
3. B
4. B
5. B
6. B
7. B

True/False Questions:

1. False
2. True
3. True
4. False
5. True
6. False
7. True
8. False
9. False
10. True

Matching Exercise:

1. C
2. D
3. A
4. E
5. B
6. F

Case Study Answers and Explanations:

1. A - Explanation: Social inappropriateness and impulsivity are hallmark features of the behavioral variant of FTNCD.
2. B - Explanation: MAPT mutations are strongly associated with familial forms of FTNCD.
3. B - Explanation: Behavioral therapy and caregiver support are essential for managing symptoms and improving quality of life.

Major or Mild Neurocognitive Disorder With Lewy Bodies

Multiple Choice Questions

1. Which of the following is a hallmark feature of Neurocognitive Disorder with Lewy Bodies?
    - A. Memory impairment as the earliest symptom.
    - B. Fluctuating cognition with variations in attention and alertness.
    - C. Progressive language deficits with apraxia.
    - D. Stepwise cognitive decline with sudden worsening.
2. A 75-year-old patient with vivid visual hallucinations and Parkinsonian features is diagnosed with Neurocognitive Disorder with Lewy Bodies. Which neuroimaging finding would most likely support this diagnosis?
    - A. Significant hippocampal atrophy on MRI.
    - B. Occipital hypometabolism on PET scan.
    - C. Diffuse white matter lesions on CT.
    - D. Enlarged ventricles on MRI.
3. Which of the following features most reliably differentiates Neurocognitive Disorder with Lewy Bodies from Alzheimer's disease?
    - A. Progressive memory impairment in early stages.
    - B. Prominent visuospatial deficits and vivid visual hallucinations.
    - C. Lack of motor symptoms in early stages.
    - D. Absence of fluctuations in alertness.
4. Which sleep-related condition is frequently associated with Neurocognitive Disorder with Lewy Bodies?
    - A. Insomnia due to generalized anxiety.
    - B. REM sleep behavior disorder.
    - C. Narcolepsy.
    - D. Obstructive sleep apnea.
5. Which treatment strategy is most appropriate for managing cognitive symptoms in Neurocognitive Disorder with Lewy Bodies?
    - A. Dopamine agonists to improve cognition and hallucinations.
    - B. Cholinesterase inhibitors to address cognitive and psychiatric symptoms.
    - C. High-dose antipsychotics to control behavioral symptoms.
    - D. Benzodiazepines for anxiety-related agitation.
6. In patients with Neurocognitive Disorder with Lewy Bodies, why should antipsychotics generally be avoided?
    - A. They worsen memory impairment.
    - B. They can cause severe motor side effects and worsen Parkinsonian features.
    - C. They are ineffective in controlling hallucinations.
    - D. They are contraindicated in all neurocognitive disorders.
7. Which factor increases the risk of developing Neurocognitive Disorder with Lewy Bodies?
    - A. Family history of frontotemporal dementia.
    - B. Long-term untreated hypertension.
    - C. Advanced age and Parkinson's disease.
    - D. Chronic alcohol use.

True/False Questions

		T	F
1	Fluctuating attention and alertness are considered a core feature of Lewy Body Neurocognitive Disorder in the DSM-5-TR.		
2	Visual hallucinations are rare and not included among the essential criteria according to the DSM-5-TR.		
3	To diagnose Major Neurocognitive Disorder with Lewy Bodies, the DSM-5-TR requires at least two key features: visual hallucinations, fluctuations, or parkinsonism.		
4	According to the DSM-5-TR, parkinsonian signs must appear before cognitive deficits to qualify for a Lewy Body diagnosis.		
5	The DSM-5-TR recognizes that REM Sleep Behavior Disorder can provide additional support for a Lewy Body diagnosis.		
6	In Lewy Body Neurocognitive Disorder, cognitive decline typically mirrors stroke-like episodes, according to the DSM-5-TR.		
7	Pronounced sensitivity to antipsychotic medications is noted as a hallmark of Lewy Body Neurocognitive Disorder.		
8	The DSM-5-TR provides specific subtypes of Lewy Body Neurocognitive Disorder, such as a cognition-focused variant or a motor-focused variant.		
9	Distinguishing Lewy Body Dementia from Parkinson's Disease Dementia partly hinges on whether motor symptoms predate or follow the onset of cognitive decline.		
10	If cognitive decline and parkinsonism arise simultaneously, the DSM-5-TR rules out Lewy Body Dementia in favor of Parkinson's Disease Dementia.		

Matching Exercise

1. Core feature involving variations in cognition and alertness. [ ]
2. Typical visual hallucination in this disorder. [ ]
3. Neuroimaging finding supporting the diagnosis. [ ]
4. Sleep disorder commonly associated with this condition. [ ]
5. Common motor symptom observed in this disorder. [ ]
6. Treatment used for cognitive and psychiatric symptoms. [ ]

Descriptions:

- A. Fluctuating attention and alertness.
- B. Vivid, well-formed hallucinations.
- C. Occipital hypometabolism.
- D. REM sleep behavior disorder.
- E. Parkinsonian features.
- F. Cholinesterase inhibitors.

Case Study

Anna, a 74-year-old woman, presents with progressive cognitive decline and recurrent vivid visual hallucinations of people and animals. Her family reports significant fluctuations in her attention and alertness, as well as episodes of rigidity and shuffling gait. Neuroimaging reveals occipital hypometabolism, and she has a history of REM sleep behavior disorder.

1. Which symptom in Anna's presentation most strongly supports the diagnosis of Neurocognitive Disorder with Lewy Bodies?
   - A. Vivid visual hallucinations.
   - B. Fluctuating alertness and attention.
   - C. Rigidity and shuffling gait.
   - D. History of REM sleep behavior disorder.
2. Which treatment would be most appropriate for managing Anna's cognitive symptoms?
   - A. Cholinesterase inhibitors.
   - B. Dopamine agonists.
   - C. High-dose antipsychotics.
   - D. Benzodiazepines.
3. Why are antipsychotics contraindicated in Anna's case?
   - A. They are ineffective for hallucinations.
   - B. They exacerbate her motor symptoms and may cause severe adverse reactions.
   - C. They interact with cholinesterase inhibitors.
   - D. They worsen fluctuations in alertness.

Answers

Multiple Choice Questions:

1. B
2. B
3. B
4. B
5. B
6. B
7. C

True/False Questions:

1. True
2. False
3. True
4. False
5. True
6. False
7. True
8. False
9. True
10. False

Matching Exercise:

1. A
2. B
3. C
4. D
5. E
6. F

Case Study Answers and Explanations:

1. B - Explanation: Fluctuating alertness and attention are hallmark features of Neurocognitive Disorder with Lewy Bodies.
2. A - Explanation: Cholinesterase inhibitors are first-line treatments for managing cognitive and psychiatric symptoms.
3. B - Explanation: Antipsychotics can worsen motor symptoms and cause severe sensitivity reactions in these patients.

Major or Mild Neurocognitive Disorder Due to Parkinson's Disease

Multiple Choice Questions

1. Which of the following mechanisms most directly links motor and cognitive decline in Neurocognitive Disorder due to Parkinson's Disease?
    - A. Loss of cholinergic neurons in the nucleus basalis of Meynert.
    - B. Alpha-synuclein accumulation in cortical and subcortical regions.
    - C. Neurofibrillary tangles in the hippocampus.
    - D. Demyelination of white matter tracts in the frontal lobe.
2. In Neurocognitive Disorder due to Parkinson's Disease, which cognitive domain is typically affected first?
    - A. Episodic memory.
    - B. Executive functioning.
    - C. Language processing.
    - D. Visuospatial abilities.
3. Which of the following criteria differentiates Neurocognitive Disorder due to Parkinson's Disease from Dementia with Lewy Bodies?
    - A. Presence of vivid visual hallucinations.
    - B. Onset of cognitive decline at least one year after motor symptoms.
    - C. Rapid progression of cognitive and motor symptoms.
    - D. Response to anticholinergic medications.
4. Which neuroimaging finding is most indicative of cognitive decline in Parkinson's Disease?
    - A. Hippocampal atrophy.
    - B. Frontal cortical hypometabolism on PET scan.
    - C. Widespread white matter hyperintensities on MRI.
    - D. Ventricular enlargement on CT.
5. Which genetic mutation is most strongly associated with Parkinson's Disease and its related neurocognitive disorders?
    - A. PSEN1.
    - B. MAPT.
    - C. LRRK2.
    - D. APOE-ε4.
6. Which pharmacological intervention is most appropriate for addressing both cognitive decline and psychiatric symptoms in this disorder?
    - A. High-dose antipsychotics.
    - B. Cholinesterase inhibitors.
    - C. Dopamine agonists.
    - D. NMDA receptor antagonists.
7. In advanced Parkinson's Disease, which of the following non-motor symptoms is most predictive of progression to Major Neurocognitive Disorder?
    - A. Orthostatic hypotension.
    - B. REM sleep behavior disorder.
    - C. Constipation.
    - D. Chronic fatigue.

True/False Questions

		T	F
1	In the DSM-5-TR, Parkinson's Disease Neurocognitive Disorder requires that motor symptoms precede cognitive decline.		
2	The DSM-5-TR includes pronounced antipsychotic sensitivity as an essential diagnostic criterion for Parkinson's Disease Neurocognitive Disorder.		
3	If cognitive deficits arise more than one year after the onset of motor symptoms, the DSM-5-TR favors Parkinson's Disease Neurocognitive Disorder over Lewy Body Dementia.		
4	The presence of isolated visual hallucinations, without cognitive decline, is sufficient for a Parkinson's Disease Neurocognitive Disorder diagnosis in the DSM-5-TR.		
5	The DSM-5-TR recognizes both Mild and Major forms of Parkinson's Disease Neurocognitive Disorder, based on functional impairment.		
6	A decline in executive functions (e.g., planning difficulties) can be an early indicator of Parkinson's Disease Neurocognitive Disorder.		
7	A Parkinson's Disease Neurocognitive Disorder diagnosis is consistent with the DSM-5-TR if cognitive symptoms emerge at least one year after motor onset.		
8	The DSM-5-TR identifies notable attention fluctuations as a hallmark of Parkinson's Disease Neurocognitive Disorder, similar to Lewy Body pathology.		
9	REM sleep behavior disorder is described as a supportive clinical marker for diagnosing Parkinson's Disease Neurocognitive Disorder in the DSM-5-TR.		
10	A gradual deterioration of visuospatial skills is listed among the possible presentations of Parkinson's Disease Neurocognitive Disorder in the DSM-5-TR.		

Matching Exercise

1. Cognitive decline occurring after motor symptoms are well established. [ ]
2. Common genetic mutation associated with Parkinson's Disease. [ ]
3. Early cognitive domain affected in this disorder. [ ]
4. Neuroimaging finding indicative of cognitive impairment. [ ]
5. Non-pharmacological strategy to address executive dysfunction. [ ]
6. Recommended pharmacological treatment for cognitive symptoms. [ ]

Descriptions:

- A. LRRK2 mutation.
- B. Executive dysfunction.
- C. Frontal cortical hypometabolism.
- D. Structured daily routines.
- E. Cholinesterase inhibitors.
- F. Cognitive decline follows motor symptoms.

Case Study

Mark, a 72-year-old man with a 12-year history of Parkinson's Disease, is evaluated for progressive cognitive decline. His wife reports increasing difficulty with planning, organizing tasks, and managing finances. He experiences vivid visual hallucinations and occasional confusion, especially in the evenings. Neuroimaging reveals frontal hypometabolism, and his symptoms began several years after the onset of motor dysfunction.

1. What aspect of Mark's history most strongly supports a diagnosis of Neurocognitive Disorder due to Parkinson's Disease?
    - A. Onset of cognitive symptoms years after motor dysfunction.
    - B. Presence of vivid visual hallucinations.
    - C. Difficulty managing finances and organizing tasks.
    - D. Frontal hypometabolism on neuroimaging.
2. Which intervention would be most appropriate to manage Mark's cognitive symptoms?
    - A. High-dose dopamine agonists.
    - B. Cholinesterase inhibitors.
    - C. Antipsychotics for visual hallucinations.
    - D. Benzodiazepines for evening confusion.
3. Why is it important to differentiate this condition from Dementia with Lewy Bodies in Mark's case?
    - A. The treatment approaches differ significantly between the two conditions.
    - B. Dementia with Lewy Bodies has a more favorable prognosis.
    - C. Parkinson's-related cognitive decline does not involve hallucinations.
    - D. Motor symptoms precede cognitive decline in Dementia with Lewy Bodies.

Answers

Multiple Choice Questions:
1. B
2. B
3. B
4. B
5. C
6. B
7. B

True/False Questions:
1. True
2. False
3. True
4. False
5. True
6. True
7. True
8. False
9. False
10. False

Matching Exercise:
1. F
2. A
3. B
4. C
5. D
6. E

Case Study Answers and Explanations:
1. A - Explanation: The temporal relationship between motor and cognitive symptoms is key to this diagnosis.
2. B - Explanation: Cholinesterase inhibitors are first-line treatments for cognitive symptoms in this condition.
3. A - Explanation: Differentiating these conditions ensures that appropriate therapies and expectations are set for the patient and caregiver.

Major or Mild Neurocognitive Disorder Due to HIV Infection

Multiple Choice Questions

1. Which of the following pathophysiological mechanisms most directly contributes to Neurocognitive Disorder due to HIV?
    - A. Neuroinflammation caused by viral proteins and infected macrophages.
    - B. Amyloid plaque deposition in cortical regions.
    - C. Autoimmune-mediated demyelination.
    - D. Alpha-synuclein aggregation in the basal ganglia.
2. What is the most common cognitive domain affected in the early stages of Neurocognitive Disorder due to HIV?
    - A. Episodic memory.
    - B. Executive functioning.
    - C. Visuospatial skills.
    - D. Language processing.
3. In a patient with HIV and mild cognitive impairment, which clinical feature would most strongly suggest progression to Major Neurocognitive Disorder?
    - A. Difficulty recalling recent events.
    - B. Impairment in managing basic activities of daily living.
    - C. Persistent fatigue and low-grade fever.
    - D. Poor adherence to antiretroviral therapy.
4. Which laboratory finding is most predictive of an increased risk of Neurocognitive Disorder in patients with HIV?
    - A. CD4 count <200 cells/μL.
    - B. Elevated liver enzymes.
    - C. Viral load suppressed to undetectable levels.
    - D. Presence of opportunistic infections.
5. Which neuroimaging finding is most commonly observed in Neurocognitive Disorder due to HIV?
    - A. Generalized brain atrophy with subcortical prominence.
    - B. White matter hyperintensities in the periventricular region.
    - C. Hippocampal atrophy.
    - D. Focal cortical infarcts.
6. Which of the following is the most effective strategy to reduce the risk of Neurocognitive Disorder in HIV-positive patients?
    - A. Early initiation and strict adherence to antiretroviral therapy.
    - B. Cognitive-behavioral therapy focusing on memory recall.
    - C. Long-term use of antipsychotics to prevent cognitive decline.
    - D. Periodic prophylaxis against opportunistic infections.
7. How does the presentation of Neurocognitive Disorder due to HIV differ from Alzheimer's Disease?
    - A. Memory impairment is the earliest symptom in both disorders.
    - B. Neurocognitive Disorder due to HIV has a more rapid progression.
    - C. Alzheimer's Disease involves significant visuospatial deficits early on.
    - D. Neurocognitive Disorder due to HIV primarily affects motor and executive functions.

True/False Questions

		T	F
1	Structural brain imaging is required to diagnose HIV Neurocognitive Disorder in the DSM-5-TR.		
2	The DSM-5-TR allows specifying whether HIV Neurocognitive Disorder is Mild or Major, based on functional independence.		
3	Once HIV viral load is suppressed, the DSM-5-TR automatically rules out HIV Neurocognitive Disorder.		
4	Motor disturbances and behavioral dysfunction can appear in HIV Neurocognitive Disorder, not only memory issues.		
5	The DSM-5-TR prohibits diagnosing HIV Neurocognitive Disorder if another psychiatric condition, such as major depression, is present.		
6	The DSM-5-TR notes that antiretroviral therapy may affect the progression of HIV Neurocognitive Disorder.		
7	HIV Neurocognitive Disorder may manifest with psychomotor slowing and reduced processing speed, even without obvious memory deficits.		
8	The DSM-5-TR requires ruling out other medical or neurological causes of cognitive decline before diagnosing HIV Neurocognitive Disorder.		
9	A fluctuating decline in attention is the most common presentation of HIV Neurocognitive Disorder, according to the DSM-5-TR.		
10	The presence of asymptomatic HIV infection, without any sign of cognitive decline, is sufficient for an HIV Neurocognitive Disorder diagnosis.		

Matching Exercise

1. Early cognitive domain most affected in this disorder. [ ]
2. Key laboratory finding predicting neurocognitive risk. [ ]
3. Neuroimaging finding commonly associated with this condition. [ ]
4. Primary strategy to reduce the risk of progression. [ ]
5. Clinical feature suggesting progression to Major Neurocognitive Disorder. [ ]
6. Mechanism contributing to cognitive decline. [ ]

Descriptions:

- A. Executive functioning.
- B. CD4 count <200 cells/μL.
- C. Generalized brain atrophy.
- D. Adherence to antiretroviral therapy.
- E. Impairment in basic daily activities.
- F. Neuroinflammation and macrophage activation.

Case Study

James, a 45-year-old man with a history of untreated HIV infection, presents with increasing forgetfulness, difficulty concentrating, and trouble completing tasks at work. His CD4 count is 150 cells/μL, and his viral load is elevated. Neuroimaging reveals generalized brain atrophy. He reports occasional confusion and struggles with daily activities such as managing finances and preparing meals.

1. What feature in James's case most strongly suggests progression to Major Neurocognitive Disorder due to HIV?
    - A. Elevated viral load.
    - B. Impairment in basic daily activities.
    - C. Forgetfulness and difficulty concentrating.
    - D. Generalized brain atrophy on neuroimaging.
2. Which intervention is most critical to managing James's condition and preventing further cognitive decline?
    - A. Initiation of antiretroviral therapy.
    - B. Prescription of cholinesterase inhibitors.
    - C. Cognitive-behavioral therapy to address memory deficits.
    - D. Antipsychotics to manage confusion.
3. Why is early initiation of antiretroviral therapy essential in preventing Neurocognitive Disorder due to HIV?
    - A. It directly repairs neuronal damage caused by the virus.
    - B. It prevents opportunistic infections, which are the primary cause of cognitive decline.
    - C. It suppresses viral replication, reducing neuroinflammation and damage.
    - D. It enhances executive functioning by increasing dopamine levels.

Answers

Multiple Choice Questions:

1. A
2. B
3. B
4. A
5. A
6. A
7. D

True/False Questions:

1. False
2. True
3. False
4. True
5. False
6. True
7. True
8. True
9. False
10. False

Matching Exercise:

1. A
2. B
3. C
4. D
5. E
6. F

Case Study Answers and Explanations:

1. B - Explanation: Impairment in basic daily activities indicates progression to Major Neurocognitive Disorder.
2. A - Explanation: Antiretroviral therapy is essential to suppress viral replication and reduce neuroinflammation.
3. C - Explanation: Suppression of viral replication reduces the neuroinflammatory response and prevents further neuronal damage.

Substance/Medication-Induced Major or Mild Neurocognitive Disorder

Multiple Choice Questions

1. Which of the following substances is most commonly associated with Neurocognitive Disorder due to chronic use?
    - A. Cannabis.
    - B. Alcohol.
    - C. Nicotine.
    - D. LSD.
2. What is the primary mechanism by which chronic alcohol use leads to Neurocognitive Disorder?
    - A. Alpha-synuclein accumulation.
    - B. Vitamin B1 (thiamine) deficiency and associated brain damage.
    - C. Dopaminergic neuron loss in the substantia nigra.
    - D. Accumulation of amyloid plaques in cortical regions.
3. A patient with a history of long-term benzodiazepine use presents with cognitive impairment. Which of the following domains is most likely to be affected?
    - A. Episodic memory.
    - B. Language processing.
    - C. Executive functioning and attention.
    - D. Visuospatial skills.
4. Which clinical feature is most indicative of Substance/Medication-Induced Neurocognitive Disorder compared to other neurocognitive disorders?
    - A. Insidious onset with progressive memory impairment.
    - B. Stepwise progression with focal neurological deficits.
    - C. Cognitive decline temporally associated with substance use or withdrawal.
    - D. Predominantly language deficits in early stages.
5. Which neuroimaging finding is most commonly associated with Neurocognitive Disorder due to chronic alcohol use?
    - A. Hippocampal atrophy.
    - B. Diffuse cortical atrophy with ventricular enlargement.
    - C. Subcortical infarcts and white matter hyperintensities.
    - D. Occipital hypometabolism.
6. A patient undergoing withdrawal from methamphetamine use exhibits cognitive deficits. Which of the following symptoms is most likely reversible with sustained abstinence?
    - A. Executive dysfunction.
    - B. Long-term memory deficits.
    - C. Severe visuospatial impairment.
    - D. Profound personality changes.
7. Which intervention is most effective for managing Substance/Medication-Induced Neurocognitive Disorder?
    - A. Cholinesterase inhibitors.
    - B. Structured abstinence programs combined with cognitive rehabilitation.
    - C. High-dose benzodiazepines to manage withdrawal symptoms.
    - D. Dopamine agonists to restore cognitive function.

True/False Questions

		T	F
1	The DSM-5-TR requires that Major Substance-Induced Neurocognitive Disorder interfere with essential daily tasks (e.g., hygiene, finances).		
2	A mild deficit in only one cognitive domain, without loss of independence, suffices for Major Substance-Induced Neurocognitive Disorder.		
3	To differentiate Mild from Major, the DSM-5-TR considers both functional impairment and social support.		
4	Ruling out other medical or psychiatric causes is mandatory before diagnosing a Substance-Induced Neurocognitive Disorder (Mild or Major).		
5	Substance-Induced Mild Neurocognitive Disorder can be diagnosed even without specific withdrawal symptoms.		
6	Impairments in complex attention or memory help determine severity in Substance-Induced Neurocognitive Disorder.		
7	If daily functioning is only partly compromised, the condition is likely Mild Substance-Induced Neurocognitive Disorder.		
8	Repeated alcohol intoxication can lead to Alcohol-Induced Major Neurocognitive Disorder even without obvious brain damage.		
9	Constant supervision needs usually indicate Major Substance-Induced Neurocognitive Disorder.		
10	One can diagnose both Substance Use Disorder and Mild Substance-Induced Neurocognitive Disorder for the same substance if all criteria are met.		

Matching Exercise

1. Primary mechanism of cognitive decline in alcohol-related cases. [ ]
2. Cognitive domain often affected by long-term benzodiazepine use. [ ]
3. Neuroimaging finding in chronic alcohol-related Neurocognitive Disorder. [ ]
4. Key reversible symptom with abstinence in methamphetamine-induced cases. [ ]
5. Effective intervention for managing this disorder. [ ]
6. Feature differentiating this disorder from other neurocognitive disorders. [ ]

Descriptions:

- A. Thiamine deficiency and associated brain damage.
- B. Executive functioning and attention.
- C. Diffuse cortical atrophy with ventricular enlargement.
- D. Structured abstinence programs.
- E. Reversal of executive dysfunction.
- F. Temporal association with substance use or withdrawal.

Case Study

Liam, a 58-year-old man with a 30-year history of alcohol use disorder, presents with memory deficits, difficulty focusing, and frequent confusion. He reports significant struggles with executive tasks, such as managing finances. Neuroimaging shows diffuse cortical atrophy and ventricular enlargement. Laboratory studies reveal a low thiamine level.

1. Which finding in Liam's case most strongly supports the diagnosis of Substance/Medication-Induced Neurocognitive Disorder?
   - A. Diffuse cortical atrophy and ventricular enlargement.
   - B. Low thiamine levels associated with chronic alcohol use.
   - C. Difficulty managing finances and executive tasks.
   - D. Frequent confusion and memory deficits.
2. What is the most appropriate first-line intervention for Liam's condition?
   - A. Initiate cholinesterase inhibitors for cognitive support.
   - B. Provide thiamine supplementation and implement an abstinence program.
   - C. Prescribe antipsychotics to address confusion.
   - D. Begin dopamine agonists to enhance executive functioning.
3. Which mechanism explains Liam's cognitive deficits?
   - A. Direct neurotoxicity from alcohol on cortical neurons.
   - B. Oxidative stress and demyelination of white matter.
   - C. Thiamine deficiency causing Wernicke-Korsakoff syndrome.
   - D. Amyloid plaque accumulation from chronic alcohol exposure.

Answers

Multiple Choice Questions:

1. B
2. B
3. C
4. C
5. B
6. A
7. B

True/False Questions:

1. True
2. False
3. True
4. True
5. True
6. True
7. True
8. True
9. True
10. True

Matching Exercise:

1. A
2. B
3. C
4. E
5. D
6. F

Case Study Answers and Explanations:

1. B - Explanation: Chronic alcohol use and thiamine deficiency directly contribute to Liam's cognitive deficits.
2. B - Explanation: Thiamine supplementation addresses the underlying nutritional deficiency, and abstinence prevents further damage.
3. C - Explanation: Thiamine deficiency leads to neuronal damage associated with Wernicke-Korsakoff syndrome.

Major or Mild Neurocognitive Disorder Due to Traumatic Brain Injury

Multiple Choice Questions

1. Which of the following findings is most commonly associated with Neurocognitive Disorder due to Traumatic Brain Injury (TBI)?
    - A. Diffuse white matter damage on neuroimaging.
    - B. Hippocampal atrophy.
    - C. Cortical amyloid plaques.
    - D. Substantia nigra degeneration.
2. In the context of TBI, which of the following symptoms is most indicative of progression to Major Neurocognitive Disorder?
    - A. Persistent headaches and dizziness.
    - B. Impaired ability to perform basic daily activities.
    - C. Episodic confusion resolving within hours.
    - D. Mild forgetfulness with preserved independence.
3. Which cognitive domain is most commonly affected in Neurocognitive Disorder due to TBI?
    - A. Language processing.
    - B. Executive functioning and attention.
    - C. Long-term memory retrieval.
    - D. Visuospatial reasoning.
4. Which factor increases the risk of developing Neurocognitive Disorder after TBI?
    - A. Presence of a mild concussion without loss of consciousness.
    - B. Repeated TBIs, as seen in contact sports.
    - C. Younger age at the time of injury.
    - D. No history of pre-existing medical conditions.
5. Which neuroimaging modality is most sensitive for detecting diffuse axonal injury in TBI?
    - A. CT scan.
    - B. PET scan.
    - C. Diffusion tensor imaging (DTI).
    - D. EEG.
6. Which of the following best differentiates Neurocognitive Disorder due to TBI from Alzheimer's Disease?
    - A. Presence of early memory impairment in both conditions.
    - B. Neuroimaging findings showing hippocampal atrophy in both.
    - C. TBI-related cognitive decline often includes emotional lability and irritability.
    - D. Alzheimer's Disease often shows sudden onset after physical trauma.
7. Which intervention is most effective in managing cognitive symptoms in Neurocognitive Disorder due to TBI?
    - A. Antipsychotics for behavioral regulation.
    - B. Structured cognitive rehabilitation programs.
    - C. High-dose benzodiazepines for anxiety.
    - D. Cholinesterase inhibitors to enhance memory.

True/False Questions

		T	F
1	The DSM-5-TR allows a diagnosis of Mild Neurocognitive Disorder due to Traumatic Brain Injury (TBI) even if the injury occurred many years ago, as long as current cognitive decline is linked to that event.		
2	If cognitive symptoms first appear two months after the injury, the DSM-5-TR automatically rules out TBI-related Neurocognitive Disorder.		
3	A single brief (under 30 minutes) loss of consciousness can still support a Major Neurocognitive Disorder diagnosis due to TBI, if functional decline is substantial.		
4	A concussion with no radiological evidence of brain lesion can never lead to a Mild Neurocognitive Disorder due to TBI, according to the DSM-5-TR.		
5	In Major Neurocognitive Disorder due to TBI, the DSM-5-TR emphasizes impairment in essential daily activities as a diagnostic criterion.		
6	The DSM-5-TR allows ruling out TBI-related Neurocognitive Disorder if there is a clear clinical recovery within the first three months post-injury, with no residual signs.		
7	TBI-related Neurocognitive Disorder can include behavioral and emotional disturbances, not just memory or attention deficits.		
8	Immediate cerebral anoxia following head trauma always indicates Major Neurocognitive Disorder due to TBI, per the DSM-5-TR.		
9	In some cases, Mild Neurocognitive Disorder due to TBI can be diagnosed even without a loss of consciousness if the clinical picture is consistent with traumatic injury.		
10	If cognitive decline is linked to multiple head injuries, the DSM-5-TR still recommends categorizing it as a TBI-related Neurocognitive Disorder, provided the traumatic events are documented.		

Matching Exercise

1. Cognitive domain commonly affected in TBI-related neurocognitive disorders. [ ]
2. Neuroimaging finding associated with diffuse axonal injury. [ ]
3. Primary intervention for cognitive rehabilitation. [ ]
4. Emotional symptom frequently observed in TBI-related cases. [ ]
5. Risk factor for developing neurocognitive disorder post-TBI. [ ]
6. Neuroimaging modality most sensitive for axonal damage. [ ]

Descriptions:

- A. Executive functioning and attention.
- B. Diffuse white matter damage.
- C. Structured cognitive rehabilitation.
- D. Emotional lability.
- E. Repeated TBIs.
- F. Diffusion tensor imaging (DTI).

Case Study

David, a 52-year-old construction worker, sustained a moderate TBI two years ago in a workplace accident. He now experiences difficulty focusing, irritability, and forgetfulness, which have begun to interfere with his ability to perform daily tasks. His family notes that he frequently forgets appointments and has become more emotionally reactive. Neuroimaging reveals evidence of diffuse axonal injury.

1. Which feature most strongly supports a diagnosis of Major Neurocognitive Disorder due to TBI in David's case?
    - A. Forgetfulness and irritability.
    - B. Difficulty focusing and performing daily tasks.
    - C. Evidence of diffuse axonal injury on neuroimaging.
    - D. Emotional reactivity.
2. What intervention would be most appropriate to address David's cognitive symptoms?
    - A. Prescribe cholinesterase inhibitors.
    - B. Initiate a structured cognitive rehabilitation program.
    - C. Use antipsychotics to manage irritability.
    - D. Begin high-dose benzodiazepines to reduce anxiety.
3. What factor in David's history most likely contributed to his persistent symptoms?
    - A. Moderate severity of initial TBI.
    - B. Delay in seeking cognitive rehabilitation.
    - C. Emotional reactivity and irritability.
    - D. Pre-existing medical conditions.

Answers

Multiple Choice Questions:

1. A
2. B
3. B
4. B
5. C
6. C
7. B

True/False Questions:

1. True
2. False
3. True
4. False
5. True
6. True
7. True
8. False
9. True
10. True

Matching Exercise:

1. A
2. B
3. C
4. D
5. E
6. F

Case Study Answers and Explanations:

1. B - Explanation: Difficulty performing daily tasks suggests progression to Major Neurocognitive Disorder.
2. B - Explanation: Cognitive rehabilitation is the cornerstone of treatment for TBI-related cognitive decline.
3. A - Explanation: Moderate TBI increases the risk of long-term cognitive deficits, especially without timely intervention.

Major or Mild Neurocognitive Disorder Due to Prion Disease

Multiple Choice Questions

1. Which of the following is the most characteristic feature of Neurocognitive Disorder due to Prion Disease?
    - A. Gradual cognitive decline over several years.
    - B. Rapidly progressive cognitive decline with myoclonus.
    - C. Prominent visuospatial deficits in early stages.
    - D. Persistent language impairment as the first symptom.
2. In Neurocognitive Disorder due to Prion Disease, which finding is most suggestive of Creutzfeldt-Jakob Disease (CJD)?
    - A. Diffuse cortical atrophy on MRI.
    - B. Periodic sharp wave complexes on EEG.
    - C. Hippocampal atrophy on neuroimaging.
    - D. Subcortical infarcts on CT.
3. Which biomarker in the cerebrospinal fluid (CSF) is most commonly associated with Prion Disease?
    - A. Elevated amyloid-beta levels.
    - B. Increased tau protein and 14-3-3 protein.
    - C. Alpha-synuclein aggregates.
    - D. Reduced acetylcholine esterase activity.
4. Which of the following symptoms is least likely in the early stages of Neurocognitive Disorder due to Prion Disease?
    - A. Rapid progression of memory impairment.
    - B. Visual hallucinations.
    - C. Ataxia and motor abnormalities.
    - D. Prominent apathy and disinhibition.
5. Which neuroimaging finding is most commonly observed in Prion Disease?
    - A. Hyperintensities in the basal ganglia and cortical ribboning on diffusion-weighted MRI.
    - B. Occipital hypometabolism on PET scan.
    - C. Ventricular enlargement on CT.
    - D. White matter hyperintensities on T2-weighted MRI.
6. Which genetic mutation is strongly associated with familial forms of Prion Disease?
    - A. PRNP gene mutation.
    - B. PSEN1 gene mutation.
    - C. APOE-ε4 allele.
    - D. MAPT gene mutation.
7. Which of the following is the most appropriate management approach for Neurocognitive Disorder due to Prion Disease?
    - A. Disease-modifying therapy targeting prion replication.
    - B. Symptomatic management and palliative care.
    - C. High-dose antipsychotics for behavioral symptoms.
    - D. Cholinesterase inhibitors to improve cognition.

True/False Questions

		T	F
1	The DSM-5-TR describes a gradual, stable onset as the typical presentation of Prion Disease Neurocognitive Disorder.		
2	Motor changes, such as myoclonus, may appear in the Major form of Prion Disease Neurocognitive Disorder.		
3	The DSM-5-TR acknowledges a Mild variant of Prion Disease Neurocognitive Disorder, even though this condition often has a rapid course.		
4	Laboratory tests (e.g., 14-3-3 protein) or imaging findings are never considered by the DSM-5-TR for diagnosis.		
5	A hallmark of prion disease is rapid progression, with marked deterioration over just a few months.		
6	If the disease course extends beyond a year, the DSM-5-TR requires ruling out other conditions like Alzheimer's Disease Neurocognitive Disorder.		
7	Prion Disease Neurocognitive Disorder can be diagnosed even when degeneration is confined solely to the motor domain.		
8	The DSM-5-TR allows specifying "Probable" or "Possible" prion disease based on clinical data, EEG, or imaging.		
9	In Major Prion Disease Neurocognitive Disorder, the decline must significantly interfere with daily functioning.		
10	According to the DSM-5-TR, Creutzfeldt-Jakob disease never presents with an acute or confusional onset.		

Matching Exercise

1. Rapid cognitive decline with myoclonus. [ ]
2. EEG finding associated with Creutzfeldt-Jakob Disease. [ ]
3. Biomarker commonly found in cerebrospinal fluid. [ ]
4. Neuroimaging finding indicative of Prion Disease. [ ]
5. Genetic mutation linked to familial forms. [ ]
6. Appropriate management approach. [ ]

Descriptions:

- A. Periodic sharp wave complexes.
- B. Increased tau protein and 14-3-3 protein.
- C. PRNP gene mutation.
- D. Hyperintensities in basal ganglia and cortical ribboning.
- E. Symptomatic and palliative care.
- F. Creutzfeldt-Jakob Disease (CJD).

Case Study

Emily, a 61-year-old woman, is brought to the clinic due to rapidly progressive cognitive decline over the past six months. Her family reports that she has difficulty remembering recent events and has developed involuntary muscle jerks. Neuroimaging reveals hyperintensities in the basal ganglia on MRI, and EEG shows periodic sharp wave complexes. CSF analysis demonstrates elevated tau protein and 14-3-3 protein.

1. Which finding in Emily's case most strongly supports a diagnosis of Creutzfeldt-Jakob Disease?
   - A. Rapid progression of cognitive decline.
   - B. Involuntary muscle jerks.
   - C. Hyperintensities in the basal ganglia on MRI.
   - D. Elevated tau protein and 14-3-3 protein in CSF.
2. What is the most appropriate management strategy for Emily's condition?
   - A. Initiate disease-modifying therapy to halt prion replication.
   - B. Provide symptomatic management and focus on palliative care.
   - C. Prescribe cholinesterase inhibitors for cognitive improvement.
   - D. Administer antipsychotics to manage behavioral symptoms.
3. What is the pathophysiological mechanism underlying Emily's symptoms?
   - A. Deposition of amyloid plaques and neurofibrillary tangles.
   - B. Misfolded prion proteins causing progressive neurodegeneration.
   - C. Alpha-synuclein aggregation in cortical regions.
   - D. Chronic neuroinflammation and demyelination.

Answers

Multiple Choice Questions:
1. B
2. B
3. B
4. D
5. A
6. A
7. B

True/False Questions:
1. False
2. True
3. True
4. False
5. True
6. False
7. False
8. True
9. True
10. False

Matching Exercise:
1. F
2. A
3. B
4. D
5. C
6. E

Case Study Answers and Explanations:
1. D - Explanation: Elevated tau protein and 14-3-3 protein in CSF are key biomarkers supporting the diagnosis of CJD.
2. B - Explanation: Palliative care focuses on managing symptoms, as there are no curative treatments for Prion Disease.
3. B - Explanation: Misfolded prion proteins cause progressive neurodegeneration, leading to rapid cognitive decline and motor symptoms.

Major or Mild Neurocognitive Disorder Due to Huntington's Disease

Multiple Choice Questions

1. Which of the following is the earliest cognitive domain affected in Neurocognitive Disorder due to Huntington's Disease?
    - A. Episodic memory.
    - B. Executive functioning.
    - C. Language processing.
    - D. Visuospatial skills.
2. What is the genetic basis of Huntington's Disease?
    - A. PRNP gene mutation.
    - B. Expansion of CAG trinucleotide repeats in the HTT gene.
    - C. APOE-ε4 allele polymorphism.
    - D. PSEN1 gene mutation.
3. Which neuroimaging finding is most commonly associated with Neurocognitive Disorder due to Huntington's Disease?
    - A. Hippocampal atrophy.
    - B. Caudate nucleus and putamen atrophy.
    - C. Occipital hypometabolism on PET.
    - D. White matter hyperintensities on MRI.
4. In addition to cognitive symptoms, which motor symptom is most characteristic of Huntington's Disease?
    - A. Resting tremor.
    - B. Chorea.
    - C. Bradykinesia.
    - D. Rigidity.
5. Which of the following features differentiates Neurocognitive Disorder due to Huntington's Disease from Parkinson's Disease?
    - A. Presence of chorea in Huntington's Disease.
    - B. Cognitive decline before motor symptoms in Huntington's Disease.
    - C. Executive dysfunction as a primary symptom in Parkinson's Disease.
    - D. Memory loss as the first symptom in Huntington's Disease.
6. Which of the following strategies is most effective in managing behavioral symptoms in Huntington's Disease?
    - A. High-dose dopamine agonists.
    - B. Antidepressants and antipsychotics.
    - C. Cholinesterase inhibitors.
    - D. Structured cognitive-behavioral therapy.
7. Which of the following factors is most predictive of disease severity in Huntington's Disease?
    - A. Age of onset of symptoms.
    - B. Length of CAG repeats in the HTT gene.
    - C. Presence of psychiatric symptoms.
    - D. Severity of motor symptoms.

True/False Questions

		T	F
1	Under the DSM-5-TR, Huntington's Disease Neurocognitive Disorder can be diagnosed even without choreiform movements if there is clear cognitive decline.		
2	The difference between Mild and Major forms depends on whether daily living activities require assistance.		
3	A negative genetic test for Huntington's automatically rules out Huntington's Disease Neurocognitive Disorder in the DSM-5-TR.		
4	Personality changes and planning difficulties are common features, in addition to motor symptoms.		
5	If motor symptoms precede cognitive decline by at least one year, the DSM-5-TR rules out Huntington's Disease Neurocognitive Disorder.		
6	The DSM-5-TR allows specifying both Mild and Major Huntington's Disease Neurocognitive Disorder.		
7	An insidious onset of cognitive symptoms is a key feature according to the DSM-5-TR.		
8	Comorbidity with depression or irritability is not considered relevant in the DSM-5-TR for diagnosing Huntington's Disease Neurocognitive Disorder.		
9	The DSM-5-TR advises assessing both executive deficits and memory problems in Huntington's.		
10	A rapid decline over a few weeks is described by the DSM-5-TR as the typical presentation of Huntington's Disease.		

Matching Exercise

1. Early cognitive domain most affected in Huntington's Disease. [ ]
2. Genetic basis of Huntington's Disease. [ ]
3. Common neuroimaging finding. [ ]
4. Primary motor symptom. [ ]
5. Management strategy for behavioral symptoms. [ ]
6. Predictor of disease severity. [ ]

Descriptions:

- A. Executive functioning.
- B. Expansion of CAG repeats in the HTT gene.
- C. Caudate nucleus atrophy.
- D. Chorea.
- E. Antidepressants and antipsychotics.
- F. Length of CAG repeats.

Case Study

John, a 42-year-old man with a family history of Huntington's Disease, presents with increasing difficulty in decision-making, frequent irritability, and involuntary movements of his arms and legs. Neuroimaging reveals caudate nucleus atrophy, and genetic testing confirms an expansion of CAG repeats in the HTT gene.

1. Which symptom in John's presentation most strongly supports the diagnosis of Huntington's Disease?
    - A. Difficulty in decision-making.
    - B. Involuntary movements of his arms and legs.
    - C. Family history of Huntington's Disease.
    - D. Caudate nucleus atrophy on neuroimaging.
2. What is the primary focus of managing John's behavioral symptoms?
    - A. Initiating high-dose dopamine agonists.
    - B. Prescribing antidepressants and antipsychotics.
    - C. Cognitive rehabilitation for decision-making.
    - D. Starting cholinesterase inhibitors.
3. Why is the length of CAG repeats important in John's case?
    - A. It determines the severity and progression of the disease.
    - B. It confirms the presence of psychiatric symptoms.
    - C. It predicts the age at which motor symptoms will resolve.
    - D. It correlates with the risk of developing memory impairment.

Answers

Multiple Choice Questions:

1. B
2. B
3. B
4. B
5. A
6. B
7. B

True/False Questions:

1. True
2. True
3. False
4. True
5. False
6. True
7. True
8. False
9. True
10. False

Matching Exercise:

1. A
2. B
3. C
4. D
5. E
6. F

Case Study Answers and Explanations:

1. B - Explanation: Chorea is a hallmark motor symptom of Huntington's Disease and supports the diagnosis.
2. B - Explanation: Antidepressants and antipsychotics are commonly used to manage behavioral symptoms in Huntington's Disease.
3. A - Explanation: The length of CAG repeats correlates with the severity and progression of Huntington's Disease.

Major or Mild Neurocognitive Disorder Due to Another Medical Condition

Multiple Choice Questions

1. Which of the following is a key criterion for diagnosing Neurocognitive Disorder due to another medical condition?
    - A. Cognitive impairment that cannot be attributed to another neurodegenerative disease or substance use.
    - B. Sudden onset of memory loss without other cognitive deficits.
    - C. Cognitive decline occurring only during episodes of acute illness.
    - D. Memory impairment as the sole symptom.
2. Which of the following medical conditions is most commonly associated with Neurocognitive Disorder?
    - A. Systemic lupus erythematosus (SLE).
    - B. Chronic obstructive pulmonary disease (COPD).
    - C. Polycystic kidney disease.
    - D. Irritable bowel syndrome.
3. In Neurocognitive Disorder due to hypothyroidism, which symptom is most likely to be prominent?
    - A. Episodic hallucinations.
    - B. Cognitive slowing and fatigue.
    - C. Chorea-like motor symptoms.
    - D. Impaired visuospatial reasoning.
4. Which of the following findings most strongly suggests Neurocognitive Disorder due to hepatic encephalopathy?
    - A. Elevated serum ammonia levels.
    - B. Hippocampal atrophy on MRI.
    - C. Normal liver function tests.
    - D. Subcortical infarcts on CT.
5. Which clinical feature best differentiates Neurocognitive Disorder due to multiple sclerosis from other medical causes?
    - A. Gradual memory loss.
    - B. Fluctuating visuospatial deficits.
    - C. Cognitive impairment with accompanying motor and sensory changes.
    - D. Persistent language deficits.
6. A patient with a recent diagnosis of syphilis presents with cognitive impairment. Which of the following is the most appropriate initial diagnostic step?
    - A. Serum creatinine levels.
    - B. MRI of the brain.
    - C. Cerebrospinal fluid (CSF) analysis for VDRL.
    - D. PET scan for metabolic abnormalities.
7. Which of the following interventions is most appropriate for managing Neurocognitive Disorder due to another medical condition?
    - A. Treating the underlying medical condition.
    - B. Cognitive-behavioral therapy to restore memory function.
    - C. Cholinesterase inhibitors to slow progression.
    - D. Antipsychotics to control behavioral symptoms.

True/False Questions

		T	F
1	A Neurocognitive Disorder due to another medical condition can be diagnosed even if the medical cause is not fully confirmed, as long as there is strong clinical suspicion.		
2	To differentiate the Mild form from the Major form in the DSM-5-TR, the degree of impairment in daily activities is crucial.		
3	Once the medical condition is successfully treated, the DSM-5-TR automatically rules out any associated Neurocognitive Disorder.		
4	Under the DSM-5-TR, ruling out delirium carefully is essential before diagnosing a Neurocognitive Disorder due to another medical condition.		
5	If cognitive symptoms are attributed to both a medical condition and a traumatic brain injury, a combined diagnosis (e.g., TBI and another medical condition) is used.		
6	A significant decline in at least one cognitive domain (e.g., memory, executive functions) can justify a Neurocognitive Disorder diagnosis related to another medical condition.		
7	The DSM-5-TR allows specifying "Probable" or "Possible" Neurocognitive Disorder due to another medical condition based on clinical evidence.		
8	The absence of a worsening (progressive) course fully excludes the diagnosis of a Neurocognitive Disorder linked to another medical condition.		
9	Endocrine or metabolic abnormalities may also qualify as "other medical conditions" causing a Neurocognitive Disorder.		
10	A mild impairment that does not significantly affect daily independence cannot be classified as a Neurocognitive Disorder due to another medical condition.		

Matching Exercise

1. Common finding in Neurocognitive Disorder due to hepatic encephalopathy. [ ]
2. Reversible cause of Neurocognitive Disorder. [ ]
3. Diagnostic test for suspected neurosyphilis. [ ]
4. Cognitive symptom typically observed in hypothyroidism. [ ]
5. Symptom differentiating multiple sclerosis-related Neurocognitive Disorder. [ ]
6. Effective management strategy. [ ]

Descriptions:

- A. Elevated serum ammonia levels.
- B. Cerebrospinal fluid (CSF) VDRL test.
- C. Treat the underlying medical condition.
- D. Cognitive slowing and fatigue.
- E. Accompanying motor and sensory changes.
- F. Vitamin B12 deficiency.

Case Study

Maria, a 56-year-old woman with a history of untreated hypothyroidism, presents with progressive cognitive slowing, fatigue, and difficulty concentrating over the past year. Blood tests reveal elevated TSH and low T3/T4 levels. She has difficulty organizing tasks and completing work-related projects but is otherwise independent in daily activities.

1. Which feature in Maria's presentation most strongly supports Neurocognitive Disorder due to hypothyroidism?
    - A. Difficulty concentrating and cognitive slowing.
    - B. Low T3/T4 levels on blood tests.
    - C. Difficulty completing work-related projects.
    - D. Independence in daily activities.
2. What is the most appropriate first step in managing Maria's condition?
    - A. Prescribe cognitive rehabilitation.
    - B. Treat her hypothyroidism with thyroid hormone replacement.
    - C. Initiate cholinesterase inhibitors for cognitive symptoms.
    - D. Order a brain MRI to exclude structural abnormalities.
3. Why is early identification of Maria's condition important?
    - A. To prevent progression to Major Neurocognitive Disorder.
    - B. To rule out neurodegenerative diseases like Alzheimer's Disease.
    - C. To assess for comorbid psychiatric symptoms.
    - D. To ensure that cognitive rehabilitation is initiated early.

Answers

Multiple Choice Questions:

1. A
2. A
3. B
4. A
5. C
6. C
7. A

True/False Questions:

1. True
2. True
3. False
4. True
5. False
6. True
7. True
8. False
9. True
10. False

Matching Exercise:

1. A
2. F
3. B
4. D
5. E
6. C

Case Study Answers and Explanations:

1. B - Explanation: Low T3/T4 levels and cognitive slowing strongly support a diagnosis related to hypothyroidism.
2. B - Explanation: Treating the underlying hypothyroidism with thyroid hormone replacement can reverse cognitive symptoms.
3. A - Explanation: Early treatment of reversible causes prevents progression to more severe neurocognitive impairment.

Major or Mild Neurocognitive Disorder Due to Multiple Etiologies

Multiple Choice Questions

1. Which of the following best defines Neurocognitive Disorder due to Multiple Etiologies?
    - A. Cognitive impairment caused by a single, identifiable medical condition.
    - B. Cognitive decline resulting from the combined effects of two or more distinct conditions.
    - C. Progressive cognitive decline without an identifiable cause.
    - D. Memory loss as the primary symptom with no other cognitive deficits.
2. Which combination of conditions is most commonly associated with this disorder?
    - A. Alzheimer's Disease and chronic kidney disease.
    - B. Vascular disease and Alzheimer's Disease.
    - C. Parkinson's Disease and substance use disorder.
    - D. Multiple sclerosis and systemic lupus erythematosus.
3. In patients with both Alzheimer's Disease and vascular contributions to cognitive impairment, which symptom is typically more prominent compared to pure Alzheimer's Disease?
    - A. Rapid progression of memory loss.
    - B. Fluctuating attention and stepwise cognitive decline.
    - C. Predominant visuospatial deficits.
    - D. Language processing impairment.
4. Which neuroimaging finding would most likely support a diagnosis of Neurocognitive Disorder due to Multiple Etiologies?
    - A. Diffuse cortical atrophy with hippocampal sparing.
    - B. Evidence of both cortical atrophy and white matter hyperintensities.
    - C. Hyperintensities in the basal ganglia and thalamus.
    - D. Unilateral hippocampal atrophy on MRI.
5. In the context of multiple etiologies, which biomarker would most likely indicate the presence of Alzheimer's Disease as a contributing factor?
    - A. Elevated amyloid-beta levels in cerebrospinal fluid.
    - B. Reduced tau protein in cerebrospinal fluid.
    - C. Elevated serum ammonia levels.
    - D. Alpha-synuclein aggregates in cortical regions.
6. Which intervention is most appropriate for managing Neurocognitive Disorder due to Multiple Etiologies?
    - A. Focus solely on treating the primary contributing condition.
    - B. Address all contributing conditions and provide cognitive rehabilitation.
    - C. Use antipsychotics to manage cognitive decline.
    - D. Implement physical therapy to address motor symptoms exclusively.
7. How does the progression of Neurocognitive Disorder due to Multiple Etiologies typically compare to single-cause disorders like Alzheimer's Disease?
    - A. It progresses more rapidly due to the interaction of contributing conditions.
    - B. It progresses more slowly due to compensatory mechanisms.
    - C. It progresses similarly to single-cause disorders but with fewer behavioral symptoms.
    - D. It does not progress, as the condition is typically static.

True/False Questions

		T	F
1	The DSM-5-TR allows a Neurocognitive Disorder Due to Multiple Etiologies when cognitive decline stems from the combined impact of two or more medical conditions (e.g., Alzheimer's disease and a stroke).		
2	If one underlying condition is resolved but cognitive decline persists due to the other condition, the DSM-5-TR no longer permits a multiple etiologies diagnosis.		
3	To distinguish Mild from Major in a Multiple Etiologies Neurocognitive Disorder, the DSM-5-TR primarily considers the level of impairment in daily functioning.		
4	The DSM-5-TR requires evidence of separate clinical events (such as a stroke plus a head injury) to support this diagnosis.		
5	Cognitive decline may be progressive or stepwise, depending on the conditions involved, yet it still qualifies under multiple etiologies.		
6	If a medical condition is present but does not significantly contribute to cognitive decline, the DSM-5-TR still counts it among the Multiple Etiologies.		
7	Substance withdrawal combined with early frontotemporal dementia can never be considered a Multiple Etiologies Neurocognitive Disorder under the DSM-5-TR.		
8	The presence of two conditions with distinct neurocognitive effects (e.g., HIV and Parkinson's disease) can justify a Multiple Etiologies diagnosis if both contribute to the decline.		
9	The DSM-5-TR requires that at least one etiological factor be confirmed (via lab tests or imaging) to justify Multiple Etiologies.		
10	If multiple causes result in only a mild deficit in one cognitive domain, the DSM-5-TR would still classify this as a Major Neurocognitive Disorder Due to Multiple Etiologies.		

Matching Exercise

1. Typical neuroimaging finding in this disorder. [ ]
2. Biomarker indicating Alzheimer's Disease contribution. [ ]
3. Key strategy for managing the condition. [ ]
4. Common symptom profile in mixed Alzheimer's and vascular cases. [ ]
5. Condition often contributing alongside vascular disease. [ ]
6. Cognitive domain frequently affected. [ ]

Descriptions:

- A. Evidence of cortical atrophy and white matter hyperintensities.
- B. Elevated amyloid-beta levels in CSF.
- C. Address all contributing conditions.
- D. Fluctuating attention and stepwise decline.
- E. Alzheimer's Disease.
- F. Executive functioning.

Case Study

Paul, a 75-year-old man, presents with progressive cognitive decline over the past three years. He has a history of hypertension and diabetes, and his family reports difficulty with memory, decision-making, and attention. Neuroimaging reveals both hippocampal atrophy and white matter hyperintensities. Cerebrospinal fluid analysis shows reduced amyloid-beta levels and elevated tau protein.

1. Which feature in Paul's case most strongly supports a diagnosis of Neurocognitive Disorder due to Multiple Etiologies?
    - A. Progressive cognitive decline with memory impairment.
    - B. History of hypertension and diabetes.
    - C. Neuroimaging showing hippocampal atrophy and white matter hyperintensities.
    - D. Difficulty with attention and decision-making.
2. What is the most appropriate management strategy for Paul?
    - A. Prescribe cholinesterase inhibitors for memory impairment.
    - B. Treat hypertension and diabetes while providing cognitive rehabilitation.
    - C. Focus on physical therapy to address cardiovascular risk factors.
    - D. Initiate antipsychotics to control behavioral symptoms.
3. Why is it important to identify multiple contributing etiologies in Paul's case?
    - A. To prioritize the treatment of primary neurodegenerative processes.
    - B. To guide a comprehensive management plan addressing all contributing factors.
    - C. To confirm the irreversibility of his cognitive decline.
    - D. To exclude vascular disease as a cause of his symptoms.

Answers

Multiple Choice Questions:

1. B
2. B
3. B
4. B
5. A
6. B
7. A

True/False Questions:

1. True
2. False
3. True
4. False
5. True
6. False
7. True
8. False
9. True
10. False

Matching Exercise:

1. A
2. B
3. C
4. D
5. E
6. F

Case Study Answers and Explanations:

1. C - Explanation: The combination of hippocampal atrophy and white matter hyperintensities supports the presence of mixed Alzheimer's and vascular contributions.
2. B - Explanation: Addressing vascular risk factors alongside cognitive rehabilitation is essential for managing multiple etiologies.
3. B - Explanation: Identifying multiple etiologies allows for a tailored management plan targeting all contributing factors.

Unspecified Neurocognitive Disorder

Multiple Choice Questions

1. Which of the following best describes Unspecified Neurocognitive Disorder?
    - A. A neurocognitive disorder with clear diagnostic criteria matching a known subtype.
    - B. A neurocognitive disorder that does not meet full criteria for a specific diagnosis but still causes significant impairment.
    - C. A temporary neurocognitive impairment related to acute medical illness.
    - D. A condition primarily affecting language processing and visuospatial skills.
2. Which clinical scenario would most likely lead to a diagnosis of Unspecified Neurocognitive Disorder?
    - A. A patient with a history of stroke and stepwise cognitive decline.
    - B. A patient with cognitive impairment and no identifiable underlying cause despite extensive testing.
    - C. A patient meeting criteria for Major Neurocognitive Disorder due to Alzheimer's Disease.
    - D. A patient with severe cognitive deficits following a traumatic brain injury.
3. In a case of Unspecified Neurocognitive Disorder, which of the following is the most appropriate initial step in management?
    - A. Prescribe cholinesterase inhibitors immediately.
    - B. Conduct further diagnostic evaluations to clarify the underlying cause.
    - C. Refer to palliative care for symptom management.
    - D. Focus solely on non-pharmacological interventions such as cognitive rehabilitation.
4. Which of the following is a common challenge in diagnosing Unspecified Neurocognitive Disorder?
    - A. Lack of patient cooperation during testing.
    - B. Overlapping symptoms with multiple neurocognitive disorders.
    - C. Difficulty identifying memory impairment.
    - D. Limited availability of pharmacological treatments.
5. What is the primary goal of managing a patient with Unspecified Neurocognitive Disorder?
    - A. Establish a definitive diagnosis through aggressive testing.
    - B. Improve quality of life and address cognitive symptoms while monitoring for progression.
    - C. Delay progression with disease-specific medications.
    - D. Focus on behavioral symptom control with antipsychotics.
6. Which diagnostic test is most useful in ruling out treatable causes of cognitive impairment in suspected Unspecified Neurocognitive Disorder?
    - A. EEG to identify cortical hyperactivity.
    - B. MRI to evaluate structural abnormalities.
    - C. Lumbar puncture to analyze cerebrospinal fluid.
    - D. PET scan for metabolic activity.
7. Which of the following is a key feature distinguishing Unspecified Neurocognitive Disorder from other specific neurocognitive disorders?
    - A. Fluctuating cognition.
    - B. Incomplete diagnostic information or inability to determine the specific etiology.
    - C. Presence of hallmark biomarkers for a known disease.
    - D. Stepwise progression of cognitive symptoms.

True/False Questions

		T	F
1	"Unspecified Neurocognitive Disorder" in the DSM-5-TR can be used when the presentation is atypical, but insufficient data prevent a more specific diagnosis.		
2	If cognitive symptoms are clearly caused by vascular lesions, the DSM-5-TR still advises using "Unspecified Neurocognitive Disorder."		
3	The DSM-5-TR allows "Unspecified Neurocognitive Disorder" when an evaluation is incomplete or conflicting.		
4	The label "Unspecified Neurocognitive Disorder" is always preferred by the DSM-5-TR over any other specific diagnosis.		
5	According to the DSM-5-TR, "Unspecified Neurocognitive Disorder" can be used in clinical settings or emergency contexts, pending further diagnostic clarification.		
6	Even without definitive evidence, the DSM-5-TR excludes "Unspecified Neurocognitive Disorder" when there is no suspicion of cognitive decline at all.		
7	The DSM-5-TR specifies that "Unspecified Neurocognitive Disorder" cannot be used if there are no cognitive symptoms whatsoever.		
8	A clinician may apply "Unspecified Neurocognitive Disorder" if it is unclear whether the impairment is Mild or Major, but cognitive deficits are suspected.		
9	Once "Unspecified Neurocognitive Disorder" is assigned, the DSM-5-TR advises against re-evaluation even if new information arises.		
10	The DSM-5-TR does not restrict how long an "Unspecified Neurocognitive Disorder" diagnosis can be maintained if data remain insufficient.		

Matching Exercise

1. Common scenario leading to this diagnosis. [ ]
2. Primary goal of management. [ ]
3. Diagnostic test for ruling out structural abnormalities. [ ]
4. Challenge in making a definitive diagnosis. [ ]
5. Cognitive symptom often observed. [ ]
6. Management approach for symptom control. [ ]

Descriptions:

- A. Overlapping symptoms with multiple neurocognitive disorders.
- B. Improve quality of life and monitor for progression.
- C. MRI to evaluate structural changes.
- D. Cognitive impairment without an identifiable cause.
- E. Memory deficits and attention difficulties.
- F. Non-pharmacological interventions such as cognitive rehabilitation.

Case Study

Sarah, a 67-year-old woman, presents with mild cognitive impairment that has gradually worsened over the past year. Extensive laboratory testing, neuroimaging, and neuropsychological evaluations fail to identify a clear etiology. Her symptoms include occasional forgetfulness, difficulty focusing, and trouble managing complex tasks, though she remains independent in daily activities.

1. Which feature in Sarah's presentation most strongly supports a diagnosis of Unspecified Neurocognitive Disorder?
   - A. Gradual cognitive decline over the past year.
   - B. Absence of a clear etiology despite extensive testing.
   - C. Difficulty managing complex tasks.
   - D. Retention of independence in daily activities.
2. What is the most appropriate next step in managing Sarah's condition?
   - A. Refer for a second opinion with a neuropsychologist.
   - B. Initiate symptomatic treatment and monitor for progression.
   - C. Perform invasive testing, such as a brain biopsy, to confirm a diagnosis.
   - D. Focus exclusively on behavioral symptom management.
3. Why is it important to continue monitoring Sarah despite the lack of a definitive diagnosis?
   - A. To identify potential progression into a specific neurocognitive disorder.
   - B. To confirm that her symptoms are not related to psychiatric comorbidities.
   - C. To evaluate her response to cholinesterase inhibitors.
   - D. To ensure that imaging abnormalities do not progress.

Answers

Multiple Choice Questions:
1. B
2. B
3. B
4. B
5. B
6. B
7. B

True/False Questions:
1. True
2. False
3. True
4. False
5. True
6. True
7. True
8. True
9. False
10. True

Matching Exercise:
1. D
2. B
3. C
4. A
5. E
6. F

Case Study Answers and Explanations:
1. B - Explanation: The absence of a clear etiology after extensive testing supports a diagnosis of Unspecified Neurocognitive Disorder.
2. B - Explanation: Symptomatic treatment and monitoring are appropriate when a definitive etiology cannot be determined.
3. A - Explanation: Monitoring ensures early identification of progression into a specific neurocognitive disorder if symptoms worsen.

Cluster A Personality Disorders

Personality disorders in Cluster A include Paranoid Personality Disorder, Schizoid Personality Disorder, and Schizotypal Personality Disorder. According to the DSM-5-TR, these conditions share "odd" or "eccentric" traits, featuring an unusual way of perceiving oneself, others, and the surrounding world. They tend to involve social withdrawal, suspicion, or unconventional beliefs, rather than the strong emotional displays or specific fears seen in other clusters. As a result, interpersonal relationships are often compromised by pervasive mistrust or limited emotional expression.

When examining typical behaviors, one may notice that individuals with Paranoid Personality Disorder tend to interpret other people's intentions as hostile or malevolent, responding with hostility or refusal to engage socially. Those with Schizoid Personality Disorder show marked emotional detachment, a lack of interest in social connections, and a narrow range of emotional expression. In Schizotypal Personality Disorder, odd beliefs, magical thinking, and pronounced social anxiety stand out, though these do not usually escalate to the level of genuine psychotic symptoms such as those seen in Schizophrenia. In any case, these personality traits appear consistently across different life situations, making it difficult for the individual to form meaningful bonds.

From a diagnostic standpoint, it's essential to distinguish these disorders from psychotic disorders, where reality testing is more deeply impaired. Though some paranoid or eccentric beliefs may appear psychotic, most people in Cluster A maintain enough contact with reality, despite a somewhat distorted or peculiar way of processing information. It's also important to differentiate them from anxiety disorders, which emphasize worry or fear. Here, the focus is more on social isolation or pervasive suspicion rather than generalized fear or preoccupation.

Comorbid conditions may include reactive depressive episodes triggered by loneliness or anxiety-related issues. In some instances, Schizotypal Personality Disorder might edge closer to subclinical psychotic features, without fulfilling the full criteria for Schizophrenia. It is also crucial to assess the potential impact of substance use or neurological factors, which could alter the clinical picture or intensify social withdrawal. The DSM-5-TR, following previous editions, keeps the cluster-based approach and underscores the importance of a thorough case history and a complete evaluation of personality traits. It also recognizes that some schizotypal features can exist along a continuum with the schizophrenia spectrum. In short, individuals with a Cluster A disorder present a distinctive relational and cognitive style, different from more severe psychotic syndromes or disorders marked by impulsivity or marked anxiety. Accurate assessment helps guide diagnosis and tailor supportive measures, considering the ingrained and enduring nature of the symptoms.

Paranoid Personality Disorder

Multiple Choice Questions

1. Which of the following characteristics is most commonly associated with paranoid personality disorder?
    - A. Lack of empathy
    - B. Pervasive suspicion and distrust
    - C. Impulsivity
    - D. Constant attention-seeking
2. A patient with paranoid personality disorder is most likely to:
    - A. Avoid social interactions due to fear of embarrassment
    - B. Challenge authority based on unrealistic suspicions
    - C. Exhibit overly dramatic behavior
    - D. Engage in manipulative behaviors
3. Which of the following is NOT a diagnostic criterion for paranoid personality disorder according to the DSM-5?
    - A. Suspecting others of plotting against them
    - B. Misinterpreting innocent remarks as threats
    - C. Expressing genuine remorse for personal mistakes
    - D. Being reluctant to confide in others out of fear the information will be used against them
4. Which therapeutic approach is generally considered most effective for patients with paranoid personality disorder?
    - A. Cognitive Behavioral Therapy (CBT)
    - B. Group therapy
    - C. Pharmacotherapy as the sole treatment
    - D. Intensive psychoanalytic interventions
5. What is the minimum age typically indicated for diagnosing paranoid personality disorder?
    - A. 12 years
    - B. 18 years
    - C. 21 years
    - D. No specific minimum age
6. A patient with paranoid personality disorder is least likely to exhibit:
    - A. Distrust of others
    - B. Reactive aggressive behaviors
    - C. A strong desire for revenge
    - D. A tendency to form deep, trusting relationships
7. Which of the following conditions is commonly comorbid with paranoid personality disorder?
    - A. Social anxiety disorder
    - B. Bipolar disorder
    - C. Obsessive-compulsive disorder
    - D. Brief psychotic disorder

True/False

		T	F
1	Individuals with Paranoid Personality Disorder (PPD) display persistent distrust and suspicion toward others.		
2	The presence of bizarre delusions is a key criterion for diagnosing PPD in the DSM-5-TR.		
3	According to the DSM-5-TR, people with PPD can experience brief psychotic episodes under high stress.		
4	Paranoid Personality Disorder belongs to Cluster C Personality Disorders, per the DSM-5-TR.		
5	PPD-related mistrust can extend even to situations where there is no concrete evidence of deceit.		
6	For a PPD diagnosis, having bizarre ideas of reference is mandatory.		
7	The likelihood of PPD is higher if there are first-degree relatives with Schizophrenia.		
8	PPD symptoms typically begin in late adulthood.		
9	Individuals with PPD readily acknowledge the unreasonableness of their suspicions when presented with contrary proof.		
10	Persistent anger and resentment toward others can characterize a paranoid personality profile.		

Matching Exercise

1. A tendency to unjustifiably suspect others [ ]
2. Interpreting neutral events as malicious [ ]
3. Reluctance to confide in others [ ]
4. Vindictive behaviors [ ]
5. Difficulties maintaining personal relationships [ ]
6. Absence of persistent hallucinations or delusions [ ]

Descriptions:

- A. Characteristic of paranoid personality disorder
- B. Not directly associated with paranoid personality disorder
- C. Often linked to extreme stress situations
- D. Typical of psychotic disorders but not this disorder
- E. A result of generalized mistrust
- F. Common trait in Cluster A disorders

Case Study

A 45-year-old man seeks therapy, reporting increasing distress at work. He believes his colleagues are conspiring to have him fired, despite lacking concrete evidence. He describes past instances where he distanced himself from close friendships due to unwarranted suspicions. He struggles to confide even in close family members, fearing they might "use the information against him." The patient exhibits no hallucinations or delusions but shows a pervasive pattern of distrust that significantly impacts his social and occupational life.

1. What is the most evident criterion for paranoid personality disorder in this case?
    - A. Episodes of hallucinations
    - B. Unfounded suspicions and distrust
    - C. Manipulative behaviors
    - D. Excessive attention-seeking
2. What could be an initial therapeutic goal for this patient?
    - A. Improving anger management
    - B. Exploring childhood trauma
    - C. Reducing excessive distrust
    - D. Addressing primary depressive symptoms
3. Which therapeutic strategy would be least appropriate for this patient?
    - A. Intensive group therapy
    - B. CBT-based approaches
    - C. Medication for secondary symptoms
    - D. Stress management education

Answers

Multiple Choice Questions

1. B
2. B
3. C
4. A
5. B
6. D
7. D

True/False Questions:

1. True
2. False
3. True
4. False
5. True
6. False
7. True
8. False
9. False
10. True

Matching Exercise

1. E
2. A
3. E
4. A
5. E
6. D

Case Study Answers and Explanations

1. B - Explanation: Unfounded suspicions are the central symptom in this clinical case.
2. C - Explanation: Reducing excessive distrust is a crucial initial step.
3. A - Explanation: Intensive group therapy may exacerbate the patient's mistrust.

Schizoid Personality Disorder

Multiple Choice Questions

1. Which of the following characteristics is most commonly associated with schizoid personality disorder?
    - A. Dramatic and theatrical behavior
    - B. Social isolation and emotional detachment
    - C. Suspiciousness toward others
    - D. Intense desire for social approval
2. A patient with schizoid personality disorder is most likely to:
    - A. Feel uncomfortable in social situations
    - B. Show disinterest in social relationships
    - C. Constantly seek to impress others
    - D. Frequently express concerns about being exploited
3. Which of the following is NOT a typical characteristic of schizoid personality disorder?
    - A. Lack of desire for close relationships
    - B. Enjoyment of many social activities
    - C. Preference for solitary activities
    - D. Indifference to praise or criticism from others
4. Which therapeutic approach is considered most effective for patients with schizoid personality disorder?
    - A. Intensive group therapy
    - B. Cognitive Behavioral Therapy (CBT)
    - C. Approaches focused on emotional expression
    - D. Pharmacological therapy as the sole treatment
5. What is the key feature that differentiates schizoid personality disorder from avoidant personality disorder?
    - A. Both include intense social anxiety
    - B. Schizoid patients avoid relationships due to indifference, while avoidant patients do so out of fear
    - C. Schizoid individuals exhibit manipulative behaviors
    - D. Schizoid individuals actively seek close relationships
6. A patient with schizoid personality disorder might exhibit:
    - A. A strong desire for attention
    - B. Marked inability to experience pleasure (anhedonia)
    - C. A tendency to be highly competitive
    - D. Highly impulsive behaviors
7. Which of the following conditions is commonly comorbid with schizoid personality disorder?
    - A. Mood disorders
    - B. Autism spectrum disorder
    - C. Somatic symptom disorders
    - D. Generalized anxiety disorder

True/False

		T	F
1	Individuals with Schizoid Personality Disorder tend to favor solitary activities and show little interest in close relationships, regardless of other circumstances.		
2	A hallmark of Schizoid Personality Disorder, according to the DSM-5-TR, is a persistent fear of persecution similar to that seen in Paranoid Personality Disorder.		
3	The DSM-5-TR includes restricted emotional expression and apparent detachment from social interactions among the criteria for Schizoid Personality Disorder.		
4	If an individual exhibits bizarre delusions or markedly disorganized thinking, Schizoid Personality Disorder is commonly diagnosed.		
5	Many people with Schizoid Personality Disorder seem indifferent to praise or criticism yet maintain an adequate daily functioning.		
6	Transient visual hallucinations are considered typical of Schizoid Personality Disorder, particularly under severe stress.		
7	In Schizoid Personality Disorder, the preference for being alone is not primarily driven by social anxiety but by a genuine desire for solitude.		
8	Those with Schizoid Personality Disorder often demonstrate a broad range of emotions in their interactions with coworkers.		
9	The DSM-5-TR suggests that individuals with Schizoid Personality Disorder may view others as sources of disturbance rather than emotional support.		
10	Schizoid Personality Disorder always results in an inability to work effectively, regardless of the nature of one's job.		

Matching Exercise

1. Preference for solitary activities [ ]
2. Indifference to praise or criticism [ ]
3. Lack of interest in close relationships [ ]
4. Reduced emotional expression [ ]
5. Avoidant behavior motivated by indifference [ ]
6. Anhedonia as a distinguishing feature [ ]

Descriptions:

- A. Characteristic of schizoid personality disorder
- B. Not associated with schizoid personality disorder
- C. Common in extreme stress situations
- D. Typical of psychotic disorders but not of this disorder
- E. Relevant in Cluster A disorders
- F. Prominent clinical feature

Case Study

A 37-year-old woman is referred to therapy by her employer, who is concerned about her social isolation and lack of engagement at work. She reports feeling indifferent toward her coworkers and states she prefers working alone. She has no close friends and avoids family gatherings. She rarely experiences strong emotions, either positive or negative, and says she doesn't care if others criticize or praise her work. She spends her free time reading or engaging in solitary hobbies and expresses no interest in romantic relationships.

1. What is the most evident symptom of schizoid personality disorder in this case?
    - A. Strong desire for social approval
    - B. Indifference toward relationships and emotional detachment
    - C. Frequent episodes of intense anger
    - D. Persistent feelings of anxiety in social situations
2. Which initial therapeutic approach might be most helpful for this patient?
    - A. Exploring childhood trauma
    - B. Gradually encouraging social engagement
    - C. Addressing intense anxiety symptoms
    - D. Focusing on developing romantic relationships
3. Which therapeutic strategy would likely be least effective?
    - A. Group therapy sessions
    - B. CBT tailored to the individual
    - C. Psychoeducation about emotional expression
    - D. Supportive psychotherapy focused on occupational functioning

Answers

Multiple Choice Questions

1. B
2. B
3. B
4. B
5. B
6. B
7. B

True/False Questions:

1. True
2. False
3. True
4. False
5. True
6. False
7. True
8. False
9. True
10. False

Matching Exercise

1. A
2. A
3. A
4. A
5. A
6. F

Case Study Answers and Explanations

1. B - Explanation: Indifference toward relationships and emotional detachment are hallmark symptoms.
2. B - Explanation: Encouraging gradual social engagement helps the patient navigate interpersonal challenges.
3. A - Explanation: Group therapy may increase discomfort for a patient who prefers solitude.

Schizotypal Personality Disorder

Multiple Choice Questions

1. Which of the following is a defining characteristic of schizotypal personality disorder?
    - A. Intense emotional outbursts
    - B. Persistent suspicion and distrust of others
    - C. Eccentric behavior and cognitive/perceptual distortions
    - D. Repeated violations of the rights of others
2. A person with schizotypal personality disorder might exhibit:
    - A. Frequent, uncontrolled physical aggression
    - B. Paranoid ideation and odd beliefs
    - C. Excessive focus on physical appearance
    - D. A strong desire for deep emotional connections
3. Which of the following best differentiates schizotypal personality disorder from schizophrenia?
    - A. Schizotypal patients have transient psychotic episodes, while schizophrenia involves persistent psychosis.
    - B. Schizotypal patients lack delusions or hallucinations.
    - C. Schizotypal patients maintain consistent interpersonal relationships, unlike schizophrenia.
    - D. Schizotypal personality disorder is not part of the DSM-5.
4. Which therapeutic approach is considered most beneficial for patients with schizotypal personality disorder?
    - A. Intensive psychodynamic therapy
    - B. Cognitive-behavioral therapy focused on social skills
    - C. High-dose antipsychotic medications as a first-line treatment
    - D. Group therapy without individual sessions
5. In schizotypal personality disorder, magical thinking refers to:
    - A. Persistent hallucinations unrelated to reality
    - B. Belief that unrelated events are causally linked
    - C. A tendency to focus on abstract philosophical ideas
    - D. Rationalizing unusual but evidence-based observations
6. Which condition is most commonly comorbid with schizotypal personality disorder?
    - A. Major depressive disorder
    - B. Narcissistic personality disorder
    - C. Obsessive-compulsive disorder
    - D. Antisocial personality disorder
7. Which of the following is a common occupational outcome for individuals with schizotypal personality disorder?
    - A. High-level executive roles due to strong interpersonal skills
    - B. Frequent job loss due to interpersonal difficulties
    - C. Consistent employment in highly social professions
    - D. Employment in roles requiring extensive teamwork

True/False

		T	F
1	Ideas of reference are common in Schizotypal Personality Disorder, though they do not necessarily rise to the level of true delusions.		
2	The constant presence of complex auditory hallucinations, similar to those in schizophrenia, is a hallmark of Schizotypal Personality Disorder.		
3	Odd beliefs or perceptual distortions are among the diagnostic criteria for Schizotypal Personality Disorder.		
4	The DSM-5-TR requires paranoia as a primary and indispensable criterion for Schizotypal Personality Disorder.		
5	Eccentric behaviors and peculiar attire can be indicative of Schizotypal Personality Disorder.		
6	Schizotypal Personality Disorder has no link whatsoever to familial risk for schizophrenia.		
7	If an individual shows ideas of reference, strange perceptions, and suspicion, the DSM-5-TR automatically indicates a primary psychotic disorder.		
8	Social isolation and reduced emotional expression are common in Schizotypal Personality Disorder.		
9	A prolonged history of recurrent psychotic episodes rules out the diagnosis of Schizotypal Personality Disorder.		
10	The lack of close relationships is solely due to fear of social judgment, as seen in Avoidant Personality Disorder.		

Matching Exercise

1. Magical thinking [ ]
2. Odd, eccentric behavior [ ]
3. Suspiciousness or paranoid ideation [ ]
4. Social anxiety unrelated to self-consciousness [ ]
5. Inappropriate or constricted affect [ ]
6. Lack of close relationships outside immediate family [ ]

Descriptions:

- A. Belief that unrelated events are causally linked
- B. Characteristic of Cluster A personality disorders
- C. Not typically associated with schizotypal personality disorder
- D. A core diagnostic feature of schizotypal personality disorder
- E. Often linked to social isolation in this disorder
- F. Commonly seen in mood disorders but not specific to this disorder

Case Study

A 29-year-old man is referred for therapy after his coworkers report discomfort with his unusual behavior. He frequently talks about having a "sixth sense" and believing he can predict future events. He avoids social gatherings and prefers to work alone. He reports seeing subtle patterns in random events that others dismiss. His affect is constricted, and he often appears awkward in conversations, avoiding eye contact. He denies experiencing hallucinations or delusions but admits to feeling that people are often "watching and judging" him.

1. What is the most likely diagnosis for this individual?
   - A. Schizophrenia
   - B. Schizotypal personality disorder
   - C. Social anxiety disorder
   - D. Narcissistic personality disorder
2. What would be the most appropriate initial therapeutic goal for this patient?
   - A. Address paranoid ideation and improve interpersonal functioning
   - B. Eliminate magical thinking entirely
   - C. Focus on reducing hallucinations and delusions
   - D. Encourage him to change his workplace environment immediately
3. Which therapeutic intervention is least likely to be effective?
   - A. Social skills training
   - B. Antipsychotic medications for transient psychotic symptoms
   - C. Intensive group therapy focused on emotional expression
   - D. Cognitive-behavioral therapy to challenge cognitive distortions

Answers

Multiple Choice Questions

1. C
2. B
3. A
4. B
5. B
6. A
7. B

True/False Questions:

1. True
2. False
3. True
4. False
5. True
6. False
7. False
8. True
9. True
10. False

Matching Exercise

1. A
2. B
3. D
4. E
5. D
6. E

Case Study Answers and Explanations

1. B - Explanation: The individual's symptoms align with schizotypal personality disorder, particularly eccentric beliefs and cognitive distortions without persistent psychosis.
2. A - Explanation: Addressing paranoia and improving interpersonal functioning are key initial goals for managing this disorder.
3. C - Explanation: Intensive group therapy may increase discomfort and is often counterproductive for individuals with this disorder.

Cluster B Personality Disorders

Cluster B personality disorders include Antisocial, Borderline, Histrionic, and Narcissistic. According to the DSM-5-TR, they share "dramatic" or "emotional" traits, often expressed through impulsivity, manipulative behaviors, or a strong need for attention. Unlike Cluster A, where isolation and distrust dominate, the focus here shifts to tumultuous interpersonal relationships, intense emotional reactions, and a more theatrical or self-centered view of social dynamics.

Observing their clinical features, Antisocial Personality Disorder is marked by a disregard for social norms, a tendency to deceive or violate others' rights, and limited empathy. Borderline Personality Disorder, by contrast, involves unstable relationships, self-image, and mood, along with self-harm or impulsive actions and deep anxiety about potential abandonment. Histrionic Personality Disorder revolves around a persistent desire for approval and attention, often accompanied by emotional displays that may appear exaggerated or insincere. Finally, Narcissistic Personality Disorder is characterized by grandiosity, a need for admiration, an inadequate concern for others' perspectives, and an expectation of special treatment.

From a diagnostic standpoint, it is important not to confuse these behavioral patterns with merely heightened personality traits. What differentiates Cluster B disorders is the pervasive nature of the symptoms and the resulting distress for both the individual and those in their environment. It is also useful to distinguish impulsive or emotionally reactive behavior seen here from similar presentations in other categories, such as anxiety or mood disorders. In Cluster B, the main emphasis lies on dysfunctional and consistent interpersonal patterns that span various life contexts. In some cases, antisocial behavior overlaps with substance use or socioeconomic disadvantage, but diagnosing Antisocial Personality Disorder requires a stable, long-term pattern of disregarding others' rights, beginning before age 15 and often preceded by Conduct Disorder.

Regarding comorbidities, Cluster B disorders frequently co-occur with mood disorders (especially in borderline presentations) or substance use disorders. Narcissistic Personality Disorder can manifest alongside reactive depressive episodes, particularly when an inflated self-image is challenged. Relational dynamics may further complicate the picture, as ongoing tension or manipulation generates conflict and affects overall mental health.

In keeping with previous editions, the DSM-5-TR maintains the cluster-based structure, underscoring that Cluster B disorders involve dramatic, impulsive, and emotionally unstable traits. Although some researchers argue for a dimensional approach to better capture these characteristics, the manual continues to rely on categorical criteria for diagnostic clarity. Nonetheless, a thorough assessment of personal history and environmental factors remains essential for distinguishing situational impulsive behavior from a deeply rooted personality pattern that leads to distress and dysfunction across multiple areas of life.

Antisocial Personality Disorder

Multiple Choice Questions

1. Which of the following is a core feature of antisocial personality disorder (ASPD)?
   - A. Persistent emotional instability
   - B. Disregard for and violation of others' rights
   - C. Excessive dependence on others for decision-making
   - D. Eccentric behavior and cognitive distortions
2. What is a distinguishing factor between antisocial personality disorder and conduct disorder?
   - A. Conduct disorder is diagnosed in childhood or adolescence, while ASPD is diagnosed in adults.
   - B. ASPD includes hallucinations, whereas conduct disorder does not.
   - C. Individuals with conduct disorder exhibit remorse, unlike those with ASPD.
   - D. ASPD primarily involves social withdrawal, unlike conduct disorder.
3. Which behavior is least likely to be associated with antisocial personality disorder?
   - A. Chronic lying and deceit
   - B. Impulsivity and poor planning
   - C. Avoidance of risk-taking
   - D. Lack of remorse for harmful actions
4. Which of the following statements about antisocial personality disorder is true?
   - A. ASPD is equally prevalent in men and women.
   - B. Substance use disorders are commonly comorbid with ASPD.
   - C. ASPD typically emerges after the age of 30.
   - D. Individuals with ASPD frequently seek help for their interpersonal difficulties.
5. Which factor is most strongly associated with the development of antisocial personality disorder?
   - A. High levels of neuroticism
   - B. Childhood history of neglect or abuse
   - C. Elevated levels of conscientiousness
   - D. Strict and supportive parenting
6. What is a key ethical concern when working with patients diagnosed with ASPD?
   - A. Maintaining the confidentiality of a patient who poses no danger
   - B. The potential for manipulation and deceit in therapeutic settings
   - C. Balancing pharmacological treatment with psychotherapy
   - D. Ensuring the patient adheres to strict behavioral guidelines
7. Which of the following is considered an evidence-based approach for managing antisocial personality disorder?
   - A. Long-term group therapy focused on emotional regulation
   - B. Psychoanalytic therapy targeting unresolved childhood trauma
   - C. Structured, goal-oriented cognitive-behavioral therapy (CBT)
   - D. Intensive family-based interventions

True/False

		T	F
1	The DSM-5-TR requires evidence of conduct disorder symptoms before age 15 to diagnose Antisocial Personality Disorder (ASPD).		
2	Lack of remorse is not listed among the diagnostic criteria for ASPD in the DSM-5-TR.		
3	The DSM-5-TR states that an individual must be at least 18 years old for an ASPD diagnosis.		
4	Illegal acts or manipulative tendencies are considered optional, non-core criteria for ASPD according to the DSM-5-TR.		
5	The DSM-5-TR disallows an ASPD diagnosis if the individual also has a substance use disorder.		
6	A pervasive pattern of disregard for and violation of others' rights is a key criterion for ASPD.		
7	Childhood ADHD is considered a risk factor for developing ASPD.		
8	An ASPD diagnosis is ruled out if the individual has Bipolar Disorder in a manic phase.		
9	Irresponsible behaviors, such as quitting jobs with no plan, can be typical of ASPD.		
10	In the DSM-5-TR, ASPD is classified under the Cluster B personality disorders.		

Matching Exercise

1. Pattern of chronic deceit [ ]
2. Impulsivity and poor self-regulation [ ]
3. Lack of remorse after harming others [ ]
4. Early evidence of conduct disorder [ ]
5. Increased risk of substance abuse [ ]
6. Difficulty maintaining long-term relationships [ ]

Descriptions:

- A. Core feature of antisocial personality disorder
- B. Frequently observed in comorbid conditions with ASPD
- C. Diagnostic precursor to antisocial personality disorder
- D. Indicates poor emotional and behavioral control
- E. Common consequence of manipulative or harmful behaviors
- F. Not directly associated with ASPD

Case Study

A 32-year-old man is referred for evaluation after a series of legal issues, including fraud and theft. He describes himself as a "survivor" who does whatever is necessary to get ahead. He shows no remorse for his actions, stating, "If people are stupid enough to get scammed, that's on them." He reports a long history of impulsive decisions, such as gambling away his earnings and repeatedly engaging in high-risk behaviors for personal gain. He acknowledges a history of skipping school and getting into fights during adolescence. Despite his charming demeanor, he struggles to maintain stable relationships and views people as tools for achieving his goals.

- Which symptom most strongly supports a diagnosis of antisocial personality disorder in this case?
  - A. Chronic interpersonal conflicts
  - B. Lack of remorse for harmful actions
  - C. Repeated risky behavior
  - D. Substance abuse
- What would be a primary therapeutic focus for this patient?
  - A. Addressing core beliefs about morality and empathy
  - B. Establishing emotional regulation skills
  - C. Building a stable support system
  - D. Encouraging participation in group therapy
- What is a key consideration for the therapist in managing this patient?
  - A. Avoiding confrontation to maintain rapport
  - B. Setting clear boundaries to mitigate manipulation
  - C. Allowing the patient to dictate the pace of therapy
  - D. Using unstructured therapy to explore root causes of behavior

Answers

Multiple Choice Questions

1. B
2. A
3. C
4. B
5. B
6. B
7. C

True/False Questions:

1. True
2. False
3. True
4. False
5. False
6. True
7. True
8. False
9. True
10. True

Matching Exercise

1. A
2. D
3. A
4. C
5. B
6. E

Case Study Answers and Explanations

1. B - Explanation: The lack of remorse and justification for harmful actions are hallmark traits of ASPD.
2. A - Explanation: Challenging the patient's distorted beliefs about morality and empathy is critical for behavior change.
3. B - Explanation: Setting firm boundaries is essential to prevent manipulation and ensure therapeutic effectiveness.

Borderline Personality Disorder

Multiple Choice Questions

1. Which of the following is a hallmark feature of borderline personality disorder (BPD)?
    - A. Persistent detachment from emotions and others
    - B. Intense and unstable interpersonal relationships
    - C. A grandiose sense of self-importance
    - D. Preoccupation with order and perfection
2. What is the term for the rapid shifts in emotional state commonly seen in individuals with BPD?
    - A. Emotional numbing
    - B. Lability
    - C. Dissociation
    - D. Catatonia
3. Which behavior is most indicative of borderline personality disorder?
    - A. Consistent, calculated manipulation of others
    - B. Frequent mood swings and impulsive self-harm
    - C. Avoidance of close relationships due to fear of criticism
    - D. Chronic suspicion of others' intentions
4. Which of the following statements about BPD is true?
    - A. It is equally prevalent in men and women.
    - B. Individuals with BPD rarely experience comorbid conditions.
    - C. BPD symptoms tend to diminish in intensity with age.
    - D. Long-term pharmacological treatment is the mainstay of management.
5. Which therapeutic approach has the most empirical support for treating BPD?
    - A. Psychoanalytic therapy
    - B. Dialectical Behavior Therapy (DBT)
    - C. Family systems therapy
    - D. Electroconvulsive therapy
6. Which of the following best describes splitting in the context of BPD?
    - A. Persistent avoidance of social interactions
    - B. Seeing people or situations as all good or all bad
    - C. Sudden detachment from reality
    - D. Recurrent, uncontrollable anger
7. Which of the following is a common risk associated with BPD?
    - A. Long-term memory loss
    - B. Cardiovascular disease
    - C. Suicidal ideation and attempts
    - D. Substance-induced psychosis

True/False

		T	F
1	A defining characteristic of Borderline Personality Disorder is self-harming behavior used solely to manipulate others.		
2	According to the DSM-5-TR, marked instability in relationships, self-image, and affect is central to the diagnosis of Borderline Personality Disorder.		
3	Fear of abandonment may lead to alternating idealization and devaluation of partners, but it is not deemed diagnostically relevant.		
4	Impulsivity in at least two potentially self-damaging areas (e.g., overspending, binge eating, reckless driving) is one of the possible criteria.		
5	The DSM-5-TR excludes the diagnosis of Borderline Personality Disorder if the person exhibits stress-related transient dissociative episodes.		
6	Intense and unstable interpersonal relationships can shift unpredictably between dependence and anger.		
7	For the DSM-5-TR, a single self-injurious act is sufficient to confirm Borderline Personality Disorder.		
8	Difficulty controlling anger is a diagnostic criterion, sometimes displayed through physical or verbal altercations.		
9	An intermittent sense of emptiness or chronic boredom can be present in Borderline Personality Disorder.		
10	The DSM-5-TR requires that symptoms begin strictly after age 30, ruling out other age groups.		

Matching Exercise

1. Splitting [ ]
2. Fear of abandonment [ ]
3. Chronic feelings of emptiness [ ]
4. Impulsive self-damaging behaviors [ ]
5. Lability [ ]
6. Suicidal threats or gestures [ ]

Descriptions:

- A. A core diagnostic feature of borderline personality disorder
- B. Instability of emotional states
- C. Attempts to manipulate or draw attention from others
- D. Related to unstable and intense interpersonal relationships
- E. Extreme fear of being left alone, even in relationships
- F. A common behavioral manifestation of impulsivity

Case Study

A 25-year-old woman seeks therapy after an argument with her boyfriend during which she threatened to harm herself. She describes a pattern of intense, unstable relationships marked by frequent breakups and reconciliations. She alternates between idealizing her partner and believing he doesn't care about her. She reports episodes of impulsive spending and substance use, as well as feelings of emptiness and intense anger when she feels ignored or misunderstood. She has a history of self-harm and says, "I feel like I'm either completely loved or completely worthless."

1. Which symptom most strongly supports a diagnosis of BPD in this case?
   - A. Persistent avoidance of social interactions
   - B. Emotional lability and fear of abandonment
   - C. Recurrent, intense anxiety unrelated to relationships
   - D. Consistent anger directed outward without self-harm
2. Which initial therapeutic goal would be most appropriate for this patient?
   - A. Improve her ability to tolerate emotional distress without self-harm
   - B. Focus on repairing her relationship with her boyfriend
   - C. Eliminate all instances of impulsive behavior
   - D. Explore deep-seated childhood trauma in detail
3. Which therapeutic technique would likely be the most effective?
   - A. Mindfulness and emotional regulation training
   - B. Group therapy with minimal individual focus
   - C. Psychoanalytic exploration of repressed memories
   - D. Pharmacological management as the primary intervention

Answers

Multiple Choice Questions

1. B
2. B
3. B
4. C
5. B
6. B
7. C

True/False Questions:

1. False
2. True
3. False
4. True
5. False
6. True
7. False
8. True
9. True
10. False

Matching Exercise

1. D
2. E
3. A
4. F
5. B
6. C

Case Study Answers and Explanations

1. B - Explanation: Emotional lability and an exaggerated fear of abandonment are hallmark symptoms of BPD.
2. A - Explanation: Teaching the patient to manage emotional distress without resorting to self-harm is a key priority in early therapy.
3. A - Explanation: Mindfulness and emotional regulation are core components of Dialectical Behavior Therapy, the gold standard for BPD.

Histrionic Personality Disorder

Multiple Choice Questions

1. Which of the following is a hallmark feature of histrionic personality disorder (HPD)?
    - A. Persistent fear of abandonment
    - B. Excessive emotionality and attention-seeking behavior
    - C. A pervasive pattern of detachment from social relationships
    - D. Recurrent aggressive and deceitful behaviors
2. What type of behavior is most characteristic of individuals with HPD?
    - A. Intense and unstable relationships with frequent breakups
    - B. Dramatic and theatrical gestures to gain attention
    - C. Persistent feelings of worthlessness and guilt
    - D. A tendency to avoid social interactions due to anxiety
3. Which of the following statements about HPD is true?
    - A. HPD is more common in males than females.
    - B. Individuals with HPD are often uncomfortable when not the center of attention.
    - C. HPD is typically characterized by rigid and inflexible behaviors.
    - D. People with HPD generally avoid expressing emotions in public.
4. Which feature differentiates HPD from narcissistic personality disorder?
    - A. Individuals with HPD exhibit attention-seeking, while narcissistic individuals have a sense of entitlement.
    - B. HPD involves emotional detachment, while narcissism involves hyperemotionality.
    - C. HPD patients avoid criticism, while narcissistic individuals thrive on feedback.
    - D. HPD is associated with a lack of empathy, whereas narcissism is not.
5. What is a common interpersonal characteristic of individuals with HPD?
    - A. Fear of forming close relationships due to mistrust
    - B. A tendency to view relationships as closer than they actually are
    - C. Avoidance of social settings due to fear of judgment
    - D. Consistent withdrawal from romantic relationships
6. Which therapeutic approach is considered most effective for individuals with HPD?
    - A. Dialectical Behavior Therapy (DBT)
    - B. Structured Cognitive Behavioral Therapy (CBT)
    - C. Long-term group therapy without individual sessions
    - D. Hypnotherapy
7. What is a common risk associated with HPD?
    - A. Chronic physical health problems
    - B. Suicidal gestures or threats aimed at gaining attention
    - C. Severe memory impairments
    - D. Total isolation from social relationships

True/False

		T	F
1	Individuals with Histrionic Personality Disorder often perceive relationships as more intimate than they actually are.		
2	According to the DSM-5-TR, those with Histrionic Personality Disorder avoid drawing attention to themselves, preferring a more understated style.		
3	A common feature is the tendency to express emotions in a theatrically exaggerated manner, even in ordinary situations.		
4	The DSM-5-TR states that seductive or sexually provocative behavior must always be present in every social setting.		
5	People with Histrionic Personality Disorder can be easily influenced by others or by external circumstances.		
6	Constantly seeking reassurance or approval is among the possible diagnostic criteria.		
7	Under the DSM-5-TR, manipulative and dramatic behaviors are ruled out in Histrionic Personality Disorder.		
8	A vague, impressionistic speech style lacking concrete details is considered a typical sign of Histrionic Personality Disorder.		
9	The DSM-5-TR notes that vulnerability to criticism and a tendency to take offense easily may appear in those with histrionic traits.		
10	Persistent superficial and theatrical attitudes do not necessarily prevent stable and functional social bonds.		

Matching Exercise

1. Attention-seeking behavior [ ]
2. Shallow and rapidly shifting emotions [ ]
3. Exaggerated sense of intimacy in relationships [ ]
4. Dramatic and theatrical gestures [ ]
5. Discomfort when not the center of attention [ ]
6. Overestimation of personal connections [ ]

Descriptions:

- A. Core characteristic of histrionic personality disorder
- B. Emotional feature commonly seen in HPD
- C. Misperception of relationship closeness
- D. Attention-focused trait
- E. Behavioral manifestation of HPD
- F. Not typically associated with HPD

Case Study

A 30-year-old woman presents for therapy, stating that her romantic relationships are often short-lived. She frequently feels unappreciated and reports going to great lengths to ensure that others notice her, such as dressing provocatively or exaggerating personal achievements. During the session, she is emotionally expressive and uses dramatic language, often redirecting the conversation to focus on herself. She perceives casual acquaintances as close friends and becomes distressed when they do not reciprocate the same level of intimacy. She describes feeling anxious and unfulfilled when she is not the center of attention in social situations.

1. Which symptom most strongly supports a diagnosis of HPD in this case?
    - A. Persistent social withdrawal due to anxiety
    - B. Excessive attention-seeking and dramatic behavior
    - C. Recurrent depressive episodes unrelated to relationships
    - D. Strong preference for solitary activities
2. What would be the most appropriate initial therapeutic goal for this patient?
    - A. Addressing distorted beliefs about relationships and intimacy
    - B. Reducing the frequency of attention-seeking behaviors
    - C. Managing co-occurring anxiety symptoms
    - D. Encouraging social withdrawal to limit distress
3. Which therapeutic approach would likely be most effective for this patient?
    - A. Psychoeducation about managing emotional intensity
    - B. Group therapy focusing on interpersonal dynamics
    - C. Structured CBT targeting attention-seeking behaviors
    - D. Pharmacotherapy to reduce emotional expression

Answers

Multiple Choice Questions

1. B
2. B
3. B
4. A
5. B
6. B
7. B

True/False Questions:

1. True
2. False
3. True
4. False
5. True
6. True
7. False
8. True
9. True
10. True

Matching Exercise

1. D
2. B
3. C
4. E
5. A
6. C

Case Study Answers and Explanations

1. B - Explanation: The patient's excessive attention-seeking and dramatic behavior are key indicators of HPD.
2. A - Explanation: Challenging the patient’s distorted beliefs about relationships is critical for improving interpersonal dynamics.
3. C - Explanation: Structured CBT provides practical tools to reduce attention-seeking behaviors and improve self-awareness.

Narcissistic Personality Disorder

Multiple Choice Questions

1. Which of the following best describes the core feature of narcissistic personality disorder (NPD)?
    - A. A pervasive pattern of disregard for others' rights
    - B. A preoccupation with fantasies of unlimited success, power, or beauty
    - C. Chronic avoidance of interpersonal relationships due to fear of rejection
    - D. Emotional instability with marked impulsivity
2. A patient with NPD is most likely to:
    - A. Display intense self-doubt and low self-esteem in social settings
    - B. Demonstrate grandiosity and a need for excessive admiration
    - C. Avoid social interactions due to fear of being embarrassed
    - D. Show pervasive suspicion and mistrust toward others
3. Which of the following traits differentiates grandiose narcissism from vulnerable narcissism?
    - A. Grandiose narcissism involves overt arrogance, while vulnerable narcissism involves hypersensitivity to criticism.
    - B. Grandiose narcissism is marked by social withdrawal, while vulnerable narcissism involves excessive social engagement.
    - C. Vulnerable narcissism includes manipulative behaviors, while grandiose narcissism does not.
    - D. Grandiose narcissism includes chronic feelings of inadequacy, while vulnerable narcissism does not.
4. Which of the following is least consistent with the presentation of NPD?
    - A. Lack of empathy toward others
    - B. Strong emotional regulation and resilience to criticism
    - C. Exploitative behavior in interpersonal relationships
    - D. Envy of others or the belief that others envy them
5. In individuals with NPD, which of the following cognitive distortions is most likely to occur?
    - A. Persistent catastrophic thinking about future events
    - B. A belief in their unique entitlement to special treatment
    - C. A pervasive fear of losing autonomy
    - D. Chronic self-doubt and insecurity
6. Which therapeutic approach is considered most effective for addressing narcissistic tendencies in NPD?
    - A. Long-term psychodynamic therapy
    - B. Cognitive Behavioral Therapy (CBT) focused on challenging grandiosity
    - C. Group therapy aimed at promoting self-awareness
    - D. Dialectical Behavior Therapy (DBT) targeting emotional regulation
7. Which of the following is a significant challenge when treating patients with NPD?
    - A. High risk of psychosis during therapy
    - B. Lack of trust in the therapeutic relationship
    - C. Excessive dependence on the therapist for decision-making
    - D. Reluctance to acknowledge personal flaws or need for change

True/False

		T	F
1	In the latest DSM-5-TR, Narcissistic Personality Disorder has been relocated to an alternative section that uses a hybrid model, abandoning the traditional categorical diagnostic criteria.		
2	The lack of empathy in individuals with Narcissistic Personality Disorder can manifest selectively, showing concern for some while ignoring others' distress.		
3	Some research suggests that, when their self-image is perceived to be threatened, individuals with Narcissistic Personality Disorder may experience episodes of depressed mood.		
4	According to the DSM-5-TR, recurrent fantasies of boundless success and power are not included among the diagnostic criteria for Narcissistic Personality Disorder.		
5	The dimensional approach introduced in the DSM-5-TR for personality disorders completely eliminates the categorical diagnosis of Narcissistic Personality Disorder.		
6	A person with Narcissistic Personality Disorder may occasionally display seemingly remorseful behavior if it helps preserve their grandiose self-image.		
7	People with Narcissistic Personality Disorder are less prone to outbursts of anger and aggressive behavior than those with Borderline Personality Disorder.		
8	Exploitative and manipulative interpersonal behaviors are frequently observed in Narcissistic Personality Disorder.		
9	The core features of Narcissistic Personality Disorder tend to diminish drastically with age in the majority of cases.		
10	A key difference between Narcissistic Personality Disorder and Antisocial Personality Disorder is a stronger need for admiration, as opposed to a disregard for social norms.		

Matching Exercise

1. Grandiosity [ ]
2. Exploitative behavior [ ]
3. Envy of others [ ]
4. Vulnerable self-esteem [ ]
5. Need for excessive admiration [ ]
6. Sense of entitlement [ ]

Descriptions:

- A. Belief in deserving special treatment regardless of context
- B. A core feature of NPD involving exaggerated self-importance
- C. Manipulation of others for personal gain
- D. Emotional instability and hypersensitivity masked by arrogance
- E. Feeling resentful of others' success or believing others feel the same toward them
- F. Desperation for validation to sustain self-image

Case Study

A 40-year-old executive is referred to therapy after receiving feedback from colleagues about their domineering and dismissive behavior. The patient describes their coworkers as "incompetent" and believes their success would be impossible without the patient's leadership. During the session, the patient boasts about their achievements but reacts defensively when questioned about areas for improvement. They report feeling frustrated when others do not recognize their contributions and often perceive criticism as a personal attack. Despite their outward confidence, the patient admits to feeling hollow and unfulfilled at times, particularly when they perceive a lack of recognition from others.

1. Which symptom most strongly supports a diagnosis of NPD in this case?
   - A. Persistent fear of criticism
   - B. Perception of being indispensable and superior
   - C. Recurrent feelings of anxiety unrelated to performance
   - D. A consistent pattern of social withdrawal
2. Which therapeutic goal would be most appropriate for this patient?
   - A. Addressing their tendency to manipulate others
   - B. Encouraging emotional validation and awareness of others' feelings
   - C. Challenging their beliefs about their superiority
   - D. Focusing exclusively on managing external conflicts
3. Which therapeutic strategy would be least effective for this patient?
   - A. Providing immediate praise to sustain engagement
   - B. Using a non-confrontational approach to explore emotional vulnerabilities
   - C. Engaging in direct confrontation about maladaptive behaviors
   - D. Encouraging reflective practices to improve self-awareness

Answers

Multiple Choice Questions

1. B
2. B
3. A
4. B
5. B
6. A
7. D

True/False Questions:

1. False
2. True
3. True
4. False
5. False
6. True
7. False
8. True
9. False
10. True

Matching Exercise

1. B
2. C
3. E
4. D
5. F
6. A

Case Study Answers and Explanations

1. B - Explanation: A persistent perception of being indispensable and superior is a hallmark of NPD.
2. C - Explanation: Challenging beliefs about superiority helps patients develop a more balanced self-image.
3. C - Explanation: Direct confrontation is often counterproductive and may lead to resistance in therapy.

Cluster C Personality Disorders

Cluster C personality disorders include Avoidant, Dependent, and Obsessive-Compulsive Personality Disorders. According to the DSM-5-TR, these conditions are defined by "anxious" or "fearful" traits, expressed through a persistent concern about criticism, a pronounced need for reassurance, or a strong tendency to maintain rigid control. Unlike Cluster B, characterized by dramatic or impulsive behavior, Cluster C is typified by insecurity, conformism, and the avoidance of situations that might cause anxiety or rejection.

In clinical practice, Avoidant Personality Disorder stands out for a fear of criticism or rejection, prompting the individual to withdraw from social contact, despite a deep desire for closeness. Dependent Personality Disorder features submissiveness and an excessive need for support, with difficulty making decisions independently and a strong fear of being abandoned or left to handle responsibilities alone. Obsessive-Compulsive Personality Disorder centers around perfectionism and control, coupled with marked rigidity regarding rules and details—a rigidity that can hinder flexibility, creativity, and relationships.

From a diagnostic standpoint, it is crucial to distinguish these patterns of functioning from ordinarily cautious or detail-oriented tendencies. Cluster C is characterized by an excessive fear of making mistakes, a constant need for approval, or an inflexible insistence on "perfect" performance. It is also important to differentiate Cluster C personality disorders from anxiety disorders like Social Anxiety Disorder or Generalized Anxiety Disorder, since in Cluster C, the anxious element is deeply ingrained in the personality structure, significantly affecting interpersonal relationships and the handling of responsibilities. Moreover, the perfectionism seen in Obsessive-Compulsive Personality Disorder can sometimes be mistaken for the obsessions and compulsions found in Obsessive-Compulsive Disorder proper, though the latter involves more recognizable intrusive thoughts or repetitive actions.

As for comorbidities, Cluster C disorders can co-occur with depressive or anxiety disorders, and symptoms may worsen under stressful or abandonment-prone circumstances. In Dependent Personality Disorder, for instance, separation events can trigger depressive symptoms or desperate behaviors. Individuals with Avoidant Personality Disorder may further withdraw when confronted with social situations they see as threatening, while those with Obsessive-Compulsive Personality Disorder can develop burnout or somatic issues when overwhelmed by a sense of responsibility.

In line with previous editions, the DSM-5-TR continues to group these personality disorders under Cluster C, emphasizing the importance of a thorough assessment of interpersonal behaviors and the automatic thoughts perpetuating avoidance, dependence, or rigid perfectionism. Exploring potential environmental or relational influences, alongside developmental history, proves essential for creating targeted treatment plans, which often integrate psychotherapeutic approaches to build self-esteem, manage fears, and develop greater flexibility.

Avoidant Personality Disorder (AvPD)

Multiple Choice Questions

1. Which cognitive distortion is most characteristic of avoidant personality disorder?
    - A. "If I make a mistake, it will confirm that I am worthless."
    - B. "Others are out to harm me, so I must remain vigilant."
    - C. "I am entitled to special treatment in all situations."
    - D. "I can manipulate others to achieve my goals."
2. Which of the following patterns distinguishes AvPD from schizoid personality disorder?
    - A. Desire for social relationships combined with avoidance due to fear of rejection
    - B. Avoidance of social interactions driven by lack of interest in relationships
    - C. Engagement in relationships only for instrumental purposes
    - D. Strong emotional detachment in interpersonal contexts
3. How does AvPD typically manifest in occupational settings?
    - A. Frequent confrontations with colleagues due to poor interpersonal skills
    - B. Reluctance to take on new responsibilities due to fear of failure
    - C. Manipulating coworkers to gain recognition
    - D. Aggressive pursuit of leadership roles to prove competence
4. Which scenario best illustrates the emotional dynamics of AvPD?
    - A. A person cancels a long-planned social event, fearing ridicule despite wanting to attend.
    - B. A person continuously seeks validation from peers and becomes angry when not praised.
    - C. A person avoids social situations entirely because they see no value in relationships.
    - D. A person creates conflict in relationships to maintain control over others.
5. In individuals with AvPD, fear of embarrassment often leads to:
    - A. Avoidance of social and occupational risks
    - B. Excessive reliance on others for decision-making
    - C. Pervasive distrust of others' motives
    - D. Frequent impulsive behaviors to escape social anxiety
6. Which therapeutic goal is most critical in the initial stages of treatment for AvPD?
    - A. Strengthening the patient's self-concept through gradual exposure to feared situations
    - B. Focusing solely on resolving early childhood trauma
    - C. Encouraging complete independence in social and occupational contexts
    - D. Minimizing discussions about fears to prevent distress
7. Which statement best captures the interpersonal perspective of someone with AvPD?
    - A. "If people see my flaws, they'll reject me completely."
    - B. "I am inherently superior, and others should respect me."
    - C. "I don't care about what others think of me."
    - D. "If I don't dominate conversations, others will think I'm weak."

True/False

		T	F
1	In the DSM-5-TR, Avoidant Personality Disorder and Social Phobia share overlapping diagnostic criteria.		
2	Individuals with Avoidant Personality Disorder do not pursue close relationships, regardless of context.		
3	Heightened sensitivity to rejection is regarded as a central aspect of Avoidant Personality Disorder.		
4	Some research points to increased amygdala activation in people with Avoidant Personality Disorder during stressful social situations.		
5	Avoidant Personality Disorder is classified within Cluster C, alongside Dependent and Obsessive-Compulsive Personality Disorders.		
6	In the DSM-5-TR, Avoidant Personality Disorder is typically associated with poor awareness of interpersonal distress.		
7	Avoidant Personality Disorder demonstrates a high comorbidity with mood disorders, particularly major depression.		
8	Certain theories propose that Avoidant Personality Disorder could be an extreme variant of Obsessive-Compulsive Personality Disorder.		
9	Most individuals with Avoidant Personality Disorder score high on measures of evaluation anxiety.		
10	An absolute inability to initiate conversations, even in perceived safe environments, is a hallmark feature of Avoidant Personality Disorder.		

Matching Exercise

1. Cognitive distortion of inferiority [ ]
2. Avoidance of occupational challenges [ ]
3. Fear of ridicule in social settings [ ]
4. Longing for relationships despite avoidance [ ]
5. Emotional response to perceived criticism [ ]
6. Reluctance to try new activities [ ]

Descriptions:

- A. Typical thought pattern in AvPD that undermines self-confidence
- B. Behavioral manifestation driven by fear of failure
- C. Emotional response that exacerbates social withdrawal
- D. Core feature of AvPD involving a paradoxical desire for connection
- E. Reflects anxiety-driven avoidance of social and occupational risks
- F. Common reaction to both real and imagined disapproval

Case Study

A 28-year-old teacher seeks therapy due to feelings of isolation and difficulty forming connections with colleagues and students. Despite positive feedback from supervisors, she doubts her abilities and avoids participating in school events, fearing judgment. She describes becoming highly anxious when asked to present at staff meetings and often experiences physical symptoms, such as sweating and nausea, in these situations. She longs to form closer relationships with coworkers but avoids socializing outside of work due to fear of rejection. She states, "It's better to stay invisible than risk being laughed at."

1. Which symptom most strongly supports a diagnosis of AvPD in this case?
   - A. Persistent feelings of distrust toward coworkers
   - B. Avoidance of professional opportunities despite a desire for connection
   - C. Chronic anger directed at authority figures
   - D. Impulsivity in interpersonal settings
2. What would be the most effective initial therapeutic approach for this patient?
   - A. Structured CBT focused on addressing cognitive distortions and exposure to feared scenarios
   - B. Long-term psychodynamic therapy to uncover the roots of her anxiety
   - C. Exclusive pharmacological treatment to manage symptoms
   - D. Group therapy to provide immediate social feedback
3. Which therapeutic technique would be least effective in treating this patient?
   - A. Exposure therapy targeting avoidance behaviors
   - B. Psychoeducation on the impact of avoidance on relationships
   - C. Direct confrontation of the patient's fears in unstructured settings
   - D. Gradual role-playing exercises to build social confidence

Answers

Multiple Choice Questions

1. A
2. A
3. B
4. A
5. A
6. A
7. A

True/False Questions:

1. True
2. False
3. True
4. False
5. True
6. False
7. True
8. False
9. True
10. False

Matching Exercise

1. A
2. B
3. E
4. D
5. F
6. C

Case Study Answers and Explanations

1. B - Explanation: Avoidance of professional opportunities due to fear of rejection, despite a desire for connection, is a hallmark of AvPD.
2. A - Explanation: Structured CBT, with a focus on challenging cognitive distortions and gradual exposure, addresses the key features of AvPD.
3. C – Explanation: Unstructured confrontation may overwhelm the patient and is less effective than a gradual, structured approach

Dependent Personality Disorder (DPD)

Multiple Choice Questions

1. Which of the following is the most defining characteristic of dependent personality disorder (DPD)?
    - A. Persistent mistrust and suspicion of others' intentions
    - B. A pervasive need to be taken care of and fear of separation
    - C. Excessive detachment and lack of interest in interpersonal relationships
    - D. A grandiose sense of self-importance and entitlement
2. How does dependent personality disorder typically manifest in interpersonal relationships?
    - A. Avoidance of relationships due to fear of rejection
    - B. Reliance on others for decision-making and excessive need for reassurance
    - C. Manipulative behaviors to maintain control over others
    - D. Intense distrust of close companions
3. Which of the following differentiates DPD from avoidant personality disorder (AvPD)?
    - A. Individuals with DPD actively seek relationships, while those with AvPD avoid them out of fear of rejection.
    - B. Individuals with DPD exhibit grandiosity, while those with AvPD do not.
    - C. AvPD involves a greater degree of manipulation than DPD.
    - D. DPD is primarily characterized by a lack of empathy, unlike AvPD.
4. Which behavior is least likely to be observed in someone with DPD?
    - A. Tolerating mistreatment in a relationship to avoid being alone
    - B. Difficulty initiating projects or making decisions independently
    - C. Persistently seeking reassurance and approval from others
    - D. Preferring solitary activities over social engagement
5. Which cognitive distortion is most typical in individuals with DPD?
    - A. "I am incompetent and cannot function without others' help."
    - B. "I am superior to others and deserve special treatment."
    - C. "Others are inherently untrustworthy and manipulative."
    - D. "I must avoid criticism at all costs, or I will fail."
6. Which therapeutic approach is most effective for treating DPD?
    - A. Long-term psychodynamic therapy focusing on dependency
    - B. Cognitive Behavioral Therapy (CBT) targeting autonomy and decision-making
    - C. Group therapy with minimal individual attention
    - D. Pharmacological management as the primary treatment
7. What is a common risk associated with dependent personality disorder?
    - A. Chronic isolation and social withdrawal
    - B. Vulnerability to abusive or exploitative relationships
    - C. Persistent delusions of persecution
    - D. Development of psychotic symptoms

True/False

		T	F
1	In the DSM-5-TR, Dependent Personality Disorder has been moved to Cluster B.		
2	Individuals with Dependent Personality Disorder may appear submissive in some relationships but exert control through passivity in others.		
3	A persistent fear of separation is listed among the principal criteria for Dependent Personality Disorder.		
4	Some individuals with Dependent Personality Disorder form multiple close relationships to avoid the anxiety of focusing on a single partner.		
5	Dependent Personality Disorder is classified in Cluster C, along with Avoidant and Obsessive-Compulsive Personality Disorders.		
6	Chronic procrastination is a fundamental diagnostic criterion for Dependent Personality Disorder in the DSM-5-TR.		
7	Some research indicates that people with Dependent Personality Disorder may oscillate between dependence and anger toward the support figure.		
8	The DSM-5-TR introduces the term "social subordination" specifically to describe Dependent Personality Disorder.		
9	Individuals with Dependent Personality Disorder can exhibit passivity along with subtle forms of relational manipulation.		
10	Those with Dependent Personality Disorder do not display anxious tendencies, only submissive behavior.		

Matching Exercise

1. Difficulty making decisions independently [ ]
2. Fear of being alone or abandoned [ ]
3. Tolerating abuse to maintain a relationship [ ]
4. Need for excessive reassurance [ ]
5. Reliance on others for responsibility [ ]
6. Avoidance of leadership roles [ ]

Descriptions:

- A. Core behavioral feature of dependent personality disorder
- B. Emotional manifestation of dependency
- C. Common cognitive distortion in DPD
- D. Result of inability to function autonomously
- E. A frequent consequence of the fear of separation
- F. Behavioral trait indicating reluctance to assert autonomy

Case Study

A 28-year-old woman presents for therapy after her partner ended their relationship. She expresses extreme distress and states, "I don't know how to manage on my own." She describes a pattern of relying heavily on her partner for decision-making, including choices about her career and daily activities. Despite feeling mistreated at times during the relationship, she says she stayed because she feared being alone. She struggles to express her own preferences and frequently seeks reassurance from friends and family, worrying they might also leave her if she becomes "too much to handle."

1. Which symptom most strongly supports a diagnosis of DPD in this case?
   - A. Persistent mistrust of her partner's intentions
   - B. Reliance on her partner for decision-making and fear of abandonment
   - C. Difficulty maintaining social relationships due to aggressive tendencies
   - D. Recurrent episodes of severe anger toward close companions
2. What would be the most appropriate initial therapeutic goal for this patient?
   - A. Developing decision-making skills and fostering autonomy
   - B. Identifying and avoiding toxic relationships entirely
   - C. Rebuilding her relationship with her former partner
   - D. Managing anger and hostility in social situations
3. Which therapeutic technique would likely be most effective for this patient?
   - A. Cognitive restructuring to challenge beliefs about dependence
   - B. Exploring repressed memories of childhood neglect
   - C. Using confrontation to address manipulative behaviors
   - D. Group therapy focused on reducing emotional intensity

Answers

Multiple Choice Questions

1. B
2. B
3. A
4. D
5. A
6. B
7. B

True/False Questions:

1. False
2. True
3. True
4. False
5. True
6. False
7. True
8. False
9. True
10. False

Matching Exercise

1. A
2. B
3. E
4. A
5. D
6. F

Case Study Answers and Explanations

1. B - Explanation: Reliance on others for decision-making and a fear of abandonment are hallmark traits of DPD.
2. A - Explanation: Helping the patient develop decision-making skills and fostering autonomy is critical for managing dependency.
3. A - Explanation: Cognitive restructuring helps the patient challenge distorted beliefs about their inability to function independently.

Obsessive-Compulsive Personality Disorder (OCPD)

Multiple Choice Questions

1. Which of the following best captures the core feature of obsessive-compulsive personality disorder (OCPD)?
    - A. Recurrent intrusive thoughts and compulsive behaviors aimed at reducing anxiety
    - B. A preoccupation with orderliness, perfectionism, and control at the expense of flexibility
    - C. A pervasive fear of contamination and excessive handwashing
    - D. Emotional instability and impulsivity in relationships
2. How does OCPD differ from obsessive-compulsive disorder (OCD)?
    - A. OCPD is characterized by intrusive thoughts, while OCD focuses on perfectionism.
    - B. OCD involves specific compulsions, while OCPD is defined by rigid personality traits.
    - C. OCPD involves repetitive rituals, while OCD involves excessive emotional detachment.
    - D. Individuals with OCPD typically exhibit a complete lack of anxiety symptoms.
3. Which of the following behaviors is least likely to be associated with OCPD?
    - A. Spending hours organizing tasks to ensure perfect execution
    - B. Difficulty delegating tasks due to fear they won't be done "correctly"
    - C. Repeated intrusive thoughts about harming others
    - D. Prioritizing work over leisure and relationships
4. What belief is most typical in individuals with OCPD?
    - A. "If everything is not perfect, it reflects poorly on me as a person."
    - B. "I must avoid rejection at all costs."
    - C. "People cannot be trusted, and I must be vigilant."
    - D. "I am entitled to special treatment and recognition."
5. How does the perfectionism in OCPD most often manifest?
    - A. Completing tasks efficiently without stress
    - B. Procrastinating or abandoning tasks due to fear they won't be perfect
    - C. Excessive focus on meeting others' emotional needs
    - D. Engaging in impulsive behaviors to reduce perfectionistic stress
6. Which therapeutic approach is most effective for addressing the rigidity and control seen in OCPD?
    - A. Exposure and Response Prevention (ERP)
    - B. Cognitive Behavioral Therapy (CBT) with a focus on cognitive flexibility
    - C. Psychoanalytic therapy to uncover unconscious conflicts
    - D. Family therapy targeting relational dynamics
7. Which of the following is a significant challenge in treating individuals with OCPD?
    - A. Their tendency to avoid structured environments
    - B. Their reluctance to engage in collaborative problem-solving
    - C. Their inability to recognize the maladaptive nature of their behaviors
    - D. Their frequent outbursts of anger and hostility

True/False

		T	F
1	Excessive criticism of others' performance is considered a possible feature in Obsessive-Compulsive Personality Disorder.		
2	Although rigidity is a central aspect, some studies suggest that individuals with Obsessive-Compulsive Personality Disorder can be flexible in contexts they deem unimportant.		
3	Some research suggests that comorbidity between Obsessive-Compulsive Personality Disorder and Obsessive-Compulsive Disorder is linked to lower symptom severity, due to more effective coping strategies.		
4	A link between Obsessive-Compulsive Personality Disorder and high levels of neuroticism has been proposed, though not formally included in the DSM-5-TR criteria.		
5	Individuals with Obsessive-Compulsive Personality Disorder typically do not experience distress or relational difficulties, as they view their habits as virtues.		
6	Perfectionism can lead to decision-making paralysis due to fear of making mistakes.		
7	The DSM-5-TR requires at least three symptoms of "extreme self-control" as a diagnostic criterion for Obsessive-Compulsive Personality Disorder.		
8	Some research shows that, despite discipline and rigidity, those with Obsessive-Compulsive Personality Disorder do not develop addictive behaviors.		
9	A common characteristic is postponing the completion of projects in order to refine every detail.		
10	According to some studies, traits of Obsessive-Compulsive Personality Disorder diminish rapidly in adulthood, unlike other personality disorders.		

Matching Exercise

1. Preoccupation with rules and order [ ]
2. Difficulty delegating tasks to others [ ]
3. Overprioritization of work over relationships [ ]
4. Reluctance to discard items with little value [ ]
5. Fear of making mistakes [ ]
6. Perfectionism leading to inefficiency [ ]

Descriptions:

- A. A core cognitive distortion in OCPD
- B. Behavioral manifestation of a need for control
- C. Reflects rigidity in interpersonal and work-related dynamics
- D. Leads to hoarding behaviors, distinct from other compulsive traits
- E. Characteristic of workaholism seen in OCPD
- F. Associated with procrastination and task incompletion

Case Study

A 42-year-old man seeks therapy after his wife threatens to leave him, citing his controlling behavior and inability to prioritize their relationship. He describes spending hours each evening reorganizing his workspace to ensure it is "just right" for the next day. At work, he is reluctant to delegate tasks, believing that no one else can meet his standards. He struggles to complete projects on time because he continually revises them, fearing they are not perfect. Despite his dedication to work, he feels unfulfilled and acknowledges that his perfectionism strains his personal and professional relationships.

1. Which symptom most strongly supports a diagnosis of OCPD in this case?
   - A. Intrusive thoughts about contamination leading to repetitive cleaning
   - B. Reluctance to delegate tasks due to perfectionistic standards
   - C. Emotional lability and impulsivity in decision-making
   - D. Frequent conflicts due to paranoia and mistrust
2. What would be the most appropriate therapeutic goal for this patient?
   - A. Teaching strategies to tolerate imperfection and delegate tasks
   - B. Exploring repressed childhood conflicts about control
   - C. Encouraging complete restructuring of his workspace habits
   - D. Focusing on repairing his relationship with his wife without addressing underlying traits
3. Which therapeutic strategy would likely be most effective for this patient?
   - A. Role-playing scenarios to confront fear of contamination
   - B. Cognitive restructuring to challenge rigid perfectionistic beliefs
   - C. Psychodynamic exploration of unconscious drives
   - D. Pharmacological intervention to reduce anxiety symptoms

Answers

Multiple Choice Questions
1. B
2. B
3. C
4. A
5. B
6. B
7. C

True/False Questions:
1. True
2. True
3. False
4. True
5. False
6. True
7. False
8. False
9. True
10. False

Matching Exercise
1. B
2. B
3. E
4. D
5. A
6. F

Case Study Answers and Explanations
1. B - Explanation: Reluctance to delegate tasks due to rigid perfectionistic standards is a hallmark of OCPD.
2. A - Explanation: Helping the patient tolerate imperfection and delegate tasks is essential for addressing the maladaptive aspects of OCPD.
3. B - Explanation: Cognitive restructuring directly addresses the rigid thought patterns that underlie OCPD behaviors.

Other Personality Disorders

Multiple Choice Questions

1. Which of the following best describes "other specified personality disorder"?
   - A. Traits causing distress that do not fully meet criteria for a specific personality disorder
   - B. A pattern of behaviors combining traits from Cluster A and B disorders
   - C. Symptoms resembling psychotic disorders
   - D. A transient response to acute stress
2. What differentiates "other specified" from "unspecified" personality disorder?
   - A. "Other specified" includes a reason why criteria are not fully met.
   - B. "Unspecified" applies only to Cluster C disorders.
   - C. "Other specified" requires psychotic symptoms.
   - D. "Unspecified" is used when traits are mild and transient.
3. Which of the following scenarios is most likely to result in a diagnosis of "unspecified personality disorder"?
   - A. The patient shows significant dysfunction, but diagnostic details are incomplete.
   - B. Traits from multiple personality disorders are equally present.
   - C. A single maladaptive trait causes distress.
   - D. The patient exhibits transient symptoms of anxiety and avoidance.
4. What is a common therapeutic focus for "other specified personality disorder"?
   - A. Addressing specific maladaptive traits that impair functioning
   - B. Reducing symptoms of anxiety and psychosis
   - C. Enhancing family dynamics exclusively
   - D. Avoiding categorization to minimize stigma
5. Which is the most common clinical context for diagnosing "unspecified personality disorder"?
   - A. Acute care settings with limited assessment time
   - B. Long-term outpatient treatment programs
   - C. Psychoanalytic therapy for unresolved trauma
   - D. Group therapy focused on relationship repair
6. Which therapeutic approach is most appropriate for individuals diagnosed with "other specified personality disorder"?
   - A. Schema therapy targeting maladaptive emotional patterns
   - B. Pharmacotherapy as a standalone treatment
   - C. Exposure-based therapy for social anxiety
   - D. Psychoeducational groups focused on symptom management
7. Which of the following is least likely to be observed in a patient with an "other specified personality disorder"?
   - A. Significant interpersonal difficulties causing distress
   - B. Consistent presentation of traits meeting criteria for a single personality disorder
   - C. Emotional instability that disrupts occupational functioning
   - D. Maladaptive traits that cause clinical impairment

True/False

		T	F
1	Unspecified Personality Disorder and Other Specified Personality Disorder in the DSM-5-TR are distinct diagnostic categories.		
2	Coexisting borderline and narcissistic traits always lead to an 'Other Personality Disorders' diagnosis.		
3	A 'Personality Change Due to Another Medical Condition' diagnosis requires clear evidence of a stable behavioral shift.		
4	The DSM-5-TR allows the use of 'Other Specified Personality Disorder' when full criteria for a single disorder are not met.		
5	Depressive symptoms are always mandatory for diagnosing a personality disorder linked to a medical condition.		
6	'Unspecified Personality Disorder' can be used when there is not enough clinical information for a more precise diagnosis.		
7	'Other Specified Personality Disorder' and 'Unspecified Personality Disorder' do not differ in terms of clinical reasoning.		
8	An atypical personality presentation, not captured by the known clusters, can be coded as 'Other Personality Disorders.'		
9	A substance-induced personality disorder cannot be coded if symptoms persist after discontinuing the substance.		
10	Having multiple traits from different clusters automatically mandates the use of the 'Other Personality Disorders' category.		

Matching Exercise

1. Traits that do not meet full criteria for a specific personality disorder [ ]
2. Lack of detailed reasoning for why criteria are not met [ ]
3. Significant distress or impairment despite subthreshold traits [ ]
4. Overlap of multiple personality traits without clear dominance [ ]
5. Diagnostic use in urgent care or limited-assessment settings [ ]
6. Explanation of the specific reasons full criteria are not met [ ]

Descriptions:

- A. Common characteristic of "other specified" personality disorder
- B. Indicates use of "unspecified" personality disorder diagnosis
- C. Behavioral and emotional patterns observed in both categories
- D. Core element requiring clinician explanation in "other specified" diagnosis
- E. Frequent context for "unspecified" personality disorder diagnoses
- F. A key consideration in determining clinical significance

Case Study

A 29-year-old woman seeks therapy, describing a pattern of intense relationships that frequently end due to perceived criticism from partners. She exhibits emotional reactivity and occasional impulsive decisions, such as quitting her job without a backup plan. However, her behaviors do not fully align with borderline personality disorder criteria due to the absence of chronic self-harm or identity disturbance. She struggles with significant distress in her interpersonal and occupational functioning but does not meet criteria for any one specific personality disorder.

1. Which symptom most strongly supports a diagnosis of "other specified" personality disorder in this case?
    - A. Persistent mistrust of her partner's intentions
    - B. Emotional reactivity and impulsivity causing distress
    - C. Difficulty maintaining relationships due to aggression
    - D. Recurrent thoughts of self-harm
2. What would be the most appropriate therapeutic focus for this patient?
    - A. Developing emotional regulation and interpersonal skills
    - B. Challenging rigid perfectionistic beliefs about herself
    - C. Addressing avoidance behaviors in social settings
    - D. Exploring childhood trauma to understand mistrust of others
3. Which therapeutic approach would likely be most effective for this patient?
    - A. Schema therapy tailored to address underlying emotional needs
    - B. Pharmacological intervention as the primary treatment
    - C. Family therapy focusing on relational dynamics
    - D. Unstructured therapy allowing the patient to guide the process

Answers

Multiple Choice Questions

1. A
2. A
3. A
4. A
5. A
6. A
7. B

True/False Questions:

1. True
2. False
3. True
4. True
5. False
6. True
7. False
8. True
9. False
10. False

Matching Exercise

1. A
2. B
3. F
4. C
5. E
6. D

Case Study Answers and Explanations

1. B - Explanation: Emotional reactivity and impulsivity causing distress are hallmark traits of this presentation.
2. A - Explanation: Emotional regulation and interpersonal skills address the patient's key areas of dysfunction.
3. A - Explanation: Schema therapy effectively targets emotional patterns and beliefs that underlie maladaptive behaviors.

Paraphilic Disorders

Paraphilic disorders involve situations in which sexual desire or gratification is tied to atypical fantasies, impulses, or behaviors that may be socially unacceptable, illegal, or distressing both for the individual and those around them. According to the DSM-5-TR, having unusual sexual interests alone does not suffice for a diagnosis: there must be clinically significant distress, impaired functioning, or a risk of harm to oneself or others. In other words, not all unusual fantasies qualify as paraphilic disorders; well-defined criteria are needed, including persistence over time, recurrence, and negative impact on the individual's life or on those involved.

From a clinical perspective, paraphilic disorders include Voyeuristic, Exhibitionistic, Frotteuristic, Sexual Masochism, Sexual Sadism, Pedophilic, Fetishistic, and Transvestic Disorders, as well as other specified or unspecified variants. Some revolve around urges directed toward objects, situations, or non-consenting individuals; others involve the need to suffer or inflict suffering as a source of pleasure. It is important to note that for a diagnosis, these fantasies or behaviors must typically persist for at least six months and be associated with real distress or impairment.

Compared to other areas—such as sexual dysfunctions, which involve a lack or malfunction of the sexual response, or personality disorders, where difficulties stem from relational and identity patterns—paraphilic disorders focus on the atypical nature of erotic drives. A common mistake is to confuse them with consensual variations of sexual behavior: the DSM-5-TR clarifies that a paraphilia becomes a disorder if it causes significant harm or disruption. It is also crucial to differentiate them from other psychiatric conditions, since in the presence of psychosis or cognitive impairments, certain behaviors might be explained by broader issues beyond paraphilic interests.

In terms of comorbidity, some studies point to links with mood or anxiety disorders, as well as substance abuse, particularly when paraphilic acts are used as a means to cope with unpleasant emotions or stress. In cases involving non-consensual paraphilias (such as Frotteurism, Voyeurism, or Pedophilic Disorder), antisocial traits or impulse-control problems may also be present, complicating the diagnostic picture and necessitating interventions aimed at protecting others from possible harm.

The DSM-5-TR continues the approach taken by previous editions, distinguishing between paraphilias that involve criminal behavior or non-consenting individuals and those limited to the private sphere of consenting adults. At the same time, it underscores the importance of assessing the individual's level of distress, any compulsion or lack of control, and the overall impact on functioning. Accurate diagnosis helps outline avenues for psychotherapeutic support and, if indicated, pharmacological treatments to manage impulses, reduce the risk of recurrence, and encourage safer, more responsible sexual behavior.

Voyeuristic Disorder

Multiple Choice Questions

1. Which of the following criteria is required for a diagnosis of Voyeuristic Disorder according to the DSM-5?
    - A. Observing sexual behaviors without consent for at least 6 months.
    - B. Experiencing clinically significant distress or functional impairment.
    - C. Repeated desire for public sexual exposure.
    - D. Absence of other psychiatric disorders.
2. What is the minimum age for diagnosing Voyeuristic Disorder?
    - A. 16 years.
    - B. 18 years.
    - C. 21 years.
    - D. No specific minimum age.
3. Which of the following is NOT a criterion for Voyeuristic Disorder?
    - A. Acting on voyeuristic urges with non-consenting individuals.
    - B. Voyeuristic interest occurs exclusively in work settings.
    - C. Symptoms persist for at least 6 months.
    - D. The behavior causes distress or interpersonal problems.
4. Which condition is often associated with Voyeuristic Disorder?
    - A. Social anxiety.
    - B. Obsessive-Compulsive Disorder.
    - C. Substance use disorders.
    - D. Schizophrenia.
5. Which therapeutic intervention is generally most appropriate for Voyeuristic Disorder?
    - A. Cognitive-behavioral therapy.
    - B. Pharmacological treatment with antipsychotics.
    - C. Electroconvulsive therapy.
    - D. Systemic-relational therapy.
6. Which of the following is a risk factor for developing Voyeuristic Disorder?
    - A. History of childhood physical abuse.
    - B. Absence of childhood trauma.
    - C. Stable family environment.
    - D. Extensive social relationships.
7. Voyeuristic Disorder can be diagnosed if:
    - A. Voyeuristic interest is the individual's only sexual behavior.
    - B. The individual observes only consenting partners.
    - C. The behavior does not cause distress or functional impairment.
    - D. Voyeuristic urges involve non-consenting individuals.

True/False Questions

		T	F
1	The DSM-5-TR requires that voyeuristic urges persist for at least six months to meet diagnostic criteria.		
2	A Voyeuristic Disorder diagnosis does not apply if the individual is 17 years old and exhibits sexual impulsivity toward unaware persons.		
3	Having both voyeuristic fantasies and significant distress, without ever acting on one's urges, can still meet diagnostic criteria.		
4	If voyeuristic behaviors occur exclusively in private settings among consenting adults, Voyeuristic Disorder is not diagnosed.		
5	For Voyeuristic Disorder, sexual arousal primarily stems from watching an unaware person, not merely from nudity itself.		
6	According to the DSM-5-TR, a diagnosis may be ruled out if the individual experiences minimal distress yet violates someone else's rights.		
7	The presence of other paraphilias rules out the possibility of diagnosing Voyeuristic Disorder.		
8	The potential for legal consequences does not affect the DSM-5-TR criteria for Voyeuristic Disorder.		
9	A hallmark of Voyeuristic Disorder is repeated exposure to possible discovery, without the victim's consent.		
10	A Voyeuristic Disorder diagnosis remains indefinitely, regardless of symptom changes over time.		

Matching Exercise

1. Minimum age for diagnosis. [ ]
2. Minimum symptom duration for diagnosis. [ ]
3. Clinically significant distress. [ ]
4. Association with substance use. [ ]
5. Prevalence in men. [ ]
6. Recommended treatment. [ ]

Descriptions:

- A. Cognitive-behavioral therapy.
- B. 6 months.
- C. 18 years.
- D. More common in men.
- E. Frequently observed.
- F. Required for diagnosis.

Case Study

A 28-year-old man reports experiencing recurring, uncontrollable urges to observe non-consenting individuals while they are undressing. These urges have been present for approximately 8 months and cause significant distress, impairing his ability to focus at work. He also reports problematic alcohol use.

1. Which DSM-5 criterion does the described case meet?
    - A. Duration of at least 6 months.
    - B. Age under 18 years.
    - C. Exclusively consensual voyeuristic interest.
    - D. Absence of clinical distress.
2. What is the most appropriate treatment in this case?
    - A. Electroconvulsive therapy.
    - B. Cognitive-behavioral therapy.
    - C. Psychodynamic psychotherapy.
    - D. Pharmacological treatment with antipsychotics.
3. What additional factor should be considered in the diagnosis?
    - A. Presence of dissociative symptoms.
    - B. Problematic alcohol use.
    - C. History of childhood trauma.
    - D. Absence of associated behaviors.

Answers

Multiple Choice Questions:

1. B
2. B
3. B
4. C
5. A
6. A
7. A

True/False Questions:

1. True
2. False
3. True
4. True
5. True
6. False
7. False
8. True
9. True
10. False

Matching Exercise:

1. C
2. B
3. F
4. E
5. D
6. A

Case Study Answers and Explanations:

1. A Explanation: The symptoms must persist for at least 6 months to meet the diagnostic criteria.
2. B Explanation: Cognitive-behavioral therapy is the most commonly recommended treatment for paraphilic disorders.
3. B Explanation: Problematic alcohol use can influence the severity of the disorder and should be addressed during the clinical evaluation.

Exhibitionistic Disorder

Multiple Choice Questions

1. Which of the following differentiates Exhibitionistic Disorder from culturally sanctioned behaviors?
    - A. The absence of non-consenting individuals.
    - B. Clinically significant distress or functional impairment caused by the behavior.
    - C. The presence of a comorbid mood disorder.
    - D. The behavior's association with a paraphilic interest cluster.
2. Exhibitionistic Disorder is often comorbid with which of the following conditions?
    - A. Borderline Personality Disorder.
    - B. Antisocial Personality Disorder.
    - C. Schizotypal Personality Disorder.
    - D. Avoidant Personality Disorder.
3. A 35-year-old man experiences recurring urges to expose himself in public settings but denies distress or impairment. Under what condition would this behavior meet DSM-5 diagnostic criteria?
    - A. If he exclusively exposes himself to consenting adults.
    - B. If his urges lead to criminal consequences.
    - C. If his behavior is part of an organized paraphilic community.
    - D. If he experiences significant distress related to the urges.
4. Which therapeutic approach is most supported by evidence for addressing the behavioral components of Exhibitionistic Disorder?
    - A. Dialectical Behavior Therapy (DBT).
    - B. Cognitive-Behavioral Therapy (CBT) with relapse prevention strategies.
    - C. Psychodynamic therapy focused on early childhood trauma.
    - D. Exposure therapy targeting distress tolerance.
5. Which of the following factors increases the likelihood of Exhibitionistic Disorder leading to legal consequences?
    - A. The individual's inability to experience guilt.
    - B. The repeated nature of the behavior despite previous warnings.
    - C. An impulsive personality with a history of rule-breaking behavior.
    - D. The lack of a formal diagnosis.
6. According to the DSM-5, which of the following is a subtype of Exhibitionistic Disorder?
    - A. Exhibitionism focused on sexual acts between others.
    - B. Exhibitionism targeting prepubescent children.
    - C. Exhibitionism focused exclusively on non-sexual nudity.
    - D. Exhibitionism without accompanying sexual arousal.
7. In the assessment of Exhibitionistic Disorder, which diagnostic tool would most effectively evaluate the presence of paraphilic interests?
    - A. Minnesota Multiphasic Personality Inventory (MMPI).
    - B. Structured Clinical Interview for DSM-5 (SCID-5).
    - C. Sexual Behavior Inventory.
    - D. Yale-Brown Obsessive Compulsive Scale (Y-BOCS).

True/False Questions

		T	F
1	Exposing one's genitals to unsuspecting individuals for at least three months meets DSM-5-TR criteria for Exhibitionistic Disorder.		
2	The DSM-5-TR allows a diagnosis of Exhibitionistic Disorder even without personal distress, if the behavior violates another's consent.		
3	Individuals with Exhibitionistic Disorder may experience sexual arousal solely from the act of exposure, without requiring further physical contact.		
4	Exposing one's genitals to a consenting acquaintance in a private setting can qualify as Exhibitionistic Disorder if the temporal criteria are met.		
5	The DSM-5-TR requires specifying whether the focus is exclusively on adults, on prepubescent children, or on both.		
6	Merely having fantasies of exposing one's genitals, without acting on them and without significant distress, leads to a diagnosis of Exhibitionistic Disorder.		
7	The individual must be at least 18 years old for Exhibitionistic Disorder to be considered.		
8	The presence of other paraphilias does not preclude an additional diagnosis of Exhibitionistic Disorder.		
9	Some research suggests the key factor is not the risk of discovery, but the reaction of the observed person.		
10	The DSM-5-TR does not distinguish severity levels of Exhibitionistic Disorder based on the age of those involved.		

Matching Exercise

1. Typical onset age for Exhibitionistic Disorder [ ]
2. Core diagnostic criterion [ ]
3. Evidence-based therapy for behavioral control [ ]
4. Common comorbidity [ ]
5. Key differential diagnosis [ ]
6. Pharmacological intervention [ ]

Descriptions:

- A. Cognitive-behavioral therapy (CBT).
- B. Selective serotonin reuptake inhibitors (SSRIs).
- C. Early adulthood.
- D. Antisocial Personality Disorder.
- E. Sexual arousal from exposing oneself to non-consenting individuals.
- F. Impulse control disorders or obsessive-compulsive spectrum disorders.

Case Study

A 42-year-old man reports recurring, intense sexual urges to expose his genitals to strangers in public. Over the past year, he has acted on these urges multiple times, leading to several arrests and increasing anxiety about his ability to control his behavior. He has a history of childhood trauma and comorbid alcohol use disorder. Despite repeated legal consequences, he continues to experience overwhelming impulses to engage in exhibitionistic acts.

1. Based on the DSM-5, what aspect of the patient's behavior confirms the diagnosis of Exhibitionistic Disorder?
   - A. Anxiety about controlling his impulses.
   - B. Repeated acts involving non-consenting individuals.
   - C. Comorbid alcohol use disorder.
   - D. History of legal issues.
2. What is the most appropriate initial intervention for this individual?
   - A. Referral to a residential treatment program for alcohol use.
   - B. Pharmacological treatment with SSRIs to reduce sexual impulsivity.
   - C. Cognitive-behavioral therapy focused on impulse control.
   - D. Psychoeducational sessions on legal consequences.
3. What additional diagnostic consideration should be prioritized?
   - A. Assessment for other paraphilic disorders.
   - B. Identification of any current mood disorder.
   - C. Evaluation of trauma-related symptoms.
   - D. Assessment of substance withdrawal symptoms.

Answers

Multiple Choice Questions:

1. B
2. B
3. D
4. B
5. B
6. B
7. C

True/False Questions:

1. False
2. True
3. True
4. False
5. True
6. False
7. True
8. True
9. True
10. False

Matching Exercise:

1. C
2. E
3. A
4. D
5. F
6. B

Case Study Answers and Explanations:

1. B Explanation: Acting on sexual urges with non-consenting individuals is a core diagnostic criterion for Exhibitionistic Disorder.
2. C Explanation: CBT is considered the most effective intervention for addressing impulse control in Exhibitionistic Disorder.
3. A Explanation: Co-occurring paraphilic disorders should be assessed to inform comprehensive treatment planning.

Frotteuristic Disorder

Multiple Choice Questions

1. Which of the following is a primary diagnostic criterion for frotteuristic disorder?
    - A. Persistent concern with hoarding objects
    - B. Recurrent and intense sexual fantasies, urges, or behaviors involving touching or rubbing against a non-consenting person
    - C. Need to dress in clothing of the opposite sex to achieve sexual arousal
    - D. Significant social avoidance due to fear of being observed
2. In which of the following situations is frotteuristic behavior most likely to occur?
    - A. Consensual intimate interactions
    - B. Crowded places like trains, buses, or stations
    - C. High-pressure workplace environments
    - D. Solitary and private settings
3. Frotteuristic disorder is classified in the DSM-5 as:
    - A. An impulse-control disorder
    - B. A personality disorder
    - C. A paraphilic disorder
    - D. An obsessive-compulsive disorder
4. Which of the following statements is correct?
    - A. Frotteuristic disorder occurs exclusively in children
    - B. Individuals with frotteuristic disorder may act impulsively without regard for legal consequences
    - C. Frotteuristic fantasies are always harmless and do not interfere with daily life
    - D. The disorder is predominantly diagnosed in women
5. Which therapeutic approach is often recommended for frotteuristic disorder?
    - A. Cognitive-behavioral therapy and, if needed, medication to reduce sexual urges
    - B. Pharmacological therapy alone
    - C. Family counseling without other interventions
    - D. No treatment needed; the disorder resolves spontaneously
6. Which of the following is true regarding the diagnosis of frotteuristic disorder?
    - A. Diagnosis can only be made with documented criminal behavior
    - B. The disorder must cause significant distress or impairment in social, occupational, or other important areas of functioning
    - C. A single frotteuristic fantasy in a lifetime is sufficient for diagnosis
    - D. The disorder develops exclusively in old age
7. Frotteuristic urges must persist for a minimum period of:
    - A. 1 month
    - B. 3 months
    - C. 6 months
    - D. 12 months

True/False Questions

		T	F
1	The DSM-5-TR requires that urges or behaviors characteristic of Frotteuristic Disorder persist for at least six months.		
2	The minimum age for diagnosing Frotteuristic Disorder is set at 18.		
3	If an individual with Frotteuristic Disorder acts on their urges without the victim's consent, the diagnosis can be made even without personal distress.		
4	Frotteuristic Disorder may be diagnosed when physical contact occurs exclusively between consenting partners.		
5	Some research suggests that behaviors seen in Frotteuristic Disorder often take place in crowded environments.		
6	If frotteuristic behaviors are infrequent and do not cause distress, the DSM-5-TR still indicates making a Frotteuristic Disorder diagnosis.		
7	The presence of another paraphilia always rules out a separate diagnosis of Frotteuristic Disorder.		
8	According to certain studies, in Frotteuristic Disorder, rubbing against an unaware victim may include fantasies of more explicit sexual involvement.		
9	The DSM-5-TR regards social isolation as a primary criterion for Frotteuristic Disorder.		
10	Sexual gratification in Frotteuristic Disorder can arise both from physical contact and from the risk of being discovered.		

Matching Exercise

1. Paraphilic disorder [ ]
2. Cognitive-behavioral therapy [ ]
3. Significant distress [ ]
4. Crowded places [ ]
5. Recurrent sexual urges [ ]
6. 6 months [ ]

Descriptions:

- A. Minimum duration for diagnostic criteria for frotteuristic disorder
- B. DSM-5 diagnostic category for frotteuristic disorder
- C. Key component of diagnosis: interference with daily functioning
- D. Common environment for frotteuristic behaviors
- E. Central impulses and fantasies in the disorder
- F. Therapy focused on behavior modification

Case Study

A 27-year-old man has been reported for inappropriate behavior in crowded places such as buses and subways. He describes recurrent fantasies and urges leading him to rub against others without their consent. The patient feels guilty but states that he cannot control his behavior, which has persisted for over six months. His distress is negatively impacting his work and social life.

1. What is the minimum duration required to diagnose this condition?
   - A. 1 month
   - B. 3 months
   - C. 6 months
   - D. 12 months
2. What is the most appropriate treatment for this patient?
   - A. No treatment; the disorder resolves spontaneously
   - B. Cognitive-behavioral therapy and medication if necessary
   - C. Family therapy alone
   - D. Pharmacological treatment without other therapies
3. Does this patient meet the criteria for frotteuristic disorder?
   - A. Yes, fully meets DSM-5 criteria
   - B. No, symptoms are not significant
   - C. No, there is no evidence of personal distress
   - D. No, lacks the appropriate context

Answers

Multiple Choice Questions:

1. B
2. B
3. C
4. B
5. A
6. B
7. C

True/False Questions:

1. True
2. False
3. True
4. False
5. True
6. False
7. False
8. True
9. False
10. True

Matching Exercise:

1. B
2. F
3. C
4. D
5. E
6. A

Case Study Answers and Explanations:

1. C - Explanation: Minimum duration required for diagnosis according to DSM-5 criteria.
2. B - Explanation: Combination of cognitive-behavioral therapy and medication is the recommended approach.
3. A - Explanation: Meets diagnostic criteria, including duration, symptoms, and significant distress.

Sexual Masochism Disorder

Multiple Choice Questions

1. Which of the following is a primary feature of sexual masochism disorder?
   - A. Recurrent fantasies about being watched by others without their consent
   - B. Intense sexual arousal from being humiliated, beaten, bound, or otherwise made to suffer
   - C. Obsessive collection of specific objects for sexual arousal
   - D. Avoidance of social interactions due to fear of embarrassment
2. For sexual masochism disorder to be diagnosed, the individual must:
   - A. Have engaged in criminal activities
   - B. Experience distress or impairment in daily functioning related to their fantasies, urges, or behaviors
   - C. Be unable to achieve sexual arousal through consensual means
   - D. Be diagnosed only if they report physical injury
3. The distinction between sexual masochism disorder and consensual masochistic practices lies in:
   - A. Whether the individual experiences distress or impairment in functioning
   - B. The frequency of masochistic fantasies
   - C. Whether the individual identifies as part of a BDSM community
   - D. The type of stimuli used to induce arousal
4. Which of the following is a potential risk associated with untreated sexual masochism disorder?
   - A. Increased criminal behavior
   - B. Engagement in high-risk activities leading to physical harm
   - C. Total withdrawal from sexual activities
   - D. Development of compulsive hoarding behaviors
5. Sexual masochism disorder falls under which diagnostic category in the DSM-5?
   - A. Paraphilic disorders
   - B. Impulse-control disorders
   - C. Personality disorders
   - D. Anxiety disorders
6. In order to meet diagnostic criteria, the symptoms of sexual masochism disorder must persist for a minimum of:
   - A. 1 month
   - B. 3 months
   - C. 6 months
   - D. 12 months
7. Which of the following therapeutic approaches is commonly used for sexual masochism disorder?
   - A. Exposure therapy
   - B. Cognitive-behavioral therapy (CBT)
   - C. Medication only
   - D. Psychoanalysis exclusively

True/False Questions

		T	F
1	The DSM-5-TR criteria for Sexual Masochism Disorder include a possible specifier "with asphyxiophilia."		
2	Sexual Masochism Disorder can be diagnosed when an individual has fantasies of suffering but reports no distress or impairment.		
3	The minimum age for diagnosing Sexual Masochism Disorder is 18.		
4	Sexual arousal may stem solely from psychological humiliation, with no physical contact involved.		
5	The DSM-5-TR requires that Sexual Masochism Disorder symptoms persist for at least six months.		
6	Simulated masochistic acts practiced only with a consenting partner always fulfill the diagnostic criteria.		
7	In some cases, Sexual Masochism Disorder can be diagnosed without actual physical suffering if the individual is significantly disturbed by the fantasies.		
8	The DSM-5-TR allows specifying whether Sexual Masochism Disorder is "in remission" or "in a controlled environment."		
9	If the act of receiving pain causes no personal distress and no social problems, the DSM-5-TR does not support the diagnosis.		
10	Sexual Masochism Disorder is classified under sexual arousal disorders rather than paraphilic disorders.		

Matching Exercise

1. Paraphilic disorder [ ]
2. 6 months [ ]
3. Impairment in daily functioning [ ]
4. High-risk behaviors [ ]
5. Cognitive-behavioral therapy [ ]
6. Distress or discomfort [ ]

Descriptions:

- A. A key criterion for the diagnosis of sexual masochism disorder
- B. Time duration required for symptoms to meet diagnostic criteria
- C. Therapy aimed at addressing problematic behaviors and thought patterns
- D. Category under which sexual masochism disorder is classified
- E. Risk associated with untreated sexual masochism disorder
- F. One of the essential components of the diagnosis

Case Study

A 32-year-old man reports recurrent fantasies and urges involving being physically restrained and humiliated, which he finds intensely sexually arousing. These thoughts and behaviors have persisted for over six months and cause him significant distress, particularly because they interfere with his ability to maintain a romantic relationship. He states that he has not acted on these urges in a consensual setting but feels compelled to do so.

1. What is the minimum duration of symptoms required for the diagnosis of sexual masochism disorder?
    - A. 1 month
    - B. 3 months
    - C. 6 months
    - D. 12 months
2. Which of the following factors supports the diagnosis of sexual masochism disorder in this case?
    - A. The patient enjoys consensual BDSM practices with a partner
    - B. The fantasies and urges cause significant distress and interfere with daily functioning
    - C. The patient has not engaged in any behaviors related to his fantasies
    - D. The patient reports no distress associated with his fantasies
3. What is the most appropriate therapeutic approach for this individual?
    - A. Cognitive-behavioral therapy
    - B. Medication only
    - C. Psychoanalysis exclusively
    - D. Group therapy

Answers

Multiple Choice Questions:

1. B
2. B
3. A
4. B
5. A
6. C
7. B

True/False Questions:

1. True
2. False
3. True
4. True
5. True
6. False
7. True
8. True
9. True
10. False

Matching Exercise:

1. D
2. B
3. F
4. E
5. C
6. A

Case Study Answers and Explanations:

1. C - Explanation: Symptoms must persist for a minimum of six months according to DSM-5 criteria.
2. B - Explanation: Significant distress and interference with functioning are key diagnostic criteria.
3. A - Explanation: Cognitive-behavioral therapy is a widely recommended treatment for paraphilic disorders.

Sexual Sadism Disorder

Multiple Choice Questions

1. Which of the following is a key distinguishing factor between sexual sadism disorder and consensual sadistic practices?
    - A. The presence of fantasies involving non-consenting individuals
    - B. The ability to achieve sexual arousal through other means
    - C. The level of physical harm caused during the act
    - D. Whether the individual identifies as part of a BDSM community
2. Which of the following criteria must be met for a diagnosis of sexual sadism disorder according to the DSM-5?
    - A. Recurrent fantasies, urges, or behaviors involving the suffering of a non-consenting individual
    - B. Regular participation in consensual BDSM activities
    - C. History of violent behavior unrelated to sexual activities
    - D. Fantasies that only occur during episodes of substance intoxication
3. A clinician is differentiating between sexual sadism disorder and other paraphilic disorders. Which of the following characteristics is unique to sexual sadism disorder?
    - A. Intense arousal derived from the physical or psychological suffering of another person
    - B. Sexual arousal primarily focused on objects rather than individuals
    - C. The presence of both arousal and distress from the individual's behavior
    - D. Impulsive sexual behaviors unrelated to specific fantasies
4. Which of the following scenarios is most consistent with sexual sadism disorder?
    - A. A person who consents to being harmed during sexual activity with a partner
    - B. An individual experiencing arousal from causing non-consensual harm to others, leading to significant distress
    - C. Someone who experiences intense arousal from observing others in private settings without their consent
    - D. An individual engaging in self-inflicted harm to achieve sexual gratification
5. Which therapeutic approach has been shown to be most effective in managing sexual sadism disorder?
    - A. Psychodynamic therapy with focus on early childhood experiences
    - B. Behavioral therapy aimed at reducing arousal to non-consensual stimuli
    - C. Medication-only approaches using selective serotonin reuptake inhibitors (SSRIs)
    - D. Group therapy exclusively for individuals with paraphilic disorders
6. Which of the following conditions can co-occur with sexual sadism disorder, complicating diagnosis and treatment?
    - A. Borderline personality disorder
    - B. Generalized anxiety disorder
    - C. Conduct disorder or antisocial personality traits
    - D. Obsessive-compulsive disorder
7. Which of the following statements about the prognosis of sexual sadism disorder is accurate?
    - A. Individuals often recover fully without intervention
    - B. Treatment success is higher when individuals voluntarily seek help
    - C. Prognosis is unrelated to comorbid conditions
    - D. Recurrence of behavior is unlikely if treated with medication alone

True/False Questions

		T	F
1	The DSM-5-TR allows specifying “in remission” or “in a controlled environment” for Sexual Sadism Disorder.		
2	To diagnose Sexual Sadism Disorder, the individual must have acted on sadistic urges with a consenting partner or experience significant distress.		
3	According to the DSM-5-TR, Sadistic Personality Disorder is officially considered a subtype of Sexual Sadism Disorder.		
4	The minimum age for a Sexual Sadism Disorder diagnosis is 18.		
5	Having sadistic fantasies without clinical distress and without involving non-consenting victims meets the criteria for Sexual Sadism Disorder.		
6	The DSM-5-TR requires at least 12 months of sadistic manifestations to confirm a Sexual Sadism Disorder diagnosis.		
7	The specifier “with extreme sexual sadism” in the DSM-5-TR mandates evidence of weapon use or intense torture.		
8	Even if the individual is undergoing treatment, the DSM-5-TR allows specifying whether Sexual Sadism Disorder is “in remission.”		
9	The DSM-5-TR states that sadistic fantasies must cause personal distress or pose a real risk to others.		
10	The presence of another coexisting paraphilia always rules out an additional Sexual Sadism Disorder diagnosis.		

Matching Exercise

1. Paraphilic disorder [ ]
2. Non-consensual suffering [ ]
3. 6 months [ ]
4. Behavioral therapy [ ]
5. Antisocial traits [ ]
6. Comorbid conditions [ ]

Descriptions:

- A. A common co-occurring issue complicating treatment and prognosis
- B. Time period required for symptoms to meet diagnostic criteria
- C. Core feature of sexual sadism disorder when distinguishing from consensual practices
- D. Therapy aimed at reducing arousal to problematic stimuli
- E. Category under which sexual sadism disorder is classified
- F. Traits often seen in individuals with a history of sexual sadism disorder

Case Study

A 40-year-old male reports recurring fantasies of causing pain and psychological distress to others in a sexual context. These fantasies have persisted for more than six months. He has acted on these urges multiple times in non-consensual scenarios, leading to legal and interpersonal consequences. The patient feels aroused by these acts but denies feeling guilt. He also exhibits antisocial traits, including a lack of empathy and disregard for others' rights.

1. What is the minimum duration required for diagnosing sexual sadism disorder?
    - A. 1 month
    - B. 3 months
    - C. 6 months
    - D. 12 months
2. What factor differentiates this case from consensual BDSM practices?
    - A. The patient feels no guilt for their actions
    - B. The acts involve non-consensual harm to others
    - C. The fantasies persist for more than six months
    - D. The patient exhibits antisocial personality traits
3. What is the most appropriate therapeutic approach for this individual?
    - A. Behavioral therapy with focus on reducing arousal to non-consensual stimuli
    - B. Psychodynamic therapy exploring early life trauma
    - C. Group therapy with individuals sharing similar traits
    - D. Pharmacological treatment only

Answers

Multiple Choice Questions:
1. A
2. A
3. A
4. B
5. B
6. C
7. B

True/False Questions:
1. True
2. True
3. False
4. True
5. False
6. False
7. False
8. True
9. True
10. False

Matching Exercise:
1. E
2. C
3. B
4. D
5. F
6. A

Case Study Answers and Explanations:
1. C - Explanation: Symptoms must persist for at least six months according to DSM-5 criteria.
2. B - Explanation: Non-consensual harm is a key distinguishing factor in sexual sadism disorder.
3. A - Explanation: Behavioral therapy is widely used to address problematic arousal patterns in paraphilic disorders.

Pedophilic Disorder

Multiple Choice Questions

1. Which of the following is a diagnostic criterion for pedophilic disorder?
    - A. Recurrent, intense sexual fantasies, urges, or behaviors involving prepubescent children
    - B. Fantasies limited to pubescent individuals between ages 12–15
    - C. Occasional sexual thoughts about minors that do not interfere with functioning
    - D. Sexual behaviors that are solely hypothetical without real-world implications
2. Pedophilic disorder is differentiated from other paraphilic disorders by:
    - A. Persistent interest in sexually mature adults
    - B. A focus on individuals under the age of 13
    - C. An absence of distress or impairment in daily functioning
    - D. A history of interpersonal trauma in adulthood
3. For a diagnosis of pedophilic disorder, the individual must:
    - A. Have acted on their urges at least once
    - B. Be at least 16 years old and at least 5 years older than the child involved in their fantasies or behaviors
    - C. Display a preference for adolescents rather than prepubescent children
    - D. Show behaviors limited to fantasy without impact on others
4. Which of the following therapeutic approaches is most commonly used for pedophilic disorder?
    - A. Insight-oriented therapy
    - B. Cognitive-behavioral therapy focusing on impulse control
    - C. Group therapy with others diagnosed with similar disorders
    - D. Psychoanalysis exploring early childhood relationships
5. What is the primary distinction between pedophilic disorder and hebephilia?
    - A. Pedophilic disorder focuses on prepubescent children, while hebephilia involves pubescent adolescents
    - B. Hebephilia is classified as a paraphilic disorder in the DSM-5
    - C. Pedophilic disorder includes a lack of remorse for behaviors
    - D. Hebephilia involves individuals over the age of 18
6. Which of the following conditions is commonly comorbid with pedophilic disorder?
    - A. Generalized anxiety disorder
    - B. Conduct disorder or antisocial personality disorder
    - C. Substance use disorder exclusively
    - D. Borderline personality disorder
7. According to research, individuals with pedophilic disorder often exhibit:
    - A. A consistent history of violent behavior towards children
    - B. No remorse for their thoughts or actions
    - C. Cognitive distortions that rationalize their fantasies or behaviors
    - D. A preference for solitary lifestyles unrelated to their paraphilic interests

True/False Questions

		T	F
1	The DSM-5-TR sets a minimum age of 16 for diagnosing Pedophilic Disorder, with at least a 5-year age difference from the child.		
2	Pedophilic Disorder cannot be diagnosed if the individual does not experience distress, even when there has been sexual contact with a non-consenting minor.		
3	Pedophilic Disorder can be diagnosed without actual abusive acts if persistent pedophilic fantasies cause significant distress.		
4	The presence of another paraphilia excludes the possibility of diagnosing Pedophilic Disorder.		
5	The DSM-5-TR requires pedophilic desires or behaviors to persist for at least six months.		
6	The DSM-5-TR does not allow specifying whether Pedophilic Disorder is in remission or if the person is in a controlled environment.		
7	The DSM-5-TR allows specifying whether the attraction is to males, females, or both.		
8	If an individual is exclusively attracted to prepubescent children, the diagnosis can be labeled as the "exclusive" type.		
9	The DSM-5-TR defines the pedophilic age range as under 10 years, regardless of the child's pubertal status.		
10	For a Pedophilic Disorder diagnosis, a minimum 10-year age gap between the individual and the child is required.		

Matching Exercise

1. Cognitive distortions [ ]
2. 6 months [ ]
3. Anti-androgen therapy [ ]
4. Prepubescent children [ ]
5. DSM-5 category [ ]
6. Conduct disorder traits [ ]

Descriptions:

- A. Common pharmacological treatment for reducing sexual urges
- B. Required duration of symptoms to meet diagnostic criteria
- C. A key feature of pedophilic disorder, involving rationalization of behaviors
- D. Comorbid condition often seen in individuals with pedophilic disorder
- E. Paraphilic disorders classification
- F. Focus of fantasies, urges, or behaviors in pedophilic disorder

Case Study

A 35-year-old male reports experiencing recurrent fantasies involving prepubescent children for over six months. He denies acting on these urges but admits to significant distress about his thoughts, which interfere with his daily life. He describes cognitive distortions, such as rationalizing these fantasies as harmless, while also expressing guilt and a desire for help. He has no history of criminal behavior or substance abuse but exhibits some antisocial traits.

1. What is the minimum duration required for diagnosing pedophilic disorder?
   - A. 1 month
   - B. 3 months
   - C. 6 months
   - D. 12 months
2. Which of the following supports the diagnosis of pedophilic disorder in this case?
   - A. The patient has acted on their urges in the past
   - B. The fantasies cause significant distress and interfere with functioning
   - C. The patient rationalizes their fantasies but expresses no guilt
   - D. The patient has antisocial traits unrelated to the disorder
3. Which treatment approach is most appropriate for this individual?
   - A. Pharmacological intervention with anti-androgen therapy
   - B. Cognitive-behavioral therapy focused on restructuring cognitive distortions
   - C. Psychoanalysis focusing on early childhood relationships
   - D. Group therapy with others who have similar symptoms

Answers

Multiple Choice Questions:
1. A
2. B
3. B
4. B
5. A
6. B
7. C

True/False Questions:
1. True
2. False
3. True
4. False
5. True
6. False
7. True
8. True
9. False
10. False

Matching Exercise:
1. C
2. B
3. A
4. F
5. E
6. D

Case Study Answers and Explanations:
1. C - Explanation: The DSM-5 requires a minimum duration of six months for diagnosis.
2. B - Explanation: Significant distress and interference with functioning are critical criteria for diagnosis.
3. B - Explanation: Cognitive-behavioral therapy is effective in addressing distorted thought patterns and managing impulses.

Fetishistic Disorder

Multiple Choice Questions

1. Which of the following is a defining characteristic of fetishistic disorder?
    - A. Sexual arousal derived from objects or non-genital body parts, leading to significant distress or impairment
    - B. Sexual fantasies involving consenting partners in unconventional scenarios
    - C. Recurrent thoughts about past relationships interfering with current functioning
    - D. Avoidance of intimacy due to fear of emotional vulnerability
2. Which of the following scenarios most accurately reflects fetishistic disorder?
    - A. An individual who collects shoes but experiences no sexual arousal from them
    - B. A person who achieves sexual gratification exclusively through contact with non-genital body parts
    - C. Someone who prefers role-play scenarios with consenting adults
    - D. A person who experiences arousal from unconventional fantasies but no distress
3. To diagnose fetishistic disorder, the individual must:
    - A. Act on their fantasies in public settings
    - B. Be unable to achieve sexual arousal in any other context
    - C. Experience significant distress or impairment due to their fetishistic interests
    - D. Demonstrate a preference for fetishistic objects over human interaction
4. Which of the following objects or body parts is most commonly associated with fetishistic disorder?
    - A. Household furniture
    - B. Shoes or feet
    - C. Facial features
    - D. General clothing preferences
5. How is fetishistic disorder classified in the DSM-5?
    - A. A personality disorder
    - B. A paraphilic disorder
    - C. An anxiety disorder
    - D. An obsessive-compulsive disorder
6. Which treatment modality is commonly recommended for fetishistic disorder?
    - A. Psychoanalysis focused on uncovering childhood trauma
    - B. Cognitive-behavioral therapy to address compulsive behaviors
    - C. Pharmacological interventions targeting anxiety
    - D. Family therapy to resolve interpersonal conflicts
7. Which of the following factors distinguishes fetishistic disorder from non-pathological fetishistic interests?
    - A. The focus of arousal being objects rather than partners
    - B. The presence of distress or significant impairment in functioning
    - C. The duration of interest in the fetishistic object
    - D. The rarity of the fetishistic preference

True/False Questions

		T	F
1	Some individuals with Fetishistic Disorder may experience distress even if their fetishistic behaviors pose no problems in their romantic relationship.		
2	The DSM-5-TR deems cultural or religious context irrelevant when evaluating a fetishistic interest, provided there is distress or functional impairment.		
3	According to certain research, the mere presence of a fetish is sufficient to rule out a Transvestic Disorder diagnosis.		
4	Fetishistic Disorder can be diagnosed when the interest involves objects that come into contact with genital areas, even if no distress is reported.		
5	In the DSM-5-TR, sexual arousal tied to nonsexual items may include body parts generally not considered erotic.		
6	A key distinction for diagnosing Fetishistic Disorder is that the fetishized object must replace the sexual stimulation derived from a human partner.		
7	If fetishistic thoughts persist for at least six months but the individual is not distressed, the DSM-5-TR still mandates considering a Fetishistic Disorder diagnosis.		
8	The DSM-5-TR includes an "exclusive" specifier to indicate when the fetishistic interest focuses on a single type of object or body part.		
9	Some forms of fetishism may present episodically rather than chronically, yet the DSM-5-TR does not allow remission periods for Fetishistic Disorder.		
10	A Fetishistic Disorder diagnosis should not be made if the interest in objects is part of consensual sexual practices that cause no psychological distress.		

Matching Exercise

1. Non-genital body parts [ ]
2. 6 months [ ]
3. Cognitive-behavioral therapy [ ]
4. Distress or impairment [ ]
5. Paraphilic disorders [ ]
6. Shoes and feet [ ]

Descriptions:

- A. Duration required for diagnosis of fetishistic disorder
- B. A focus of sexual arousal commonly associated with the disorder
- C. Therapy designed to address compulsive or distressing behaviors
- D. Key component of diagnosis distinguishing pathological from non-pathological interests
- E. Classification of fetishistic disorder in the DSM-5
- F. Common targets of fetishistic interests

Case Study

A 28-year-old male reports experiencing recurrent, intense sexual arousal exclusively from leather gloves, which he has collected over the past year. He states that he cannot achieve sexual satisfaction without the presence of these objects and feels ashamed about his behavior, which is beginning to interfere with his romantic relationship. The individual denies any history of substance use or other psychiatric disorders.

1. What is the required duration of symptoms to meet the diagnostic criteria for fetishistic disorder?
   - A. 1 month
   - B. 3 months
   - C. 6 months
   - D. 12 months
2. What factor supports the diagnosis of fetishistic disorder in this case?
   - A. The patient has acted on his fantasies in public settings
   - B. The fetishistic interest causes significant distress and relationship issues
   - C. The patient collects leather gloves but feels no shame or distress
   - D. The fetishistic interests have been present for less than six months
3. Which treatment approach is most appropriate for this individual?
   - A. Cognitive-behavioral therapy focused on managing distress and compulsive behaviors
   - B. Psychoanalysis exploring childhood influences on fetishistic interests
   - C. Family therapy to resolve interpersonal conflicts related to the fetish
   - D. Group therapy with others who share similar interests

Answers

Multiple Choice Questions:

1. A
2. B
3. C
4. B
5. B
6. B
7. B

True/False Questions:

1. True
2. True
3. False
4. False
5. True
6. True
7. False
8. True
9. False
10. False

Matching Exercise:

1. F
2. A
3. C
4. D
5. E
6. B

Case Study Answers and Explanations:

1. C - Explanation: Symptoms must persist for at least six months according to DSM-5 criteria.
2. B - Explanation: Significant distress and impairment are key components of the diagnosis.
3. A - Explanation: Cognitive-behavioral therapy is effective in addressing compulsive behaviors and distress associated with fetishistic disorder.

Transvestic Disorder

Multiple Choice Questions

1. Which of the following criteria is essential for diagnosing transvestic disorder?
   - A. Sexual arousal derived from cross-dressing that causes significant distress or impairment
   - B. Persistent desire to transition to another gender
   - C. Frequent use of clothing associated with another gender in non-sexual contexts
   - D. Participation in theatrical performances requiring cross-dressing
2. How does transvestic disorder differ from non-pathological cross-dressing?
   - A. It involves only male individuals
   - B. It is associated with distress, impairment, or compulsive behavior
   - C. It always co-occurs with gender dysphoria
   - D. It requires a history of non-consensual actions
3. Which of the following might indicate transvestic disorder rather than other paraphilic disorders?
   - A. Persistent sexual arousal from the humiliation of others
   - B. Intense sexual arousal related to wearing clothing of another gender
   - C. Sexual fantasies involving non-consenting individuals
   - D. Preference for specific objects unrelated to clothing
4. Which term describes the added component when sexual arousal involves imagining oneself as a female (if biologically male)?
   - A. Gender dysphoria
   - B. Autoandrophilia
   - C. Autogynephilia
   - D. Transgenderism
5. Which of the following therapeutic approaches is most appropriate for transvestic disorder?
   - A. Cognitive-behavioral therapy focusing on managing distress and reducing compulsive behavior
   - B. Psychoanalysis to explore childhood trauma
   - C. Gender-affirming therapy to support identity transitions
   - D. Family therapy to resolve interpersonal conflicts
6. Which of the following is a common comorbidity with transvestic disorder?
   - A. Generalized anxiety disorder
   - B. Borderline personality disorder
   - C. Major depressive disorder
   - D. Obsessive-compulsive disorder
7. What distinguishes transvestic disorder with fetishism from the standard presentation of the disorder?
   - A. The individual collects clothing without wearing it
   - B. Sexual arousal derives from specific fabrics or garments
   - C. The distress is focused solely on societal rejection
   - D. The behavior occurs only in private, non-sexual contexts

True/False Questions

		T	F
1	The DSM-5-TR states that diagnosing Transvestic Disorder requires clinically significant distress or functional impairment.		
2	The presence of nonsexual cross-dressing automatically rules out a Transvestic Disorder diagnosis in the DSM-5-TR.		
3	The DSM-5-TR includes a "with autogynephilia" specifier for Transvestic Disorder, referring to fantasies of oneself in a female role.		
4	A man who cross-dresses solely for drag shows, without focusing on sexual arousal, meets the criteria for Transvestic Disorder.		
5	The DSM-5-TR sets 18 as the minimum age for diagnosing Transvestic Disorder.		
6	The DSM-5-TR allows a diagnosis of Transvestic Disorder even in the absence of sexual fantasies, provided the cross-dressing is accompanied by distress.		
7	Among the criteria for Transvestic Disorder, there is no mention of whether the individual agrees to be filmed while cross-dressing.		
8	The DSM-5-TR does not require a minimum duration of six months for Transvestic Disorder symptoms.		
9	It is possible to specify whether Transvestic Disorder is accompanied by fetishism, autogynephilia, or both.		
10	The DSM-5-TR allows a Transvestic Disorder diagnosis even when there is no sexual arousal, as long as the person experiences mere curiosity about cross-dressing.		

Matching Exercise

1. Sexual arousal [ ]
2. 6 months [ ]
3. Cognitive-behavioral therapy [ ]
4. Distress or impairment [ ]
5. Paraphilic disorders [ ]
6. Autogynephilia [ ]

Descriptions:

- A. Component required for the diagnosis of transvestic disorder
- B. Duration required for symptoms to meet diagnostic criteria
- C. Therapy aimed at addressing distress and compulsive behaviors
- D. Classification of transvestic disorder in the DSM-5
- E. Condition involving arousal from imagining oneself as the opposite gender
- F. Key factor distinguishing pathological cross-dressing

Case Study

A 42-year-old male reports experiencing intense sexual arousal when wearing women's lingerie. These behaviors have persisted for over a year and have begun to interfere with his relationship with his spouse, who feels uncomfortable with the practice. The individual states that he feels significant shame and distress about his behavior, which he attempts to suppress unsuccessfully. He denies any desire to transition to another gender.

1. What is the required duration of symptoms to diagnose transvestic disorder?
   - A. 1 month
   - B. 3 months
   - C. 6 months
   - D. 12 months
2. What factor supports the diagnosis of transvestic disorder in this case?
   - A. The individual denies any shame or distress about his behavior
   - B. The cross-dressing is associated with significant sexual arousal and distress
   - C. The behavior does not interfere with relationships or functioning
   - D. The individual wishes to transition to another gender
3. What is the most appropriate therapeutic approach for this individual?
   - A. Cognitive-behavioral therapy focused on managing distress and compulsions
   - B. Psychoanalysis to explore early life influences
   - C. Family therapy to address relationship issues
   - D. Group therapy with others who share similar experiences

Answers

Multiple Choice Questions:

1. A
2. B
3. B
4. C
5. A
6. C
7. B

True/False Questions:

1. True
2. True
3. True
4. False
5. True
6. False
7. False
8. False
9. True
10. False

Matching Exercise:

1. A
2. B
3. C
4. F
5. D
6. E

Case Study Answers and Explanations:

1. C - Explanation: Symptoms must persist for at least six months according to DSM-5 criteria.
2. B - Explanation: Significant sexual arousal and distress are core components of the diagnosis.
3. A - Explanation: Cognitive-behavioral therapy is effective for managing distress and compulsive behaviors associated with transvestic disorder.

Other Paraphilic Disorders

Multiple Choice Questions

1. Which of the following would most likely fall under the category of Other Specified Paraphilic Disorder?
    - A. Sexual arousal exclusively from consensual adult relationships
    - B. Intense sexual arousal from non-consenting voyeuristic acts that do not meet full voyeurism criteria
    - C. Fantasies involving prepubescent children with significant distress or impairment
    - D. Persistent sexual arousal involving genital pain during intercourse
2. The primary distinction between Specified and Unspecified paraphilic disorders lies in:
    - A. The severity of distress or impairment
    - B. Whether the clinician chooses to specify the nature of the paraphilic focus
    - C. The individual's ability to control their impulses
    - D. Whether the disorder is explicitly listed in the DSM-5
3. Which of the following is an example of an Unspecified Paraphilic Disorder?
    - A. Persistent sexual arousal from dead bodies without associated distress
    - B. Sexual arousal from behaviors involving consenting adults
    - C. Paraphilic behaviors causing significant distress but not specified in the DSM-5
    - D. Sexual arousal exclusively from wearing clothing of another gender
4. A key diagnostic criterion for all paraphilic disorders, including Other Specified and Unspecified types, is:
    - A. Distress or impairment caused by the paraphilic interest
    - B. Repeated criminal activity related to the paraphilic behavior
    - C. The presence of fantasies involving harm to others
    - D. A preference for non-consensual scenarios
5. Which of the following situations would qualify as an Other Specified Paraphilic Disorder rather than another DSM-5 paraphilic disorder?
    - A. Recurrent sexual arousal from exposing oneself in public
    - B. Persistent arousal from non-genital body parts, such as feet
    - C. Sexual arousal from obscene phone calls that causes significant distress
    - D. Sexual arousal from observing others in private settings
6. Why might a clinician use the Unspecified Paraphilic Disorder category?
    - A. The specific nature of the paraphilia cannot be communicated due to limited information
    - B. The clinician wants to avoid stigmatizing the patient with a specific diagnosis
    - C. The patient's symptoms meet criteria for multiple paraphilic disorders
    - D. The patient does not meet the full criteria for any paraphilic disorder
7. Which of the following treatments is commonly recommended for Other Specified and Unspecified Paraphilic Disorders?
    - A. Psychoanalysis exclusively focused on childhood experiences
    - B. Behavioral therapy and pharmacological interventions
    - C. Group therapy to normalize the behavior
    - D. No treatment, as these disorders typically resolve spontaneously

True/False Questions

		T	F
1	The DSM-5-TR uses the "Other Paraphilic Disorders" category for atypical sexual behaviors that do not fully meet criteria for any specific paraphilic disorder.		
2	If someone exhibits violent sexual fantasies without personal distress or potential harm to others, the DSM-5-TR still recommends an "Other Paraphilic Disorders" diagnosis.		
3	The coexistence of two well-defined paraphilias (e.g., voyeurism and fetishism) prevents the use of the "Unspecified Paraphilic Disorder" diagnosis.		
4	The DSM-5-TR does not allow specifying whether "Other Paraphilic Disorders" are in remission or present in a controlled environment.		
5	A sexual interest focused on another person's scars, causing significant distress, may fall under "Other Paraphilic Disorders."		
6	The DSM-5-TR requires a minimum of 12 months of symptoms to consider an "Other Paraphilic Disorders" diagnosis.		
7	If an individual shows multiple paraphilic features but does not fully meet criteria for any one disorder, "Other Specified Paraphilic Disorder" may be used.		
8	The DSM-5-TR states that any form of psychological humiliation experienced by the individual must be classified under "Other Paraphilic Disorders."		
9	Certain rare paraphilic fantasies that cause marked distress can be coded as "Other Paraphilic Disorders."		
10	A diagnosis of "Unspecified Paraphilic Disorder" always requires the clinician to give a detailed explanation of the clinical reasons.		

Matching Exercise

1. Significant distress [ ]
2. Behavioral therapy [ ]
3. Specified category [ ]
4. Pharmacological interventions [ ]
5. Unspecified category [ ]
6. Non-consensual acts [ ]

Descriptions:

- A. A common treatment approach for managing paraphilic disorders
- B. Causes impairment in social, occupational, or other areas of functioning
- C. Used when the clinician provides a reason why the paraphilia does not meet standard criteria
- D. Involves reduced sexual arousal through medication
- E. Applied when the specific nature of the paraphilia is not described or clarified
- F. Behaviors violating the rights of others, often associated with paraphilic disorders

Case Study

A 45-year-old male reports recurrent sexual arousal from making anonymous obscene phone calls. These behaviors have persisted for over a year and cause significant distress, particularly as they interfere with his ability to form romantic relationships. The individual denies any criminal record but expresses guilt and embarrassment over his actions. He seeks help to reduce these urges, which he finds uncontrollable.

1. What is the required duration of symptoms to diagnose Other Specified Paraphilic Disorder?
   - A. 1 month
   - B. 3 months
   - C. 6 months
   - D. 12 months
2. What factor supports the diagnosis of Other Specified Paraphilic Disorder in this case?
   - A. The behaviors involve non-consensual actions causing distress to others
   - B. The distress and interference in functioning caused by the behaviors
   - C. The individual denies guilt about his actions
   - D. The symptoms meet criteria for voyeurism
3. Which treatment approach is most appropriate for this individual?
   - A. Behavioral therapy to manage compulsive urges
   - B. Psychoanalysis focused on childhood influences
   - C. Pharmacological treatment without therapy
   - D. Group therapy with others who share similar symptoms

Answers

Multiple Choice Questions:

1. B
2. B
3. C
4. A
5. C
6. A
7. B

True/False Questions:

1. True
2. False
3. False
4. False
5. True
6. False
7. True
8. False
9. True
10. False

Matching Exercise:

1. B
2. A
3. C
4. D
5. E
6. F

Case Study Answers and Explanations:

1. C - Explanation: Symptoms must persist for at least six months according to DSM-5 criteria.
2. B - Explanation: Significant distress and interference with functioning are key components of the diagnosis.
3. A - Explanation: Behavioral therapy is effective in addressing compulsive behaviors and managing distress in paraphilic disorders.

Other Mental Disorders

The "Other Mental Disorders" category encompasses conditions that, while not fitting neatly into the more common diagnostic groups, still feature symptoms or patterns of behavior or thought that significantly interfere with personal, social, or occupational functioning. In the DSM-5-TR, the designations "Specified" or "Unspecified" are often used for clinical presentations that do not fully meet the criteria of a clearly defined disorder, or that exhibit overlapping features from multiple categories without clearly belonging to any of them. This flexibility acknowledges the reality that clinical presentations can be highly variable, and that the complexity of symptoms sometimes goes beyond set diagnostic boundaries.

When classifying conditions that do not align with more structured categories (such as mood disorders, anxiety disorders, or neurocognitive disorders), clinicians need to carefully evaluate the overall symptom profile, its duration, and its pervasiveness. In some cases, "Specified" indicates the presence of key features from a particular group of disorders but missing some requirement related to duration, severity, or the number of criteria. In others, "Unspecified" signals the inability to define a more precise diagnosis—though it is clear that the issue exists and requires intervention. The advantage of these designations is that they allow for a functional diagnosis even when a clear-cut category has not emerged or when available information is incomplete.

A central consideration is distinguishing these presentations from other disorders with clearer defining criteria. For example, brief psychotic symptoms not convincingly attributed to Brief Psychotic Disorder or Schizoaffective Disorder may be placed in this category if they do not neatly fit an established diagnosis but still demand clinical attention. Similarly, subthreshold symptoms of depression or anxiety that do not meet the full criteria for a mood or anxiety disorder can be classified as "Specified" or "Unspecified" if they still significantly affect a person's quality of life.

Comorbidities often arise when an "Unspecified" diagnosis coexists with more clearly defined conditions, such as personality disorders, medical issues, or substance use. The difficulty in categorizing such symptoms precisely can reflect a particularly complex interplay of environmental, relational, or biological factors. The DSM-5-TR, in line with the more dimensional ideas hinted at in some sections, encourages a comprehensive assessment that takes into account the person's full clinical picture and how it develops over time.

The usefulness of this category lies in its ability to provide a "hybrid" option for those forms of mental distress that do not fit established classifications but nonetheless require clinical attention. In this sense, it serves as a reminder that clinicians should not overlook presentations that do not match rigid criteria, but still have a substantial impact on an individual's psychological well-being.

Other Specified and Unspecified Mental Disorders

Multiple Choice Questions

1. Which of the following best describes the purpose of the "Other Specified Mental Disorder" category?
    - A. To diagnose mild symptoms that do not cause distress or impairment
    - B. To identify disorders not listed in the DSM-5 that cause significant distress or impairment
    - C. To provide a placeholder diagnosis until a full evaluation is completed
    - D. To classify disorders that meet criteria for multiple DSM-5 diagnoses
2. When is the "Unspecified Mental Disorder" category most appropriately used?
    - A. When the symptoms align with multiple DSM-5 diagnoses
    - B. When the clinician cannot specify the nature of the disorder due to insufficient information
    - C. When the patient does not experience any distress or impairment
    - D. When the disorder is related to cultural or situational factors
3. Which of the following is an example of an "Other Specified Mental Disorder"?
    - A. Symptoms of anxiety lasting for less than four weeks
    - B. Symptoms of depression occurring exclusively during the winter months
    - C. Symptoms of psychosis caused by substance intoxication
    - D. Symptoms of bereavement lasting longer than culturally expected norms
4. What distinguishes the "Specified" category from the "Unspecified" category?
    - A. The presence of a specific explanation for why the symptoms do not meet criteria for a standard diagnosis
    - B. The absence of impairment in functioning
    - C. The inclusion of subclinical symptoms in the diagnosis
    - D. The exclusion of temporary or situational factors
5. Which of the following is a common reason to use the "Unspecified Mental Disorder" category?
    - A. The patient's symptoms resolve before a definitive diagnosis can be made
    - B. The clinician identifies a new disorder not currently listed in the DSM-5
    - C. The patient refuses to provide information necessary for diagnosis
    - D. The clinician lacks sufficient time or data to provide a more specific diagnosis
6. What is the minimum requirement for both "Specified" and "Unspecified" mental disorders to be diagnosed?
    - A. The symptoms must last at least six months
    - B. The symptoms must cause significant distress or impairment
    - C. The symptoms must occur in the context of a recognized medical condition
    - D. The symptoms must involve multiple areas of functioning
7. Which of the following treatment approaches is most appropriate for these categories?
    - A. Standardized protocols based on similar cases
    - B. Tailored interventions focusing on the individual's symptoms and distress
    - C. Pharmacological treatments applied uniformly across all patients
    - D. Group therapy sessions designed for broad diagnostic categories

True/False Questions

		T	F
1	In the DSM-5-TR, the Other Specified Mental Disorder category requires clarifying why the		
2	full criteria for another disorder are not met.		
3	Unspecified Mental Disorder is used when there is evidence of psychopathology, but the clinician opts not to specify due to insufficient information.		
4	The two categories Other Specified Mental Disorder and Unspecified Mental Disorder include rigid additional criteria that significantly limit their use.		
5	Other Specified Mental Disorder allows describing atypical presentations with subthreshold symptoms, provided there is clinically significant distress.		
6	According to the DSM-5-TR, Unspecified Mental Disorder can only be assigned in psychiatric emergency settings where no time is available for a complete assessment.		
7	In research settings, Unspecified Mental Disorder is often preferred to study symptom constellations not yet classified under a defined disorder.		
8	The DSM-5-TR criteria suggest that a diagnosis of Other Specified Mental Disorder should be periodically reassessed to see if it evolves into a more specific disorder.		
9	Some experts argue that overreliance on the Other Specified and Unspecified categories may mask more precise differential diagnoses.		
10	The DSM-5-TR advises using Unspecified Mental Disorder when the presentation is highly atypical, but a detailed clinical history is lacking.		

Matching Exercise

1. Short-duration depressive episode [ ]
2. Emergency use [ ]
3. Significant distress or impairment [ ]
4. Symptom-focused therapy [ ]
5. Clinician-specified explanation [ ]
6. Time constraints [ ]

Descriptions:

- A. Common reason for assigning "Unspecified Mental Disorder"
- B. Diagnosis under the "Specified" category when symptoms do not fully meet criteria for a DSM-5 disorder
- C. A key requirement for diagnosing both Specified and Unspecified categories
- D. Treatment approach focusing on alleviating presenting symptoms
- E. Rationale provided for symptoms not meeting full diagnostic criteria
- F. Typical context in which the "Unspecified" category is applied

Case Study

A 38-year-old male presents with symptoms of irritability, disrupted sleep, and difficulty concentrating. These symptoms began after a significant work-related stressor and have persisted for three weeks. The symptoms are distressing and interfere with his job performance but do not meet full criteria for generalized anxiety disorder or major depressive disorder. The clinician documents the diagnosis as "Other Specified Anxiety Disorder."

1. What feature supports the use of the "Specified" category in this case?
   - A. The clinician specifies the symptoms as subthreshold anxiety lasting less than one month
   - B. The patient meets criteria for generalized anxiety disorder
   - C. The symptoms are related to substance use
   - D. The clinician cannot determine the underlying cause of the symptoms
2. How would the "Unspecified" category differ in this case?
   - A. It would not specify the reason the symptoms do not meet full diagnostic criteria
   - B. It would require the patient to meet criteria for multiple disorders
   - C. It would focus exclusively on cultural factors influencing the symptoms
   - D. It would be applied only in cases involving severe distress
3. Which treatment approach is most appropriate for this individual?
   - A. Short-term therapy targeting anxiety symptoms and coping mechanisms
   - B. Immediate pharmacological treatment without further evaluation
   - C. Group therapy designed for individuals with generalized anxiety disorder
   - D. Referral for psychoanalysis to explore underlying unconscious conflicts

Answers

Multiple Choice Questions:

1. B
2. B
3. D
4. A
5. D
6. B
7. B

True/False Questions:

1. True
2. True
3. False
4. True
5. False
6. False
7. True
8. True
9. True
10. False

Matching Exercise:

1. B
2. A
3. C
4. D
5. E
6. F

Case Study Answers and Explanations:

1. A - Explanation: The clinician specifies that the symptoms are subthreshold anxiety lasting less than one month, fitting the "Specified" category.
2. A - Explanation: The "Unspecified" category would not include a specific reason why the symptoms fail to meet full diagnostic criteria.
3. A - Explanation: Short-term, symptom-focused therapy is most appropriate to address the distress and impairment caused by anxiety symptoms.

Medication-Induced Movement Disorders and Other Adverse Effects of Medication

Medication-induced movement disorders and other adverse effects hold a unique position in the DSM-5-TR, as they do not stem from a "primary" psychopathological condition but rather arise from reactions or secondary conditions triggered by particular substances, medications, or treatments. What unifies them is the alteration of motor functions and/or behaviors that appears after exposure to an external agent, with symptoms ranging from mild restlessness to severe dyskinesia or extrapyramidal syndromes.

Clinically, the most widely recognized manifestations are linked to older-generation antipsychotics (and, to a lesser extent, newer antipsychotics), which can cause effects such as akathisia (restlessness and an inability to remain still), drug-induced parkinsonism (muscle rigidity, slowed movements, tremors), and tardive dyskinesia (repetitive, often facial, involuntary movements). However, other drugs—such as certain antiemetics or dopamine antagonists—may produce similar outcomes, highlighting the specific neurochemical mechanisms involved. Beyond movement disorders, the DSM-5-TR also covers additional adverse effects, including allergic reactions, problematic drug interactions, or significant metabolic changes (for example, marked weight gain or alterations in glucose levels).

It is important to differentiate these disorders from primary neurological conditions (such as Parkinson's disease or genetic choreas), since the role of the medication in the individual's clinical history is traceable and verifiable. Likewise, they should not be confused with true psychiatric disorders, even though some symptoms—particularly akathisia—can resemble the anxiety or psychomotor agitation seen in manic episodes. The timeline is key: symptoms emerge or worsen following medication use (or dosage increases) and often diminish or disappear if the medication is tapered or discontinued under medical supervision.

Comorbidities are common, since people receiving antipsychotics, antidepressants, or other psychiatric medications typically already have a primary disorder (e.g., schizophrenia, bipolar disorder, severe depression). Drug-induced symptoms may overlap with the underlying condition, making diagnosis and treatment management more complex. Certain patients also present risk factors (such as older age or a history of adverse reactions) that predispose them to develop movement disorders.

Medication-Induced Movement Disorders

Multiple Choice Questions

1. Which of the following is an example of a medication-induced movement disorder?
   - A. Essential tremor
   - B. Tardive dyskinesia caused by long-term antipsychotic use
   - C. Idiopathic Parkinson's disease
   - D. Huntington's chorea
2. Which type of movement disorder is commonly associated with the use of antipsychotic medications?
   - A. Tics
   - B. Akathisia
   - C. Restless legs syndrome
   - D. Myoclonus
3. Which of the following medications is most likely to cause dystonia as a side effect?
   - A. Benzodiazepines
   - B. Antipsychotics
   - C. Beta blockers
   - D. Antidepressants
4. Tardive dyskinesia typically presents with:
   - A. Slow, rhythmic tremors in the hands
   - B. Involuntary, repetitive movements of the face, tongue, or extremities
   - C. Muscle rigidity and bradykinesia
   - D. Sudden, brief jerking movements
5. Which of the following best describes neuroleptic malignant syndrome (NMS)?
   - A. A disorder characterized by progressive muscle weakness
   - B. A life-threatening reaction to antipsychotic medications, including rigidity and hyperthermia
   - C. An allergic reaction to psychotropic medications presenting with skin rash
   - D. A syndrome of involuntary tics triggered by stimulants
6. Which treatment is most appropriate for akathisia caused by antipsychotic medication?
   - A. Increase the dose of the antipsychotic
   - B. Discontinue the medication or lower the dose, and consider beta blockers or benzodiazepines
   - C. Introduce a second antipsychotic to counterbalance the symptoms
   - D. Use anticholinergic agents exclusively
7. Which of the following is a preventive strategy for medication-induced movement disorders?
   - A. Avoiding all antipsychotic medications
   - B. Regularly monitoring for side effects and using the lowest effective dose
   - C. Only prescribing medications without any risk of movement disorders
   - D. Treating with prophylactic benzodiazepines in all patients

True/False Questions

		T	F
1	The DSM-5-TR lists Tardive Dyskinesia among medication-induced movement disorders, typically linked to long-term antipsychotic use.		
2	Medication-induced akathisia appears exclusively within the first 48 hours of treatment and never at a later stage.		
3	Antipsychotic-induced parkinsonism can mimic Parkinson's disease, presenting with tremor, bradykinesia, and rigidity.		
4	Tardive Dyskinesia may arise even after discontinuation of the medication, making it hard to distinguish from a primary movement disorder.		
5	In the DSM-5-TR, Neuroleptic Malignant Syndrome is classified as a variant of Tardive Dyskinesia.		
6	Serotonin Syndrome is classified under medication-induced movement disorders in the DSM-5-TR.		
7	Some Tardive Dyskinesia cases include tooth grinding as a clinical sign.		
8	The DSM-5-TR requires at least 3 months of continuous antipsychotic treatment to diagnose Tardive Dyskinesia.		
9	Akathisia always resolves spontaneously once the antipsychotic dose is lowered.		
10	According to the DSM-5-TR, using anticholinergic agents can help alleviate some symptoms of medication-induced parkinsonism.		

Matching Exercise

1. Tardive dyskinesia [ ]
2. Neuroleptic malignant syndrome [ ]
3. Akathisia [ ]
4. Dystonia [ ]
5. Anticholinergic agents [ ]
6. Beta blockers [ ]

Descriptions:

- A. A life-threatening reaction involving hyperthermia, muscle rigidity, and autonomic dysregulation
- B. Subjective restlessness and inability to remain still, often caused by antipsychotics
- C. Involuntary repetitive movements, commonly affecting the face and tongue
- D. Sudden, sustained muscle contractions causing abnormal postures
- E. Medications used to treat dystonia or Parkinsonism caused by antipsychotics
- F. Often used to manage symptoms of akathisia

Case Study

A 54-year-old female with a history of schizophrenia presents with involuntary facial grimacing and tongue movements that have been gradually worsening over the past six months. She has been on a high-dose antipsychotic for five years. The symptoms cause her embarrassment and interfere with her social interactions. The clinician suspects tardive dyskinesia.

1. Which diagnostic feature is most consistent with tardive dyskinesia in this case?
    - A. Symptoms that develop soon after starting antipsychotics
    - B. Involuntary, repetitive movements affecting the face and tongue
    - C. Muscle rigidity and generalized weakness
    - D. Sudden, jerking movements without a clear pattern
2. What is the best initial approach to managing this patient's symptoms?
    - A. Increase the dose of the current antipsychotic to reduce movement symptoms
    - B. Switch to a second-generation antipsychotic with a lower risk of tardive dyskinesia
    - C. Start benzodiazepines to reduce involuntary movements
    - D. Discontinue antipsychotics entirely and start anticholinergic therapy
3. What is a preventive strategy for tardive dyskinesia in patients taking antipsychotics?
    - A. Avoiding the use of antipsychotics in all patients
    - B. Prescribing anticholinergic medications to all patients on antipsychotics
    - C. Using the lowest effective dose of antipsychotics and regularly monitoring for symptoms
    - D. Avoiding second-generation antipsychotics

Answers

Multiple Choice Questions:

1. B
2. B
3. B
4. B
5. B
6. B
7. B

True/False Questions:

1. True
2. False
3. True
4. True
5. False
6. False
7. True
8. False
9. False
10. True

Matching Exercise:

1. C
2. A
3. B
4. D
5. E
6. F

Case Study Answers and Explanations:

1. B - Explanation: Tardive dyskinesia is characterized by involuntary, repetitive movements, particularly of the face and tongue.
2. B - Explanation: Switching to a second-generation antipsychotic with a lower risk profile is an effective approach to manage tardive dyskinesia.
3. C - Explanation: Using the lowest effective dose of antipsychotics and regular monitoring helps prevent tardive dyskinesia.

Other Adverse Effects of Medication

Multiple Choice Questions

1. Which of the following adverse effects is commonly associated with long-term corticosteroid use?
    - A. Hair loss
    - B. Hyperglycemia and osteoporosis
    - C. Improved cardiovascular function
    - D. Reduced risk of infection
2. Which medication class is most commonly associated with serotonin syndrome?
    - A. Antipsychotics
    - B. Selective serotonin reuptake inhibitors (SSRIs)
    - C. Beta blockers
    - D. Benzodiazepines
3. What is a common adverse effect of ACE inhibitors?
    - A. Sedation
    - B. Persistent dry cough
    - C. Hypoglycemia
    - D. Increased heart rate
4. Which of the following symptoms is most consistent with neuroleptic malignant syndrome?
    - A. Increased appetite and weight gain
    - B. Rigidity, hyperthermia, and autonomic instability
    - C. Drowsiness and confusion
    - D. Nausea and vomiting
5. Which adverse effect is associated with prolonged use of proton pump inhibitors (PPIs)?
    - A. Increased bone density
    - B. Vitamin B12 deficiency
    - C. Enhanced liver function
    - D. Weight loss
6. Stevens-Johnson syndrome is a rare but serious adverse effect most commonly triggered by which class of drugs?
    - A. Antiepileptics and sulfonamides
    - B. Antibiotics like penicillin
    - C. Nonsteroidal anti-inflammatory drugs (NSAIDs)
    - D. Beta blockers
7. Which approach is most appropriate for managing drug-induced adverse effects?
    - A. Discontinuing the offending medication, if possible, and providing symptomatic treatment
    - B. Continuing the medication while treating the adverse effects with additional drugs
    - C. Ignoring the symptoms unless they worsen significantly
    - D. Reducing the dose of the medication without monitoring

True/False Questions

		T	F
1	Other Adverse Effects of Medication also covers brief but clinically significant reactions not explained by other disorders.		
2	If a mild side effect does not cause emotional distress, it should still be coded as Other Adverse Effects of Medication.		
3	A transient delusional reaction, not meeting criteria for a substance-induced psychotic disorder, may be placed under Other Adverse Effects of Medication.		
4	Concomitant use of multiple medications that trigger atypical symptoms always belongs in Other Adverse Effects of Medication.		
5	The DSM-5-TR requires physiological markers to diagnose Other Adverse Effects of Medication.		
6	A paradoxical effect (e.g., sedation-induced agitation) that resolves upon discontinuation can still be considered in this category.		
7	A temporary personality shift from steroid use, without mood disorder criteria, can be included under Other Adverse Effects of Medication.		
8	Mild discomfort from drug-induced hyperprolactinemia warrants evaluating Other Adverse Effects of Medication.		
9	Withdrawal symptoms following a gradual taper are not included in Other Adverse Effects of Medication.		
10	If a non-psychoactive medication causes behavioral changes not classifiable elsewhere, Other Adverse Effects of Medication is a valid diagnosis.		

Matching Exercise

1. Hyperglycemia and bone loss [ ]
2. Serotonin syndrome [ ]
3. Persistent dry cough [ ]
4. Stevens-Johnson syndrome [ ]
5. Neuroleptic malignant syndrome [ ]
6. Vitamin B12 deficiency [ ]

Descriptions:

- A. Adverse effect commonly linked to ACE inhibitors
- B. Triggered by proton pump inhibitors with long-term use
- C. Life-threatening reaction to antipsychotics characterized by rigidity and hyperthermia
- D. Adverse effect of corticosteroids with long-term use
- E. Condition caused by excessive serotonergic activity, often drug-induced
- F. Rare, severe skin reaction associated with antiepileptics and sulfonamides

Case Study

A 62-year-old male with a history of hypertension presents with persistent dry cough and mild swelling of the lips. He has been taking an ACE inhibitor for three months. His symptoms have been bothersome enough to interfere with his sleep and daily activities.

1. What adverse effect is most likely responsible for the patient's symptoms?
    - A. Drug-induced lupus
    - B. Angioedema and persistent cough caused by ACE inhibitor use
    - C. Stevens-Johnson syndrome caused by an unknown medication
    - D. Neuroleptic malignant syndrome due to psychotropic medications
2. What is the best initial step in managing this patient's condition?
    - A. Increase the dose of the ACE inhibitor to counteract the side effects
    - B. Discontinue the ACE inhibitor and consider an alternative medication class, such as ARBs
    - C. Continue the ACE inhibitor and monitor the symptoms over time
    - D. Add a corticosteroid to manage the swelling and cough
3. What is a key preventive strategy when prescribing medications with known adverse effects?
    - A. Prescribing the highest dose possible to ensure efficacy
    - B. Avoiding medications with any potential adverse effects
    - C. Regularly monitoring for side effects and educating patients about early warning signs
    - D. Only prescribing medications in combination to reduce individual drug dosages

Answers

Multiple Choice Questions:

1. B
2. B
3. B
4. B
5. B
6. A
7. A

True/False Questions:

1. True
2. False
3. True
4. False
5. False
6. True
7. True
8. True
9. True
10. True

Matching Exercise:

1. D
2. E
3. A
4. F
5. C
6. B

Case Study Answers and Explanations:

1. B - Explanation: ACE inhibitors are known to cause persistent cough and angioedema as adverse effects.
2. B - Explanation: Discontinuing the ACE inhibitor and switching to an ARB is the most appropriate step.
3. C - Explanation: Monitoring and patient education help detect and manage adverse effects early.

Other Conditions That May Be a Focus of Clinical Attention

This category brings together situations and concerns that may not qualify as full-fledged mental disorders but still warrant clinical attention or targeted support from professionals. The core idea is that certain life circumstances, complicated interpersonal relationships, or social, occupational, or academic issues can undermine psychological well-being and daily functioning—even if they do not align with traditional diagnostic categories.

A common example involves relational difficulties, such as marital conflict, family communication problems, or ongoing tension between parents and children. Occupational-related challenges—harassment in the workplace, prolonged unemployment, or high levels of professional stress—can also lead to significant distress, increasing the likelihood of developing a bona fide mental disorder if not addressed properly. Similarly, academic environments sometimes become a source of concern, for instance in cases of bullying or poor performance linked to learning difficulties, necessitating intervention from psychologists, pedagogues, or other specialists.

Another point is that these factors do not always operate independently of more classical psychiatric conditions. They often act as contributing or aggravating factors for anxiety, depression, or behavioral symptoms. Recognizing their relevance—even in the absence of a precise diagnosis—helps deliver more targeted support and can prevent progression toward more complex clinical issues. An acute marital crisis or sudden job loss, for example, may destabilize an individual's emotional balance enough to trigger an Adjustment Disorder or even a Major Depressive Episode.

The distinction from actual mental disorders stems from the fact that, in this category, the focus lies on life circumstances or relational patterns that do not present a structured clinical picture (as with anxiety or mood disorders) but that nonetheless impair relationship quality, workplace performance, or academic progress. Thus, interventions might include brief psychological counseling, family mediation, or career guidance, depending on the nature of the problem.

When it comes to comorbidities, it is not unusual for individuals with job- or relationship-related difficulties to also exhibit anxiety symptoms or low self-esteem. Likewise, a chronic medical condition in the family can spark emotional struggles that fall under this category, requiring support that addresses both practical and psychological aspects. It is crucial for clinicians to consider the broader life context, rather than focusing solely on a diagnosable disorder and overlooking challenging circumstances that affect overall well-being.

The DSM-5-TR underscores the importance of having a dedicated space for classifying these issues, emphasizing the need for clinical or psychosocial attention. In other words, intervention may be aimed at improving relational, work, or academic conditions, thereby preventing further complications and promoting more balanced, adaptive functioning in everyday life.

Relational Problems

Multiple Choice Questions

1. Which of the following is a key feature of relational problems according to the DSM-5?
    - A. Significant distress or impairment in social, occupational, or other important areas of functioning due to interpersonal difficulties
    - B. Presence of psychotic symptoms affecting the relationship
    - C. Complete absence of communication in all social contexts
    - D. A persistent desire to avoid all social interactions
2. Which of the following best describes parent-child relational problems?
    - A. Behavioral patterns where the child consistently displays high academic achievement
    - B. Difficulty in communication, emotional involvement, or disciplinary approaches between the parent and child
    - C. A parental inability to provide financial support for the child
    - D. Mutual satisfaction with the relationship despite external stressors
3. Partner relational problems often involve which of the following?
    - A. Physical symptoms without emotional involvement
    - B. Persistent conflict, poor communication, or lack of emotional intimacy
    - C. A unilateral decision to avoid the relationship without reason
    - D. Stable but distant interactions in the relationship
4. Which term best describes relational problems influenced by cultural or societal expectations?
    - A. Relationship avoidance disorder
    - B. Relational mismatch syndrome
    - C. Relationship distress with cultural context
    - D. Sociocultural relational conflicts
5. Which type of relational problem is typically addressed in therapy when caregiving burdens are excessive?
    - A. Family communication difficulties
    - B. Relational problems associated with caregiving for an individual with a chronic condition
    - C. Parent-child conflicts over autonomy
    - D. Peer relationship stress
6. Which therapeutic approach is most commonly used to address relational problems?
    - A. Psychoanalysis exclusively
    - B. Family or couple therapy focusing on communication and conflict resolution
    - C. Pharmacological intervention to improve emotional regulation
    - D. Behavioral therapy targeting individual emotional responses
7. Which of the following is a preventive strategy for relational problems?
    - A. Avoid addressing interpersonal conflicts to minimize stress
    - B. Encourage open communication and establish clear boundaries
    - C. Isolate individuals to reduce relational strain
    - D. Delay addressing issues until they become severe

True/False Questions

		T	F
1	The DSM-5-TR categories for Relational Problems do not address bullying at school.		
2	In Parent-Child Relational Problem, conflicts can revolve around household rules without other psychopathology.		
3	Relationship Distress With Spouse is only diagnosable when one partner has a mental disorder.		
4	The DSM-5-TR considers Sibling Relational Problem if there is a marked breakdown in communication between siblings.		
5	Relational Problems can be listed as a secondary diagnosis when they affect the management of a primary disorder.		
6	Upbringing Away From Parents is not included under Relational Problems since it is separately coded.		
7	In the DSM-5-TR, problematic family dynamics may impact adherence to medical treatments.		
8	If a parent with a personality disorder struggles with emotional regulation, the DSM-5-TR deems it sufficient for Child Affected by Parental Relationship Distress.		
9	Relational Problems are included in treatment plans only within family therapy settings.		
10	According to the DSM-5-TR, a relational problem can exist even in the absence of verbal or physical conflict.		

Matching Exercise

1. Parent-child relational problems [ ]
2. Partner relational problems [ ]
3. Caregiving relational issues [ ]
4. Communication difficulties [ ]
5. Cultural conflicts [ ]
6. Emotional intimacy [ ]

Descriptions:

- A. Commonly observed in individuals responsible for caring for chronically ill family members
- B. Conflicts related to autonomy, discipline, or emotional support in parent-child dynamics
- C. Involves poor communication, frequent conflicts, or lack of closeness between romantic partners
- D. Challenges influenced by societal or cultural expectations in relationships
- E. Core issue in many types of relational problems, often addressed in therapy
- F. Often characterized by a lack of mutual understanding and emotional closeness

Case Study

A 35-year-old woman and her 37-year-old husband present for therapy, reporting frequent arguments about financial decisions and a lack of emotional intimacy. The wife feels unsupported in her efforts to balance work and family responsibilities, while the husband feels unappreciated for his contributions to the household. They both express a desire to improve their communication and strengthen their relationship.

1. Which of the following issues is most likely contributing to the relational problems in this case?
   - A. Parent-child conflict
   - B. Partner relational problems involving communication and emotional intimacy
   - C. Caregiving relational stress due to chronic illness
   - D. Sociocultural relational mismatches
2. Which therapeutic approach is most appropriate for this couple?
   - A. Family therapy focused on the dynamics between extended family members
   - B. Couple therapy aimed at improving communication and addressing emotional needs
   - C. Individual therapy for the wife to address her work-life balance
   - D. Behavioral therapy for the husband to focus on his contributions
3. What is a key goal for therapy in this case?
   - A. To resolve financial stressors without addressing emotional intimacy
   - B. To foster open communication and rebuild emotional connection
   - C. To establish separate financial responsibilities for each partner
   - D. To encourage one partner to take full responsibility for resolving conflicts

Answers

Multiple Choice Questions:

1. A
2. B
3. B
4. C
5. B
6. B
7. B

True/False Questions:

1. False
2. True
3. False
4. True
5. True
6. True
7. True
8. False
9. False
10. True

Matching Exercise:

1. B
2. C
3. A
4. E
5. D
6. F

Case Study Answers and Explanations:

1. B - Explanation: The primary issues involve poor communication and lack of emotional intimacy, common in partner relational problems.
2. B - Explanation: Couple therapy is the most appropriate approach to improve communication and address emotional needs.
3. B - Explanation: Therapy aims to foster open communication and rebuild emotional connection, addressing the couple's relational issues.

Work-Related Problems

Multiple Choice Questions

1. Which of the following best describes work-related problems according to the DSM-5?
    - A. Significant distress or impairment in functioning due to interpersonal or task-related challenges in the workplace
    - B. Persistent inability to find employment despite appropriate skills
    - C. Absence of motivation to engage in leisure activities
    - D. Conflicts with family members caused by work-life imbalance
2. What is a common feature of interpersonal work-related problems?
    - A. Overachievement in all assigned tasks
    - B. Frequent conflicts with supervisors, coworkers, or subordinates
    - C. Complete withdrawal from social relationships outside of work
    - D. Consistently high levels of job satisfaction
3. Which of the following scenarios best reflects work-related stress?
    - A. A high-performing employee consistently meets deadlines without complaints
    - B. A worker experiences persistent anxiety, irritability, and difficulty concentrating due to excessive workload
    - C. An individual is satisfied with their job but wishes for a promotion
    - D. A team celebrates its successful completion of a challenging project
4. Which of the following could contribute to work-related problems?
    - A. Lack of appropriate training or resources for assigned tasks
    - B. Strong interpersonal relationships with colleagues
    - C. High levels of work engagement and motivation
    - D. Consistent recognition and reward for performance
5. Which term describes a prolonged response to workplace stress that has not been successfully managed?
    - A. Job satisfaction
    - B. Professional growth
    - C. Burnout syndrome
    - D. Work-life balance
6. What therapeutic approach is most commonly used to address work-related problems?
    - A. Psychoanalysis focusing on early childhood experiences
    - B. Cognitive-behavioral therapy targeting stress management and coping strategies
    - C. Pharmacological intervention to enhance job performance
    - D. Group therapy with colleagues experiencing similar challenges
7. Which of the following is a preventive strategy for work-related problems?
    - A. Avoid addressing stressors to minimize workplace conflicts
    - B. Encouraging open communication and fostering a supportive work environment
    - C. Replacing employees experiencing stress with new hires
    - D. Allowing employees to work without supervision to promote autonomy

True/False Questions

		T	F
1	The DSM-5-TR codes a Work-Related Problem (V62.29) even without psychiatric symptoms, provided work functioning is impaired.		
2	A latent conflict with coworkers, not affecting productivity, still falls under Work-Related Problems.		
3	Performance-related anxiety that does not meet full criteria for an anxiety disorder may be considered a Work-Related Problem.		
4	A mandatory department change that causes distress excludes a Work-Related Problem diagnosis if a more significant mental condition is present.		
5	The DSM-5-TR differentiates between a work issue tied to relational factors and one due to poor organizational conditions.		
6	An employee facing discrimination who shows no notable emotional reaction is not included in the definition of a Work-Related Problem.		
7	If a worker exhibits subthreshold depressive symptoms related to job stress, the clinician may code a Work-Related Problem.		
8	Difficulty adapting to night shifts, causing significant distress, could lead to a Work-Related Problem code.		
9	When a workplace issue co-occurs with a diagnosed anxiety disorder, a Work-Related Problem cannot be added as a contributing factor.		
10	DSM-5-TR guidelines allow noting a Work-Related Problem if it affects adherence to treatment for a primary disorder.		

Matching Exercise

1. Burnout syndrome [ ]
2. Work-related stress [ ]
3. Interpersonal conflict [ ]
4. Preventive strategies [ ]
5. Cognitive-behavioral therapy [ ]
6. Lack of training or resources [ ]

Descriptions:

- A. Prolonged exposure to unmanaged workplace stress leading to emotional exhaustion and reduced performance
- B. Persistent anxiety, irritability, or difficulty concentrating due to work pressures
- C. Common source of work-related problems involving disagreements with coworkers or supervisors
- D. Includes fostering supportive environments and encouraging communication
- E. Therapy approach focused on managing stress and improving coping strategies
- F. Factor contributing to task-related problems in the workplace

Case Study

A 42-year-old man reports increasing irritability, fatigue, and difficulty concentrating at work over the past six months. He attributes these symptoms to an excessive workload and lack of recognition for his contributions. He has begun to withdraw from interactions with coworkers and feels demotivated about his job. His performance has recently declined, and he is considering leaving his position.

1. What is the most likely diagnosis in this case?
    - A. Generalized anxiety disorder unrelated to workplace stress
    - B. Work-related stress contributing to burnout syndrome
    - C. Interpersonal relational problems with coworkers
    - D. Task-related difficulties due to lack of skills
2. Which intervention would be most effective in managing this individual's symptoms?
    - A. Cognitive-behavioral therapy focused on stress management and coping skills
    - B. Immediate pharmacological treatment to reduce symptoms of anxiety
    - C. Group therapy with other employees experiencing workplace dissatisfaction
    - D. Psychoanalysis to explore past traumatic experiences
3. What is a key preventive measure to reduce the risk of burnout in similar cases?
    - A. Encouraging employees to work longer hours to complete tasks
    - B. Providing regular recognition and feedback for employee contributions
    - C. Avoiding discussions about stress to maintain a professional environment
    - D. Reassigning the individual to a different department without addressing the root cause

Answers

Multiple Choice Questions:

1. A
2. B
3. B
4. A
5. C
6. B
7. B

True/False Questions:

1. True
2. False
3. True
4. False
5. True
6. False
7. True
8. True
9. False
10. True

Matching Exercise:

1. A
2. B
3. C
4. D
5. E
6. F

Case Study Answers and Explanations:

1. B - Explanation: The symptoms are consistent with work-related stress and burnout syndrome, characterized by emotional exhaustion and reduced performance.
2. A - Explanation: Cognitive-behavioral therapy can help manage stress and develop effective coping mechanisms.
3. B - Explanation: Regular recognition and feedback can reduce stress and improve motivation, preventing burnout.

Academic Problems

Multiple Choice Questions

1. Which of the following is a common feature of academic problems?
    - A. Significant difficulties in academic performance due to lack of access to educational resources
    - B. Complete disinterest in any form of learning or education
    - C. A consistent pattern of overachievement and perfectionism
    - D. Conflicts with family members unrelated to school performance
2. Which of the following is an example of task-related academic problems?
    - A. Poor time management and difficulty completing assignments
    - B. Strong academic performance but dissatisfaction with grades
    - C. Enjoyment of learning but difficulty understanding complex material
    - D. Positive relationships with peers and teachers
3. What is a potential cause of academic problems in children and adolescents?
    - A. Access to advanced learning resources
    - B. Unaddressed learning disabilities or attention deficits
    - C. High levels of parental involvement in school activities
    - D. Consistent positive feedback from teachers
4. Which of the following best describes interpersonal academic problems?
    - A. Conflicts with peers or teachers affecting classroom participation
    - B. Struggles with understanding abstract concepts
    - C. Inability to focus due to external distractions at home
    - D. Lack of access to transportation to attend school
5. What type of intervention is commonly recommended for academic problems related to learning disabilities?
    - A. General therapy without a specific focus on education
    - B. Educational accommodations and individualized education plans (IEPs)
    - C. Punitive measures to encourage better performance
    - D. Removal from traditional educational settings
6. Which therapeutic approach is most effective for addressing academic problems linked to anxiety?
    - A. Psychoanalysis exploring unconscious conflicts
    - B. Cognitive-behavioral therapy targeting performance anxiety and stress management
    - C. Pharmacological interventions exclusively
    - D. Group therapy with other students experiencing similar challenges
7. Which strategy is best for preventing academic problems in students with attention deficits?
    - A. Ignoring symptoms unless they become severe
    - B. Implementing structured routines and providing positive reinforcement
    - C. Focusing on disciplinary actions for poor performance
    - D. Encouraging competition among peers

True/False Questions

		T	F
1	In the DSM-5-TR, Academic Problems can be noted even if a student shows a mild drop in grades without other clinical symptoms.		
2	A conflict with a teacher, with no impact on study habits or mood, is categorized under Academic Problems.		
3	Significant difficulty in one subject area, accompanied by notable concern, fits Academic Problems if no neurocognitive conditions are present.		
4	If a student exhibits persistent demotivation and sadness linked to performance, the DSM-5-TR labels it as an Academic Problem.		
5	The DSM-5-TR rules out Academic Problem when a Specific Learning Disorder is diagnosed.		
6	A mild attention deficit not meeting criteria for ADHD may be coded as an Academic Problem.		
7	The DSM-5-TR always requires formal IQ testing to document Academic Problems.		
8	Excessive family pressure regarding grades, causing subthreshold performance anxiety, can be considered an Academic Problem.		
9	If academic struggles occur in the context of bullying, the DSM-5-TR suggests coding only a Relational Problem.		
10	The DSM-5-TR allows an Academic Problem diagnosis when it influences adherence to ongoing psychological treatment.		

Matching Exercise

1. Learning disabilities [ ]
2. Performance anxiety [ ]
3. Task-related issues [ ]
4. Interpersonal conflicts [ ]
5. Structured routines [ ]
6. Individualized education plans (IEPs) [ ]

Descriptions:

- A. Poor time management and difficulty completing assignments
- B. Tailored accommodations for students with specific academic challenges
- C. Stress and fear of failure impacting academic performance
- D. Conflicts with teachers or peers affecting classroom behavior
- E. Common factor contributing to academic problems, such as dyslexia or ADHD
- F. Preventive strategy to support students with attention deficits

Case Study

A 10-year-old boy is referred for evaluation due to declining academic performance and conflicts with his teacher. His parents report that he struggles to complete assignments and often appears frustrated with schoolwork. His teacher states that he frequently interrupts the class and has difficulty staying focused. The boy enjoys playing video games but expresses low confidence in his academic abilities.

1. What is the most likely factor contributing to this boy's academic problems?
   - A. Interpersonal issues with peers unrelated to classroom behavior
   - B. A learning disability or attention deficit impacting task completion and focus
   - C. Poor intellectual ability preventing success in school
   - D. Lack of parental involvement in his education
2. Which intervention would be most effective for this student?
   - A. Educational accommodations, such as extra time for assignments, and behavioral strategies to improve focus
   - B. Immediate pharmacological treatment to address his frustration
   - C. Group therapy to address his interpersonal conflicts with teachers
   - D. Assigning additional homework to improve his academic confidence
3. What preventive measure could help reduce the risk of similar academic problems in other students?
   - A. Ignoring signs of learning difficulties until they become severe
   - B. Providing individualized support plans and fostering a positive learning environment
   - C. Removing students with academic challenges from traditional classrooms
   - D. Focusing on punitive measures to improve classroom behavior

Answers

Multiple Choice Questions:

1. A
2. A
3. B
4. A
5. B
6. B
7. B

True/False Questions:

1. True
2. False
3. True
4. True
5. False
6. True
7. False
8. True
9. False
10. True

Matching Exercise:

1. E
2. C
3. A
4. D
5. F
6. B

Case Study Answers and Explanations:

1. B - Explanation: The boy's symptoms suggest a learning disability or attention deficit, as evidenced by his difficulty focusing and completing tasks.
2. A - Explanation: Educational accommodations and behavioral strategies are effective for managing learning difficulties and attention deficits.
3. B - Explanation: Individualized support and a positive learning environment can prevent academic problems and build confidence in students.

Other Conditions of Clinical Relevance

Multiple Choice Questions

1. Which of the following best defines conditions of clinical concern according to the DSM-5?
    - A. Diagnosable mental disorders that meet full DSM-5 criteria
    - B. Non-diagnosable situations or events that significantly impact mental health and functioning
    - C. Physical illnesses with no psychological impact on the patient
    - D. Situations limited to occupational and educational settings
2. Which of the following scenarios could be classified under conditions of clinical concern?
    - A. A recent divorce leading to significant distress and impaired social functioning
    - B. Persistent depressive symptoms lasting for over a year
    - C. Frequent anxiety attacks with no identifiable cause
    - D. Unexplained fatigue and weight loss
3. Which of the following is an appropriate clinical intervention for conditions of clinical concern?
    - A. Comprehensive pharmacological treatment targeting core symptoms
    - B. Brief, solution-focused therapy to address specific stressors
    - C. Long-term psychodynamic therapy with no focus on the identified concern
    - D. Avoidance of any clinical intervention due to lack of a formal diagnosis
4. A patient experiencing interpersonal conflicts following a traumatic event without meeting PTSD criteria would most likely fall under which classification?
    - A. Generalized anxiety disorder
    - B. Adjustment disorder or other conditions of clinical concern
    - C. Major depressive disorder
    - D. Unspecified mental disorder
5. Which of the following is a critical component of assessing conditions of clinical concern?
    - A. Identifying whether the situation meets DSM-5 diagnostic criteria for a mental disorder
    - B. Understanding the patient's context, including cultural, social, and situational factors
    - C. Focusing solely on physical symptoms to rule out medical conditions
    - D. Ignoring the patient's subjective experience unless they meet diagnostic thresholds
6. Which term best describes the goal of therapy for conditions of clinical concern?
    - A. Symptom eradication through medication
    - B. Restoring functioning and reducing distress associated with the situation
    - C. Avoiding clinical involvement until a full diagnosis is reached
    - D. Long-term therapeutic engagement to prevent recurrence
7. In which scenario would the clinician document the case under "other conditions of clinical concern"?
    - A. A patient meets the criteria for a specific mood disorder
    - B. A patient struggles to adapt to a new job, resulting in moderate social withdrawal
    - C. A patient exhibits persistent psychotic symptoms without insight
    - D. A patient reports no significant distress or impairment despite recent stressors

True/False Questions

		T	F
1	The DSM-5-TR allows listing "Other Conditions of Clinical Relevance" for issues that do not constitute a mental disorder but do affect treatment.		
2	If a person has Major Depressive Disorder, adding a "Housing Problem" under "Other Conditions of Clinical Relevance" is not permitted.		
3	V/Z codes (e.g., V60.0, Z59.0) may be used to classify difficult socioeconomic circumstances within "Other Conditions of Clinical Relevance."		
4	Cultural or religious factors do not appear in this section, as they are placed elsewhere in the DSM-5-TR.		
5	A child experiencing distress due to parental conflicts can be classified as "Child Affected by Parental Relationship Distress" (if no other criteria are met) under "Other Conditions of Clinical Relevance."		
6	The DSM-5-TR excludes any general medical conditions from "Other Conditions of Clinical Relevance," similar to the old multi-axial system.		
7	An instance of psychological, physical, or sexual abuse can be documented here if the individual does not display a specific related disorder.		
8	A social exclusion issue without a matching psychiatric disorder cannot appear in "Other Conditions of Clinical Relevance."		
9	If a patient fails to adhere to medical treatment in the absence of diagnosable mental symptoms, the clinician may note it under "Other Conditions of Clinical Relevance."		
10	This section cannot serve as the principal diagnosis if there is no confirmed psychiatric disorder.		

Matching Exercise

1. Adjustment difficulties [ ]
2. Cultural considerations [ ]
3. Loss of a loved one [ ]
4. Solution-focused therapy [ ]
5. Restoring functioning [ ]
6. Social withdrawal [ ]

Descriptions:

- A. A therapeutic approach effective in addressing specific, situational concerns
- B. A common consequence of stressors, often impacting interpersonal relationships
- C. Goal of therapy in conditions of clinical concern
- D. A situational stressor that may cause grief or emotional challenges without meeting depression criteria
- E. Key factor in understanding the patient's reaction to stressors or events
- F. Often seen in individuals struggling to adapt to new situations or environments

Case Study

A 30-year-old woman presents with feelings of isolation and sadness after moving to a new city for work. She reports difficulty forming social connections and adapting to her new environment. She denies symptoms of major depression or anxiety but feels that her struggles are interfering with her ability to focus at work and enjoy her personal life.

1. What is the most appropriate clinical classification for this patient's situation?
   - A. Generalized anxiety disorder
   - B. Adjustment difficulties under conditions of clinical concern
   - C. Major depressive disorder with situational triggers
   - D. Unspecified mental disorder
2. Which therapeutic approach would be most effective in this case?
   - A. Psychoanalysis focused on exploring early life experiences
   - B. Solution-focused therapy addressing adaptation challenges and promoting coping strategies
   - C. Pharmacological treatment targeting her sadness
   - D. Group therapy for individuals with major depression
3. What is the primary goal of intervention in this case?
   - A. Symptom eradication through intensive therapeutic engagement
   - B. Immediate resolution of all emotional challenges through pharmacological means
   - C. Restoring her ability to function effectively in her work and personal life
   - D. Identifying a long-term diagnosis to guide future interventions

Answers

Multiple Choice Questions:

1. B
2. A
3. B
4. B
5. B
6. B
7. B

True/False Questions:

1. False
2. True
3. False
4. True
5. True
6. True
7. False
8. False
9. True
10. True

Matching Exercise:

1. F
2. E
3. D
4. A
5. C
6. B

Case Study Answers and Explanations:

1. B - Explanation: The patient's situation involves adjustment difficulties due to a situational stressor, without meeting criteria for a DSM-5 mental disorder.
2. B - Explanation: Solution-focused therapy is an effective approach to address adaptation challenges and promote coping strategies.
3. C - Explanation: The primary goal of intervention is to restore functioning and address the situational challenges impacting her work and personal life.

Your Opinion Can Make a Difference

"Small acts, when multiplied by many people, can transform the world."

This workbook was designed to help clinicians enhance their practice and refine their skills through thought-provoking exercises and case studies. If you've found it helpful, you have the opportunity to make a difference for someone else.

Would you take a moment to share your experience? Your honest review—whether it's about what you appreciated, what surprised you, or what you think could be better—helps other clinicians discover a resource that could be valuable to them.

Your feedback can:

- Guide a student preparing for exams.
- Help a professional choose tools to enhance their practice.
- Improve future editions of this workbook.

It takes less than a minute to leave a review, but the impact can last a lifetime. Thank you for your time and for being part of a community that strives to elevate clinical care.

Scan to leave a review on Amazon

Conclusion

As we reach the end of this workbook, take a moment to reflect on the path you've traveled. Studying the DSM-5-TR and engaging with its concepts is no small feat. The manual itself is a cornerstone in the understanding of mental health, and its richness and depth can feel overwhelming at times. Yet, by completing the exercises and activities in this workbook, you've taken significant steps to make these concepts more accessible, practical, and meaningful in your own learning journey.

This workbook was not designed to replace the DSM-5-TR, but rather to complement it—offering a structured, interactive approach to break down complex material into manageable and actionable steps. Through this process, you've gained tools that help you bridge the gap between theory and practice. Whether you're a student, a mental health professional, or simply someone eager to better understand the intricacies of mental health, you've developed valuable skills that will serve you in a variety of contexts.

Over the course of this workbook, you've honed key skills that extend beyond memorizing diagnostic criteria. You've practiced:

- **Critical Thinking:** By analyzing case studies and reflecting on diagnostic challenges, you've built a stronger ability to evaluate complex information.
- **Application:** Through exercises that encourage you to use theoretical knowledge in practical scenarios, you've strengthened your ability to make meaningful connections between the DSM-5-TR and real-world contexts.
- **Confidence:** Perhaps most importantly, you've grown more comfortable engaging with material that might have once seemed daunting. This confidence will propel you as you continue to explore and deepen your understanding of mental health.

Remember, learning is an ongoing journey, especially in a field as dynamic and evolving as mental health. The DSM-5-TR is a living document, reflecting the latest research and perspectives, and it is likely to continue evolving. Your commitment to staying informed, asking questions, and seeking new perspectives will keep you adaptable and prepared for the challenges ahead.

If you've felt moments of doubt or frustration along the way, know that this is a natural part of the process. Growth often comes from confronting challenges and pushing through them. By working through this workbook, you've demonstrated resilience, curiosity, and determination—qualities that are essential not only in understanding the DSM-5-TR but in any endeavor.

Now that you've completed this workbook, you may be wondering, "What's next?" The answer depends on your goals and aspirations:

- **For students:** Continue exploring related materials, attend lectures or workshops, and engage with peers to discuss and debate your interpretations.

- **For professionals in training:** Apply the concepts you've learned to real-world scenarios, whether in clinical practice, internships, or collaborative projects.
- **For lifelong learners:** Consider delving deeper into specific topics that interest you, such as particular disorders, therapeutic approaches, or the social and cultural contexts of mental health.

No matter your path, the key is to keep building on the foundation you've created. The DSM-5-TR is not a static reference—it's a tool for understanding the complexities of human behavior and mental health. As you continue to learn, you'll find new ways to integrate its insights into your studies, practice, or personal growth.

Thank you for allowing this workbook to be part of your learning journey. It has been an honor to accompany you through this process. My hope is that this resource has not only made the DSM-5-TR more accessible but also inspired a deeper curiosity and passion for the study of mental health.

If this workbook has been helpful to you, consider sharing your feedback or even recommending it to others who might benefit from its approach. The learning process is enriched when shared, and your insights might spark someone else's journey toward greater understanding.

In closing, I want to remind you of something simple yet powerful: progress, not perfection. The study of mental health is vast, and it's normal to feel like there's always more to learn. Embrace this fact as part of the beauty of the field—you're not alone in this journey, and the effort you've put in today will continue to pay dividends in the future.

Thank you for trusting this workbook as your guide. Wherever your path leads next, I wish you clarity, confidence, and continued growth.

www.ingramcontent.com/pod-product-compliance
Ingram Content Group UK Ltd.
Pitfield, Milton Keynes, MK11 3LW, UK
UKHW050942290926
15470UKWH00005B/1588

9 781803 626062